T0227261

Cardiac Arrhythmias in Adults with Congenital Heart Disease

Editors

SESHADRI BALAJI
RAVI MANDAPATI
KALYANAM SHIVKUMAR

CARDIAC ELECTROPHYSIOLOGY CLINICS

www.cardiacEP.theclinics.com

Consulting Editors
RANJAN K. THAKUR
ANDREA NATALE

June 2017 • Volume 9 • Number 2

ELSEVIER

1600 John F. Kennedy Boulevard • Suite 1800 • Philadelphia, Pennsylvania, 19103-2899

http://www.theclinics.com

CARDIAC ELECTROPHYSIOLOGY CLINICS Volume 9, Number 2
June 2017 ISSN 1877-9182, ISBN-13: 978-0-323-52999-0

Editor: Stacy Eastman
Developmental Editor: Susan Showalter

Cardiac Electrophysiology Clinics (ISSN 1877-9182) is published quarterly by Elsevier Inc., 360 Park Avenue South, New York, NY 10010-1710. Months of issue are March, June, September, and December. Subscription prices are $215.00 per year for US individuals, $331.00 per year for US institutions, $236.00 per year for Canadian individuals, $373.00 per year for Canadian institutions, $299.00 per year for international individuals, $399.00 per year for international institutions and $100.00 per year for US, Canadian and international students/residents. To receive student/resident rate, orders must be accompanied by name of affiliated institution, date of term, and the signature of program/residency coordinator on institution letterhead. Orders will be billed at individual rate until proof of status is received. Foreign air speed delivery is included in all Clinics subscription prices. All prices are subject to change without notice. **POSTMASTER:** Send address changes to Cardiac Electrophysiology Clinics, Elsevier Health Sciences Division, Subscription Customer Service, 3251 Riverport Lane, Maryland Heights, MO 63043. **Customer Service: 1-800-654-2452 (US and Canada). From outside of the US and Canada, call 314-477-8871. Fax: 314-447-8029. E-mail: JournalsCustomerService-usa@elsevier.com (for print support); JournalsOnlineSupport-usa@elsevier.com (for online support).**

Reprints. For copies of 100 or more of articles in this publication, please contact the Commercial Reprints Department, Elsevier Inc., 360 Park Avenue South, New York, NY 10010-1710. Tel.: 212-633-3874; Fax: 212-633-3820; E-mail: reprints@elsevier.com.

Cardiac Electrophysiology Clinics is covered in *MEDLINE/PubMed (Index Medicus)*.

Contributors

CONSULTING EDITORS

RANJAN K. THAKUR, MD, MPH, MBA, FACC, FHRS
Professor of Medicine and Director, Arrhythmia Service, Thoracic and Cardiovascular Institute, Sparrow Health System, Michigan State University, Lansing, Michigan

ANDREA NATALE, MD, FACC, FHRS, FESC
Department of Cardiology, Texas Cardiac Arrhythmia Institute, St. David's Medical Center, Department of Biomedical Engineering, Cockrell School of Engineering, Department of Internal Medicine, Dell Medical School, University of Texas, Austin, Texas; Department of Cardiology, MetroHealth Medical Center, Case Western Reserve University School of Medicine, Cleveland, Ohio; Atrial Fibrillation and Arrhythmia Center, California Pacific Medical Center, San Francisco, California; Division of Cardiology, Stanford University, Stanford, California; Interventional Electrophysiology, Scripps Clinic, La Jolla, California

EDITORS

SESHADRI BALAJI, MBBS, FRCP(UK), PhD
Professor, Pediatrics (Cardiology), Director, Pediatric Arrhythmia, Doernbecher Children's Hospital, Oregon Health & Science University, Portland, Oregon

RAVI MANDAPATI, MD, FHRS, FACC
Professor of Medicine and Pediatrics, Director, Loma Linda University International Heart Institute, Director, Cardiac Electrophysiology, Loma Linda University Health, Loma Linda, California

KALYANAM SHIVKUMAR, MD, PhD, FHRS
Professor of Medicine and Radiology, Director, UCLA Cardiac Arrhythmia Center and EP Programs, Director and Chief, Interventional CV Programs, UCLA Cardiac Arrhythmia Center, David Geffen School of Medicine, University of California Los Angeles, Los Angeles, California

AUTHORS

PABLO ÁVILA, MD
Department of Cardiology, Instituto de Investigación Sanitaria, Hospital Gregorio Marañón, Universidad Complutense, Madrid, Spain

JAMIL A. ABOULHOSN, MD, FACC
Associate Professor of Medicine, Department of Cardiology, UCLA Medical Center, Ahmanson/UCLA Adult Congenital Heart Disease Center, David Geffen School of Medicine at University of California Los Angeles, Los Angeles, California

DOMINIC J. ABRAMS, MD, MRCP
Division of Cardiac Electrophysiology, Boston Children's Hospital, Assistant Professor, Harvard Medical School, Boston, Massachusetts

SHERRIE JOY BAYSA, MD
Fellow, Pediatric Electrophysiology, Nicklaus Children's Hospital, Miami, Florida

AD J.J.C. BOGERS, MD, PhD
Department of Cardiothoracic Surgery, Erasmus Medical Center, Rotterdam, The Netherlands

STEVEN K. CARLSON, MD
Fellow, Clinical Cardiac Electrophysiology, Keck Hospital of USC, Keck School of Medicine of the University of Southern California, Los Angeles, California

FRANK CECCHIN, MD
Andrall E. Pearson Professor of Pediatric Cardiology, Professor of Internal Medicine, Division Director, Pediatric Cardiology, Director of Pediatric and Congenital Electrophysiology, New York University Langone Medical Center, New York, New York

MARIE-A. CHAIX, MD, MS
Adult Congenital Heart Center, Montreal Heart Institute, Université de Montréal, Montreal, Canada

PHILIP M. CHANG, MD
Assistant Professor of Clinical Medicine and Pediatrics, Medical Director, USC Adult Congenital Heart Disease Care Program, Keck Hospital of University of Southern California, Keck School of Medicine of the University of Southern California, Los Angeles, California

TAHMEED CONTRACTOR, MD
Assistant Professor of Medicine, Department of Cardiology, Arrhythmia Center, Loma Linda University International Heart Institute, Loma Linda, California

NATASJA M.S. DE GROOT, MD, PhD
Department of Cardiology, Erasmus Medical Center, Rotterdam, Netherlands

BARBARA J. DEAL, MD
Getz Professor of Cardiology, Feinberg School of Medicine, Northwestern University, Chicago, Illinois

SABINE ERNST, MD, PhD, FESC
Consultant Cardiologist/Electrophysiologist, Reader in Cardiology, Cardiology Department, National Heart and Lung Institute, Royal Brompton and Harefield Hospital, Imperial College, London, United Kingdom

DANIEL G. HALPERN, MD
Assistant Professor of Internal Medicine, Director of Adult Congenital Heart Disease Program, New York University Langone Medical Center, New York, New York

LOUISE HARRIS, MD, FRCPC
Professor of Medicine, Department of Cardiology, Peter Munk Cardiac Centre, University Health Network, University of Toronto, Toronto, Ontario, Canada

CHRISTOPHER M. JANSON, MD
Attending Physician, Division of Cardiology, The Children's Hospital at Montefiore, Assistant Professor of Pediatrics, Albert Einstein College of Medicine, Bronx, New York

RONALD J. KANTER, MD
Director of Electrophysiology, Nicklaus Children's Hospital, Miami, Florida; Professor Emeritus, Duke University, Durham, North Carolina

PAUL KHAIRY, MD, PhD
Adult Congenital Heart Center, Montreal Heart Institute, Université de Montréal, Montreal, Canada

VADIM LEVIN, MD
Consultant Electrophysiologist, Phoenixville Hospital, Pottstown, Pennsylvania

RAVI MANDAPATI, MD, FHRS, FACC
Professor of Medicine and Pediatrics, Director, Loma Linda University International Heart Institute, Director, Cardiac Electrophysiology, Loma Linda University Health, Loma Linda, California

CONSTANTINE MAVROUDIS, MD
Professor of Surgery, Johns Hopkins School of Medicine, Site Director, Johns Hopkins Children's Heart Surgery, Florida Hospital for Children, Orlando, Florida

BLANDINE MONDÉSERT, MD
Adult Congenital Heart Center, Montreal Heart
Institute, Université de Montréal, Montreal,
Canada

JEREMY P. MOORE, MD, MS, FHRS
Assistant Professor of Pediatrics, UCLA
Medical Center, Ahmanson/UCLA Adult
Congenital Heart Disease Center, David Geffen
School of Medicine at University of California
Los Angeles, Los Angeles, California

KRISHNAKUMAR NAIR, MBBS, MD, DM
Assistant Professor of Medicine, Cardiac
Electrophysiology Fellowship Program
Director, Peter Munk Cardiac Centre,
University Health Network, University of
Toronto, Toronto, Ontario, Canada

MELISSA OLEN, ARNP
Clinical Coordinator of Electrophysiology and
Remote Device Monitoring, Nicklaus
Children's Hospital, Miami, Florida

AKASH R. PATEL, MD
Assistant Professor of Pediatrics, University
of California San Francisco Benioff Children's
Hospital, University of California San Francisco
School of Medicine, San Francisco, California

**GNALINI SATHANANTHAN, MBBS,
BSc (Med), FRACP**
Adult Congenital Heart Disease Fellow,
Department of Cardiology, Peter Munk Cardiac
Centre, University Health Network, University
of Toronto, Toronto, Ontario, Canada

MAULLY J. SHAH, MBBS
Director, Cardiac Electrophysiology, Division of
Cardiology, The Children's Hospital of
Philadelphia, Professor of Pediatrics, Perelman
School of Medicine at the University of
Pennsylvania, Philadelphia, Pennsylvania

ELIZABETH D. SHERWIN, MD
Division of Cardiology, Children's National
Medical Center, George Washington University
School of Medicine, Washington, DC

ADRIANUS P. WIJNMAALEN, MD, PhD
Department of Cardiology, Leiden University
Medical Center, Leiden, The Netherlands

KATJA ZEPPENFELD, MD, PhD
Department of Cardiology, Leiden University
Medical Center, Leiden, The Netherlands

Contents

Mechanisms, Diagnosis and Clinical Aspects

> The position and course of the conduction system in congenital heart disease are intricately tied to the underlying congenital malformation. Although only subtle differences exist between the anatomy of the conduction axis for simple congenital heart lesions and normal anatomy, almost every patient with congenital heart disease harbors some important anatomic variation. This article summarizes the body of literature by retaining original classical concepts and by attempting to translate the available knowledge into useful points for the congenital heart disease specialist. This discussion spans the entire spectrum of simple to complex congenital heart disease.

> Bradyarrhythmias in adults with congenital heart disease (CHD) comprise a complex group of arrhythmia disorders with congenital and acquired origins, highly variable long-term sequelae, and complicated treatment options. They can develop across the spectrum of CHD defects and can be encountered at all ages. Although permanent pacing is effective in treating bradyarrhythmias, it is associated with many complications and morbidity, where it is often used early in life. This section discusses the incidence and prevalence of bradyarrhythmias in the CHD population, their timing of occurrence with respect to specific disease entities and interventions, and their short- and long-term clinical sequelae.

> Supraventricular arrhythmias represent a major source of morbidity in adults with congenital heart disease (ACHD). Anatomic variants and post-operative changes contribute to a unique electrophysiologic milieu ripe for the development of supraventricular tachycardia. Intra-atrial reentrant tachycardia is the most prevalent mechanism. Atrioventricular reciprocating tachycardia is common in lesions associated with accessory pathways. Abnormal anatomy complicates the management of atrioventricular nodal reentrant tachycardia. Tachycardia mediated by twin atrioventricular nodes is rare. Focal tachycardias are considerations in the ACHD population. Each of these tachycardia mechanisms is reviewed, focusing on the inherent diagnostic and therapeutic challenges.

The risk of ventricular arrhythmias in the adult congenital heart disease population increases with age. The mechanism, type, and frequency vary depending on the complexity of the defect, whether it has been repaired, and the type and timing of repair. Risk stratification for sudden death in patients with congenital heart disease is often challenging. Current recommendations provide a useful guide for management of these patients and risk stratification continues to evolve. Internal cardiac defibrillator implantation is often challenging due to limited transvenous access, often resulting in the need for epicardial or subcutaneous devices.

Sudden death of presumed arrhythmic etiology is a leading cause of mortality in adults with congenital heart disease. Anticipated benefits of the implantable cardioverter-defibrillator (ICD) must be weighed against high complication rates. Without robust evidence from randomized trials, caregivers face difficult decisions in selecting appropriate candidates. Although secondary prevention indications are often clear-cut, risk stratification for primary prevention ICDs is more challenging. Factors associated with sudden death in patients with tetralogy of Fallot are reasonably consistent across studies. In contrast, identification of high-risk patients with systemic right ventricles or univentricular hearts remains controversial.

Specific Congenital Heart Defects: Clinical Aspects and Ablation

Atrial arrhythmias are common in patients with atrial septal defects. A myriad of factors are responsible for these that include remodeling related to the defect and scar created by the repair or closure. An understanding of potential arrhythmias, along with entrainment and high-density activation mapping can result in accurate diagnosis and successful ablation. Atrial fibrillation is being seen increasingly after patent foramen ovale closure and may be the primary etiology of recurrent stroke in these patients.

Ebstein anomaly is a rare form of congenital heart disease with a uniquely high prevalence of arrhythmias. The most prevalent arrhythmia mechanisms are intrinsic to the underlying embryologic defects and may manifest at any stage. Current electrophysiological and surgical strategies are well equipped to address these arrhythmia mechanisms, yet despite available technology and a robust understanding of the mechanisms, these cases remain challenging. Surgical techniques that render arrhythmia substrates unreachable mandate comprehensive presurgical electrophysiological assessment and potential ablation. As the population ages, the need to address atrial fibrillation management and risk stratification for sudden cardiac death becomes ever more pertinent.

The atrial switch operations, the Mustard and Senning procedures, performed for dextro-transposition of the great arteries, have largely been supplanted by the arterial switch operation. As such, affected patients will only exist for approximately 30 more years. The main arrhythmias in these patients include sinoatrial node dysfunction, intraatrial reentry tachycardia, and sudden death. Device therapy for these patients is well-established, and catheter ablation for atrial tachycardias is highly efficacious. The application of meticulous procedural planning, customization of catheter courses, and electrophysiologic principles to this patient group may be extended to all postoperative complex congenital heart patients.

Patients with a Fontan circulation are at a high risk of developing a variety of cardiac dysrhythmias after cardiac surgery. These dysrhythmias are most often supraventricular tachyarrhythmias (SVT), but ventricular tachyarrhythmias (VT) may also occur. Mechanisms underlying SVT are variable, including both ectopic activity and reentry. Over time, successive SVT may be caused by different mechanisms. The acute success rate of ablative therapy of atrial tachyarrhythmias is considerably high yet during long-term follow-up 'recurrences' frequently occur. It is most likely that these 'recurrences' are caused by a progressive atrial cardiomyopathy instead of arrhythmogeneity of prior ablative lesions.

Life expectancy of patients with rToF has considerably improved due to refined surgical interventions. Monomorphic fast VTs are frequently encountered in adult patients with rToF. The dominant substrate of VT is anatomical isthmuses bordered by surgical incisions, patch material and valve annuli. Substrate based ablation strategies aim to transect all slow conducting anatomical isthmuses (SCAI) as identified by electroanatomical mapping. Procedural success is defined as non-inducibility of VT and confirmed conduction block over the SCAI resulting in long-term VT free survival in most patients. The identification of SCAIs in rToF may have important implications for risk stratification and preventive treatment.

Management

Adults with congenital heart disease are at risk for atrial and ventricular arrhythmias that can lead to an increased morbidity as well as mortality. When catheter ablation is not an option or unsuccessful, antiarrhythmic drugs are the mainstay of treatment.

There is limited data on the use of antiarrhythmics in this population. The purpose of this article is to discuss the practical aspects of the use of antiarrhythmics in adults with congenital heart disease. Several tables have been provided to provide clinicians a reference for daily use.

Catheter Ablation: General Principles and Advances   311

Sabine Ernst

Besides antiarrhythmic medication, there are now very good options for a potentially curative therapy by catheter ablation targeting the origin of the underlying arrhythmias in patients with complex congenital heart disease. Three-dimensional (3D) reconstruction of tomographic imaging (MRI or computed tomography) is helpful to understand the underlying cardiac anatomy, identify the most likely target chamber, and help with planning access. Use of the available 3D mapping systems (sequential or simultaneous acquisition) and (if available) more advanced navigation systems, such as remote magnetic navigation, can improve the acute and long-term outcomes of catheter ablation in congenital heart disease.

Cardiac Arrhythmias in Adults with Congenital Heart Disease: Pacemakers, Implantable Cardiac Defibrillators, and Cardiac Resynchronization Therapy Devices   319

Frank Cecchin and Daniel G. Halpern

Implanting cardiac rhythm medical devices in adults with congenital heart disease requires training in congenital heart disease. The techniques and indications for device implantation are specific to the anatomic diagnosis and state of disease progression. It often requires a team of physicians and is best performed at a specialized adult congenital heart center.

Arrhythmia Surgery for Adults with Congenital Heart Disease   329

Barbara J. Deal and Constantine Mavroudis

Patients with repaired or unrepaired congenital heart anomalies are at increased risk for arrhythmia development throughout their lives, often paralleling the need for reoperations for hemodynamic residua. The ability to incorporate arrhythmia surgery into reoperations can result in improvement in functional class and decreased need for antiarrhythmic medications. Every reoperation for congenital heart disease can be viewed as an opportunity to assess the electrical and arrhythmia substrates and to intervene to improve the arrhythmias and the hemodynamic condition of the patient. The authors review and summarize the operative techniques for arrhythmia surgery that are based on the arrhythmia mechanisms.

CARDIAC ELECTROPHYSIOLOGY CLINICS

CARDIAC ELECTROPHYSIOLOGY CLINICS

FORTHCOMING ISSUES

September 2017
Normal Electrophysiology, Substrates, and the Electrocardiographic Diagnosis of Cardiac Arrhythmias: Part I
Luigi Padeletti and Giuseppe Bagliani, Editors

December 2017
Contemporary Challenges in Sudden Cardiac Death
Mohammad Shenasa, N. A. Mark Estes III, and Gordon F. Tomaselli, Editors

March 2018
Contemporary Issues in Patients with Implantable Devices
Raymond Yee, Mark Link, and Amin Al-Ahmad, Editor

RECENT ISSUES

March 2017
Ventricular Tachycardia in Structural Heart Disease
Amin Al-Ahmad and Francis E. Marchlinski, Editors

December 2016
Pathophysiology of the Human His-Purkinje System
Masood Akhtar, Editor

September 2016
Ventricular Arrhythmias in Apparently Normal Hearts
Frank M. Bogun, Thomas C. Crawford, and Rakesh Latchamsetty, Editor

ISSUE OF RELATED INTEREST

Interventional Cardiology Clinics October 2016 (Vol. 5, No. 4)
Controversies in the Management of STEMI
Timothy D. Henry, Editor
Available at: http://www.Interventional.theclinics.com/

Foreword

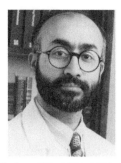

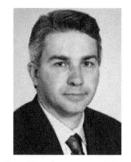

Ranjan K. Thakur, MD, MPH, MBA, FACC, FHRS   Andrea Natale, MD, FACC, FHRS

Consulting Editors

The human heart likes a little disorder in its geometry
— Louis de Bernières, Captain Corelli's Mandolin

We are pleased to introduce this issue of *Cardiac Electrophysiology Clinics*, which focuses on the fascinating topic of congenital heart disease (CHD) and its related arrhythmias.

Thanks to the advances in surgery, many children with CHD reach adulthood, and arrhythmias become an important issue in management of these patients. CHDs can predispose to both bradyarrhythmias and tachyarrhythmias, due to the congenital anomaly itself or as a result of the corrective surgery. Each arrhythmia is unique, and knowing the peculiar substrate is a key to understand the distinctive mechanism and choosing the appropriate therapy.

Multiple right-sided accessory pathways sustaining atrioventricular reentrant tachycardias are the hallmark of patients with Ebstein anomaly and can be successfully eliminated with ablation. Sinus node dysfunction and atrioventricular block can be both congenital and postoperative; when symptomatic, patients with CHD require pacemaker implantation, which might be particularly challenging given the associated venous return anomalies, surgical obstacles, or unusual heart anatomies. Patients with surgical scars have incisional macro-reentrant arrhythmias, in both the atria and the ventricles, which respond well to ablation. Some patients might develop myopathy secondary to the hemodynamic consequences of the congenital anatomy, predisposing to complex arrhythmias, which are more difficult to manage and require an integrated approach. Of note, the risk of sudden cardiac death in patients with CHDs involving the ventricle, although low, is still not negligible, and the debate on primary prevention ICD is still wide open.

We thank Drs Balaji, Mandapati, and Shivkumar, for thoughtfully editing this issue covering important aspects of common CHDs seen by adult electrophysiologists. We hope you will enjoy reading it as much as we did.

Ranjan K. Thakur, MD, MPH, MBA, FACC, FHRS
Sparrow Thoracic and Cardiovascular Institute
Michigan State University
1200 East Michigan Avenue, Suite 580
Lansing, MI 48912, USA

Andrea Natale, MD, FACC, FHRS
Texas Cardiac Arrhythmia Institute
Center for Atrial Fibrillation at
St. David's Medical Center
1015 East 32nd Street, Suite 516
Austin, TX 78705, USA

E-mail addresses:
thakur@msu.edu (R.K. Thakur)
andrea.natale@stdavids.com (A. Natale)

1877-9182/17/© 2017 Published by Elsevier Inc.

cardiacEP.theclinics.com

Preface

Cardiac Arrhythmias in Adults with Congenital Heart Disease

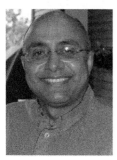
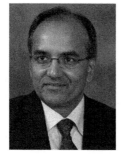
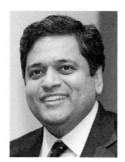

Seshadri Balaji, MBBS, FRCP(UK), PhD

Ravi Mandapati, MD, FHRS, FACC

Kalyanam Shivkumar, MD, PhD, FHRS

Editors

This issue of *Cardiac Electrophysiology Clinics* is entirely devoted to Arrhythmias in Adults with Congenital Heart Disease. It is intended to be a comprehensive and up-to-date review of the state of this rapidly growing field. The material is aimed toward adult and pediatric cardiologists who come across older children and adults with congenital heart disease.

As more and more children survive heart surgery and their life expectancy improves, there are now more adults than children alive with congenital heart disease, and most of them have repaired congenital heart disease. Rhythm disorders are among the most prominent complications encountered by adults with congenital heart disease. Arrhythmias are the leading cause of mortality and morbidity in this population.

The range of complexity of congenital heart disease and the innovative surgeries that have been performed create challenges for the future management of these patients. For one, it is hard to see homogenous cohorts with similar disease that can be systematically studied. While there are a few defects like transposition of the great arteries and tetralogy of Fallot that tend to be relatively homogenous, others, particularly more complex defects like single ventricle, tend to be

highly variable in the range and complexity of the anomaly from one patient to another. The lack of a homogeneous group that can be studied leads to the problem of most rare diseases: namely, that clinical research tends to be based on small case collections rather than large-scale studies. Thus, the management of these patients tends to vary from center to center based on local experience and expertise. Also, many of the management protocols are based on similar diseases and conditions studied in larger populations. Electrophysiologists who care for such patients develop opinions and dogmas based on our understanding of the underlying pathophysiology of arrhythmias in such complex patients. Given this problem, it is not hard to see why there are multiple approaches to the same condition and some repetition and even disagreement among experts.

Advances in catheter ablation technologies, image integration, and so forth, have revolutionized management for many arrhythmias. An important aspect of the care of adults with congenital heart disease is the nonuniform transition of care from pediatrics to adult cardiology. The growth of adult congenital heart disease as a subspecialty has been patchy and variable from center to center. This has created the tendency for patients to

Card Electrophysiol Clin 9 (2017) xv–xvi
http://dx.doi.org/10.1016/j.ccep.2017.04.001
1877-9182/17/© 2017 Published by Elsevier Inc.

cardiacEP.theclinics.com

"fall off the radar" when they reach college age. Many of them then show up in emergency rooms (ERs) far away from their primary place of care with poor records and a poor self-understanding of their heart condition. When they show up in such an ER with an arrhythmia, the local ER physicians tend to be placed in a highly unfavorable position in caring for these patients. It is beyond the scope of this issue to deal with such transitions of care. It is our hope, however, that this issue becomes a reference manual for practitioners in such a place.

We have been fortunate to have some of the world's experts agree to and expeditiously write articles on their topics of expertise. We, the editors, are extremely indebted to the authors for doing such a terrific job under a stressful deadline.

We dedicate this issue to the countless patients with congenital heart disease, who have taught us valuable lessons and endured our ignorance as we painfully learned about the best ways to care for them over the past few decades.

Seshadri Balaji, MBBS, FRCP(UK), PhD
Pediatric Arrhythmia, Doernbecher
Children's Hospital
Oregon Health and Science University
Portland, OR 97239, USA

Ravi Mandapati, MD, FHRS, FACC
Cardiac Electrophysiology
Loma Linda University
International Heart Institute
Loma Linda University Health
11234 Anderson Street
Loma Linda, CA 92354, USA

Kalyanam Shivkumar, MD, PhD, FHRS
UCLA Cardiac Arrhythmia Center
David Geffen School of Medicine
UCLA Health System
Los Angeles, CA 90025, USA

E-mail addresses:
balajis@ohsu.edu (S. Balaji)
rmandapati@llu.edu (R. Mandapati)
KShivkumar@mednet.ucla.edu (K. Shivkumar)

Mechanisms, Diagnosis and Clinical Aspects

Introduction to the Congenital Heart Defects
Anatomy of the Conduction System

Jeremy P. Moore, MD, MS, FHRS*, Jamil A. Aboulhosn, MD

KEYWORDS

- Congenital heart disease • Conduction system • AV node • His-Purkinje system • Heart block
- Supraventricular tachycardia • Atrioventricular reciprocating tachycardia • Heterotaxy syndrome

KEY POINTS

- Knowledge of the location of the conduction tissue is essential for safe and effective arrhythmia management for patients with congenital heart disease.
- The sinus node complex is located in the usual position for most forms of congenital heart disease with the notable exception of the heterotaxy syndromes.
- The location of the compact atrioventricular node and His bundle vary significantly according to the type of congenital heart malformation.
- There are scarce histologic data on the location of transitional cell inputs to the atrioventricular node in congenital heart disease.
- Knowledge of both histologic and clinical data of the location of the conduction system should improve the safety and efficacy of ablation procedures in this population.

INTRODUCTION

The conduction system in congenital heart disease has been studied extensively with notable publications emerging in the early 20th century.[1] The nature of the conduction system in congenital heart disease is intricately related to the underlying lesion, and no description can occur without reference to the unique structural anatomy of this population. Although only subtle differences between simple congenital heart lesions and normal may exist, almost every patient with congenital heart disease harbors an important variation in the conduction system anatomy.

Studies of the conduction system based on histopathology techniques are generally limited to identification of the sinus node complex, the compact atrioventricular (AV) node, and the His-Purkinje system in relation to the identifiable gross anatomic structures as visualized by the pathologist or cardiac surgeon. As a consequence, application of this information to the electrophysiology laboratory is not necessarily straightforward. Perhaps more importantly, because of the focused nature of these studies, there are limited data on the location of the transitional cell inputs to the compact AV node. This finding may be clinically relevant, for instance, when attempting to modify the slow pathway for AV node reentry tachycardia in patients with complex congenital heart disease.

This article summarizes the vast body of literature by keeping to the original classical concepts and by attempting to translate the available

Disclosure Statement: The authors have nothing to disclose.
UCLA Medical Center, Ahmanson/UCLA Adult Congenital Heart Disease Center, David Geffen School of Medicine at UCLA, 100 Medical Plaza Drive, Suite 770, Los Angeles, CA 90095, USA
* Corresponding author.
E-mail address: jpmoore@mednet.ucla.edu

Card Electrophysiol Clin 9 (2017) 167–175
http://dx.doi.org/10.1016/j.ccep.2017.02.001

knowledge into useful points for the practicing interventionalist and electrophysiologist. Greater focus is placed on those lesions with the most significant departure from normal, where an in-depth understanding of the conduction system is essential for safe and effective treatment of cardiac arrhythmia. This discussion spans the entire spectrum ranging from simple to complex congenital heart disease.

SIMPLE DEFECTS
Atrial Septal Defect

The embryologic location of the conduction tissue in atrial septal defect is generally not altered by the congenital heart disease, except for the primum atrial septal defect, which is described extensively in the section on atrioventricular septal defect. With right heart enlargement caused by augmented pulmonary blood flow, however, there may be significant right atrial and ventricular enlargement with distortion of the landmarks for the conduction system anatomy.

Ventricular Septal Defect

There are multiple anatomic types of ventral septal defect (VSD), all of which have important implications for the anatomy of the conduction system. In general, the compact AV node together with the transitional cell inputs are expected to be located in their normal location at the apex of the triangle of Koch for all of the various subtypes, whereas the AV bundle and bundle branches are located variably. These issues are generally of greatest importance to the cardiac surgeon, who must repair these defect without incurring AV block. With the increasing frequency of transcatheter interventions for VSD closure, however, this anatomy must also be increasingly understood by the interventional cardiologist.

There are various classification schemes for VSD, generally derived for their surgical significance.[2,3] The most common type of VSD is the perimembranous (also referred to as *membranous*, *conoventricular*, or *subaortic*) defect, which involves a deficiency in the membranous portion of the interventricular septum and the surrounding muscular tissue.[4] The defect may extend into the inlet, trabecular, or infundibular portions of the ventricular septum, and is named according to the type and degree of extension. Although the precise relationship between the AV bundle and the defect varies with the type of extension, all perimembranous defects share the quality that the AV bundle passes posterior and inferior to them (or rightward as viewed by the surgeon). The portion of the bundle that is at highest risk

for surgically-induced AV block is located at the posteroinferior edge of the defect where it is encased in a thin rim of fibrous tissue (**Fig. 1**).[5] In general, defects with extension into the inlet septum are most closely related to the AV bundle whereas defects with outlet extension are the most remote. Defects with muscular trabecular extension are intermediate with respect to their proximity to the conduction tissue but are generally considered to be at low risk for surgically-induced AV block.

Of the other types of VSD, isolated muscular inlet defects are important to recognize. These are the only VSDs in which the conduction tissue is located in an anterosuperior position relative to the defect (or leftward as viewed by the surgeon). Fortunately, these defects are typically remote from the AV bundle.[6] The final category of defects, the muscular outlet defects and the so-called doubly committed or subarterial defects, are also remote from the conduction tissue. In these cases, the AV bundle and bundle branches travel posterior and inferior to the defect, but at a distance.

MODERATELY COMPLEX DEFECTS
Atrioventricular Septal Defect

The gross and histologic anatomy of the AV conduction system in atrioventricular septal defect

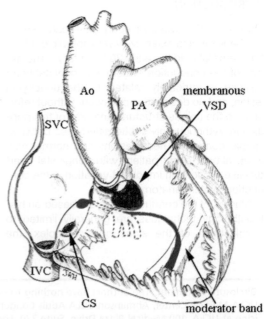

Fig. 1. Perimembranous septal defect. Ao, aorta; CS, coronary sinus; IVC, inferior vena cava; PA, pulmonary artery; SVC, superior vena cava; VSD, ventricular septal defect.

(AVSD) has been described primarily with reference to the major anatomic landmarks for surgical repair. Because the primum atrial septum is deficient and does not make contact with the inlet ventricular septum, the AV node and penetrating AV bundle are displaced inferiorly toward the crux of the heart.[7–10]

The usual surgical landmarks that mark Koch's triangle are still present in AVSD but no longer contain the conduction tissues. Rather, there is a second, more inferior triangle that indicates the site of the compact AV node. This nodal triangle is formed by unique borders that include (1) the thickened edge of the atrial septum (referred to as the *bridging tendon*), (2) the inferior bridging leaflet of the atrioventricular valve, and (3) the ostium of the coronary sinus (**Fig. 2**).[8]

The exact position of the AV node may vary in relation to the ostium of the coronary sinus, depending on the development of the atrial septum. For example, in partial AVSD, the septum tends to be more developed and the apex of the nodal triangle more remote from the coronary sinus. This finding has significant surgical implications, because the atrial septal patch may need to be placed around the coronary sinus ostium in some cases, resulting in its drainage to the left atrium.

Because of the variable relation between the coronary sinus ostium and the compact AV node, alternative landmarks for identification of the compact AV node have been recommended.

For example, regardless of the development of the atrial septum and size and location of the coronary sinus ostium,[11] the compact AV node is most consistently related to the point of contact between the bridging tendon and the attachment of the inferior bridging leaflet. Here, the His bundle is located superficially as it descends on the "scooped out" ventricular septum.

Pathologic study of the transitional cell zones has not been performed in cases of AVSD, so that knowledge of fast and slow pathway inputs to the AV node is derived from a limited number of clinical reports. Case reports describe successful slow pathway modification inferior and usually posterior to the location of the His bundle electrogram[12–15] and, more rarely, superior the His bundle electrogram (so-called *inverted AV nodal inputs*).[16] It can be inferred that the slow pathway is most commonly located in a posteroinferior position relative to the displaced location of the compact AV node in the setting of AVSD. For cases of septal patch placement that incorporate the coronary sinus ostium into the left atrium, the His bundle electrogram and therefore the compact AV node and transitional inputs may not be attainable from the right side. In these cases, a transseptal puncture and left-sided slow pathway modification may be necessary.[13]

Congenitally Corrected Transposition of the Great Arteries

The conduction system in congenitally corrected transposition of the great arteries (CCTGA) was a subject of intense investigation in the early era of congenital pathology, and current knowledge of the anatomy is a result of many years of careful histologic dissection. Initial reports were somewhat conflicted, describing both posterior and anterior AV nodes but without a clear consensus on the dominant route of AV conduction.[17–19] Current understanding is probably best attributed to Anderson and colleagues,[20,21] who described their findings in large series of hearts with CCTGA.

Despite the presence of a normally positioned posterior AV node at the apex of the triangle of Koch as in the normal heart, the posterior node in CCTGA is generally hypoplastic without a true connection to the AV bundle.[18,20,21] Instead, a well-formed anterior node serves as the principal conduction pathway. This anterior node is located at the atrial aspect of the pulmonary-mitral continuity where it connects to a penetrating AV bundle. From here, a long nonbranching AV bundle extends anteriorly around the pulmonary valve annulus to reach the superior margin of the VSD

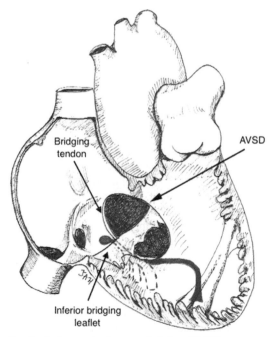

Bridging tendon

AVSD

Inferior bridging leaflet

Fig. 2. Atrioventricular septal defect (AVSD).

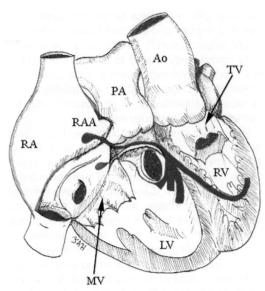

Fig. 3. Congenitally corrected transposition of the great arteries. Ao, aorta; LV, left ventricle; MV, mitral valve; PA, pulmonary artery; RA, right atrium; RAA, right atrial appendage; RV, right ventricle; TV, tricuspid valve.

if present (**Fig. 3**). The bundle then travels along the left ventricular (right-hand) side of the VSD and bifurcates as inverted bundle branches (the fanlike left bundle along its course to the rightward morphologic left ventricle and the cordlike right bundle distally to the leftward morphologic right ventricle). The bundle is most tenuous at its proximal connection with the AV node and along its course around the pulmonary valve annulus where it may become extensively infiltrated by fibrous tissue.[18,21] This is believed to explain the high rate of spontaneous AV block in this patient population. Rarely, both the anterior and the posterior AV nodes may give rise to separate AV conduction systems in CCTGA, with the potential for a conduction sling.[1,21,22] This seems most likely to occur when CCTGA coexists with an AV septal defect. In this situation, AV reciprocating tachycardia mediated by twin AV nodes may develop.[23]

A complete histologic description of the transitional cell inputs to the AV node in CCTGA does not exist. Although there are various descriptions from the catheter ablation literature, these are also limited. In general, successful slow pathway modification has been achieved from the right atrial septum, most commonly from the posterior and midseptal regions.[24,25] Less commonly, slow pathway modification can be achieved from the anteroseptal mitral annulus or even from the posterior aspect of the pulmonary annulus, presumably targeting a leftward extension of the anterior

AV node.[26,27] Unfortunately, because there is an opportunity for ≥1 AV node to exist in the setting of CCTGA, the precise relationship between the site of slow pathway modification and the location of the culprit AV node(s) is not always clear.

CCTGA can occasionally be observed in the setting of atrial situs inversus, which has unique implications. Unlike the situs solitus situation, the posterior node located at the apex of the triangle of Koch in this case almost always serves as the principal conduction pathway. It connects with an AV bundle that descends on the inferior aspect of the VSD (when present) and similarly bifurcates to the bundle branches much as with the situation for isolated VSD.[28–31] Although an anterior node may also be present, this node is generally hypoplastic, ending blindly without connection to the ventricular myocardium.[31] It is of surgical importance that the proximal AV bundle in cases of situs inversus may pass to the right side of the fibrous annulus and septum before coursing along the VSD,[29,31] potentially placing the proximal bundle at risk during tricuspid valve surgery.[30] Slow pathway modification seems to be possible at sites along the left-sided posterior or midseptal mitral annulus with this anomaly, although reports to date are scarce.[25,32]

Tetralogy of Fallot

In general, the conduction system in tetralogy of Fallot follows the anatomic rules noted previously for isolated ventricular septal defects, as discussed previously. The compact AV node is located in the usual position at the apex of the triangle of Koch, and the AV nodal transitional inputs are expected to be located normally. The proximal AV bundle penetrates the central fibrous body to travel inferior to the remnant of the membranous septum.[33]

In approximately 85% of cases of tetralogy of Fallot, the VSD is closely related to the membranous septum and is therefore most appropriately referred to as a *perimembranous defect*.[34,35] However, as the defect is embryologically formed by anterior deviation of the conal septum, the muscular borders of the defect include the anterior and posterior limbs of the septomarginal trabeculation (inferiorly) and the ventriculo-infundibular fold (superiorly).[36] The posteroinferior border in this case consists of remnants of the membranous septum with fibrous continuity between the tricuspid and aortic valve. In this situation, the penetrating AV bundle is variably exposed superficially at the posteroinferior border of the defect in the region of the membranous septum. Although

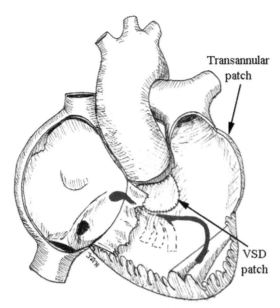

Fig. 4. Repaired Tetralogy of Falalot. VSD, ventricular septal defect.

the posterior limb of the septomarginal trabeculation may occasionally protect this portion of the proximal bundle, this region is generally considered most susceptible to surgically induced AV block. From here, the AV bundle travels on the leftward aspect of the septum, giving off the ramifications of the left bundle midway and then the right bundle branch from left to right near the apical portion of the VSD, where it may be also be susceptible to trauma from surgical patch placement (**Fig. 4**).[33,37]

In approximately 15% of cases of tetralogy of Fallot, the VSD is instead a true muscular outlet defect. This occurs when the ventriculo-infundibular fold merges with the posterior limb of the septomarginal trabeculation, forming a complete muscular rim.[34–36] In this situation, the proximal bundle at the posteroinferior border is remote from the crest of the ventricular septum. The nature of the VSD and the course of the conduction system have important ramifications for surgical repair as well as for catheter ablation of reentrant monomorphic ventricular tachycardia, especially with regard to the posterior muscular rim. These issues are discussed more extensively in other texts.[38,39]

COMPLEX DEFECTS
Tricuspid Atresia

Tricuspid atresia can be described as either a membranous form in which there is an imperforate tricuspid valve that connects to a morphologic

right ventricle (membranous atresia) or, alternatively, complete absence of the tricuspid valve and any anatomic connection to the right ventricle. The specialized conduction system in *membranous* atresia is similar to that of isolated ventricular septal defect.[40] On the other hand, in the more common form of tricuspid atresia with complete absence of the tricuspid valve, there is no right ventricular inlet septum, and an anomalous AV node forms at the junction of the inlet atrial and trabecular septae.[41]

Despite the altered right atrial anatomy for the common form of tricuspid atresia, the AV node is still grossly found in relation to the coronary sinus and the insertion of the tendon of Todaro as in the normal heart.[41,42] The AV node is adjacent to the central fibrous body, which is usually identified as a dimple in the floor of the right atrium (**Fig. 5**).[41–43] When present, transillumination of the dimple shows that it connects directly to the left ventricle.[41] Similarly, the AV bundle leaves the compact AV node in the region of the central fibrous body and passes to the leftward aspect of the ventricular septum. It is for this reason that His bundle electrograms are most easily obtained from the septal mitral annulus at electrophysiological study.[44]

The transitional inputs to the AV node in tricuspid atresia are generally described as normal in classic histologic studies; however, detailed characterization of their location is absent.[42] Moreover, clinical reports of slow pathway modification suggest that

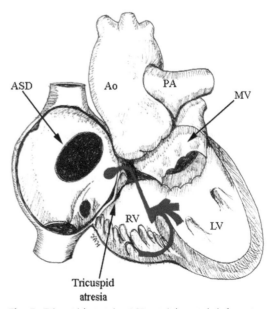

Fig. 5. Tricuspid atresia. ASD, atrial septal defect; Ao, aorta; LV, left ventricle; MV, mitral valve; PA, pulmonary artery; RV, right ventricle.

the transitional cell inputs may be found inferior to the compact AV node within the blind-ending right atrium, much as in the normal heart.[45,46] Alternatively, slow pathway modification has also been described at the inferior aspect of the septal mitral annulus below this bundle deflection, usually after careful mapping of the fast pathway location during tachycardia.[47–49]

After exiting onto the inferior and leftward aspect of the ventricular septum, the AV bundle promptly gives rise to the left bundle branches. This early branching is similar to the situation for AVSD and explains the counter-clockwise vector loop for both congenital lesions.[43]

Double Inlet Left Ventricle

Despite major differences in the congenital anatomy, the conduction system in double inlet left ventricle is often similar to that observed for cases of CCTGA as described previously. Both posterior and anterior AV nodes are also observed with this congenital heart defect but with only the anterior node making a connection with a penetrating AV bundle.[50,51] The course of the bundle then depends on the location of the rudimentary outlet chamber.[52] For the more common left-sided outlet chamber, the His bundle has a prolonged course, passing anterior to the posterior great vessel as in cases of CCTGA. From here, it enters the superior rim of the VSD extending along the left ventricular aspect of the VSD before bifurcating into the bundle branches. For cases of right-sided outlet chambers, the His bundle takes a much shorter course to the inferior rim of the VSD, again extending along the left side before bifurcating. This difference is principally of surgical importance, as enlargement of the VSD must be undertaken inferiorly for cases of left-sided outlet chambers and superiorly for right-sided outlet chambers.[52]

Heterotaxy Syndromes

Of the various forms of congenital heart disease, the heterotaxy syndromes are often considered the most complex in terms of cardiac morphology. This is equally true for the nature of the AV conduction system. Initially described in terms of the presence or absence of a normally appearing spleen, it is now realized that atrial morphology is the key determinant for the classification of these syndromes.[53] Therefore, the terms *right* and *left atrial isomerism* are used in the following text to denote the 2 major classes of heterotaxy syndrome.

The sinus node in heterotaxy syndrome is nearly always abnormal in terms of number, morphology, or location. Because the sinus node is inherently an atrial structure, its structural variations are linked to the type of atrial isomerism. For patients with left atrial isomerism for instance, the sinus node has been described as either absent, or hypoplastic and ectopic in location. Absence of the sinus node despite a careful search for this structure has been noted in greater than 50% of cases.[54] Other described locations include lateral displacement within the atrial wall or inferiorly near the posterior septum.[55] On the other hand, bilateral sinus nodes are always encountered in cases of right atrial isomerism either at the junction of the superior vena cavae with the atrium on both sides, or at these expected locations when only one is present.[54]

The anatomic routes of AV conduction in heterotaxy syndrome are also highly variable. Clinically speaking, AV block is associated with left atrial isomerism.[56,57] On the other hand, cases of atrioventricular reciprocating tachycardia mediated by twin AV nodes in patients with heterotaxy syndrome are most often associated with right atrial isomerism,[58–60] (although left atrial isomerism is also occasionally implicated).[61]

Duplication of the AV node and conduction system is one of the striking features of heterotaxy syndrome with right atrial isomerism. The histologic description is that of an anterior and posterior AV node that each give rise to a separate AV bundle that join together distally, forming a conduction sling" (**Fig. 6**).[54,55,62–64] Alternatively, the AV bundles may less commonly give rise to

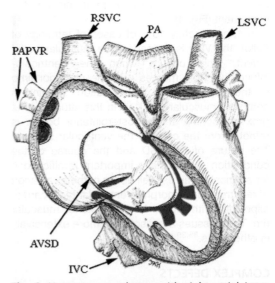

Fig. 6. Heterotaxy syndrome with right atrial isomerism. AVSD, atrioventricular septal defect; IVC, inferior vena cava; LSVC, left superior vena cava; PA, pulmonary artery; PAPVR, partial anamolous pulmonary venous return; RSVC, right superior vena cava.

separate bundle branches that end individually in the myocardium without establishing a true connection (**Fig. 6**). This form in particular has been noted to occur in association with asplenia in the setting of a hypoplastic anterior AV node.[65] Perhaps the least common variety is duplication of the posterior AV nodes, which connect via an unusual sling of conduction tissue, giving rise to a solitary cordlike bundle branch, which then enters an indeterminate ventricle.[54,55,64]

Attempts to predict that nature of the conduction system in heterotaxy syndrome have been fraught with difficulty, given the extreme heterogeneity of this population. However, some general rules exist. Although the hallmark of left atrial isomerism is the clinical association with AV block, dual AV nodes and a connecting sling of conduction tissue have been noted to occur in one-third of cases of biventricular AV connections.[54] This occurrence is especially likely if the ventricles are *l*-looped.[54,55] Despite duplicated AV nodes however, patients with left atrial isomerism may have interruption of one or both of the AV bundles in approximately one-third of these cases, typically at the site of connection with the node to the AV bundle, so that a continuous conduction sling is not formed.[54,65,66] On the other hand, in the setting of right atrial isomerism, duplicated AV nodes and conduction systems are the rule.[54,55,62,64–66] Again, the cardiac looping seems to be contributory, as cases of right atrial isomerism with biventricular AV connection and *l*-looping appear to most often possess an uninterrupted conduction sling.[54]

SUMMARY

Abnormalities in the conduction system are highly prevalent in the population with congenital heart disease. Although only minor variations may be present for many of the simple congenital heart defects, these can still have important ramifications for successful management of rhythm disturbances in this population. For the defects with more significant departure from normal, a thorough understanding of the disposition of the conduction system is vital for anyone caring for these patients. These issues are pertinent for all congenital practitioners, ranging from the interventional cardiologist to the electrophysiologist to the congenital cardiac surgeon. This review represents only a limited summary of the congenital heart disease spectrum, and the reader is encouraged to seek other excellent reviews describing these congenital conduction system abnormalities in their entirety.[67]

REFERENCES

1. Mönckeberg JG. Zur Entwicklungsgeschichte des Atrioventrikularsystems. Verhandl Deutsch Path Gesellsch 1913;16:228–49.
2. Soto B, Becker AE, Moulaert AJ, et al. Classification of ventricular septal defects. Br Heart J 1980;43:332–43.
3. Donald DE, Edwards JE, Harshbarger HG, et al. Surgical correction of ventricular septal defect: anatomic and technical considerations. J Thorac Surg 1957;33:45–59.
4. Becu LM, Burchell HB, Dushane JW, et al. Anatomic and pathologic studies in ventricular septal defect. Circulation 1956;14:349–64.
5. Milo S, Ho SY, Wilkinson JL, et al. Surgical anatomy and atrioventricular conduction tissues of hearts with isolated ventricular septal defects. J Thorac Cardiovasc Surg 1980;79:244–55.
6. Latham RA, Anderson RH. Anatomical variations in atrioventricular conduction system with reference to ventricular septal defects. Br Heart J 1972;34:185–90.
7. Feldt RH, DuShane JW, Titus JL. The atrioventricular conduction system in persistent common atrioventricular canal defect: correlations with electrocardiogram. Circulation 1970;42:437–44.
8. Thiene G, Wenink AC, Frescura C, et al. Surgical anatomy and pathology of the conduction tissues in atrioventricular defects. J Thorac Cardiovasc Surg 1981;82:928–37.
9. Ho SY, Rossi MB, Mehta AV, et al. Heart block and atrioventricular septal defect. Thorac Cardiovasc Surg 1985;33:362–5.
10. Lev M. The architecture of the conduction system in congenital heart disease. I. Common atrioventricular orifice. AMA Arch Pathol 1958;65:174–91.
11. Seo JW, Zuberbuhler JR, Ho SY, et al. Surgical significance of morphological variations in the atrial septum in atrioventricular septal defect for determination of the site of penetration of the atrioventricular conduction axis. J Card Surg 1992;7:324–32.
12. Kriebel T, Schneider H, Sigler M, et al. Slow pathway ablation in a 5-year-old boy with atrioventricular septal defect: value of cryoenergy application. Clin Res Cardiol 2006;95:668–70.
13. Stoyanov MK, Shalganov TN, Protich MM, et al. Selective slow pathway ablation using transseptal approach in a patient with surgically corrected partial atrioventricular canal defect and atrioventricular nodal reentrant tachycardia of the common type. Europace 2010;12:756–7.
14. Rausch CM, Runciman M, Collins KK. Cryothermal catheter ablation of atrioventricular nodal reentrant tachycardia in a pediatric patient after atrioventricular canal repair. Congenit Heart Dis 2010;5:66–9.

15. Upadhyay S, Marie Valente A, Triedman JK, et al. Catheter ablation for atrioventricular nodal reentrant tachycardia in patients with congenital heart disease. Heart Rhythm 2016;13:1228–37.

16. Khairy P, Mercier LA, Dore A, et al. Partial atrioventricular canal defect with inverted atrioventricular nodal input into an inferiorly displaced atrioventricular node. Heart Rhythm 2007;4:355–8.

17. Lev M, Licata RH, May RC. The conduction system in mixed levocardia with ventricular inversion (corrected transposition). Circulation 1963;28:232–7.

18. Lev M, Fielding RT, Zaeske D. Mixed levocardia with ventricular inversion (corrected transposition) with complete atrioventricular block. A histopathologic study of the conduction system. Am J Cardiol 1963;12:875–83.

19. Hudson RE. Surgical pathology of the conducting system of the heart. Br Heart J 1967;29:646–70.

20. Anderson RH, Arnold R, Wilkinson JL. The conducting system in congenitally corrected transposition. Lancet 1973;1:1286–8.

21. Anderson RH, Becker AE, Arnold R, et al. The conducting tissues in congenitally corrected transposition. Circulation 1974;50:911–23.

22. Hosseinpour AR, McCarthy KP, Griselli M, et al. Congenitally corrected transposition: size of the pulmonary trunk and septal malalignment. Ann Thorac Surg 2004;77:2163–6.

23. Epstein MR, Saul JP, Weindling SN, et al. Atrioventricular reciprocating tachycardia involving twin atrioventricular nodes in patients with complex congenital heart disease. J Cardiovasc Electrophysiol 2001;12:671–9.

24. Eisenberger M, Fox DJ, Earley MJ, et al. Atrioventricular node reentrant tachycardia ablation in a patient with congenitally corrected transposition of the great vessels using the CARTO mapping system. J Interv Card Electrophysiol 2007;19: 129–32.

25. Liao Z, Chang Y, Ma J, et al. Atrioventricular node reentrant tachycardia in patients with congenitally corrected transposition of the great arteries and results of radiofrequency catheter ablation. Circ Arrhythm Electrophysiol 2012;5:1143–8.

26. Tada H, Nogami A, Naito S, et al. Selected slow pathway ablation in a patient with corrected transposition of the great arteries and atrioventricular nodal reentrant tachycardia. J Cardiovasc Electrophysiol 1998;9:436–40.

27. Noheria A, Asirvatham SJ, McLeod CJ. Unusual atrioventricular reentry tachycardia in congenitally corrected transposition of great arteries: a novel site for catheter ablation. Circ Arrhythm Electrophysiol 2016;9:e004120.

28. Dick M 2nd, Van Praagh R, Rudd M, et al. Electrophysiologic delineation of the specialized atrioventricular conduction system in two patients with corrected transposition of the great arteries in situs inversus (I, D,D). Circulation 1977;55:896–900.

29. Anderson RH, Arnold R, Jones RS. D-bulboventricular loop with L-transposition in situs inversus. Circulation 1972;46:173–9.

30. Thiene G, Nava A, Rossi L. The conduction system in corrected transposition with situs inversus. Eur J Cardiol 1977;6:57–70.

31. Wilkinson JL, Smith A, Lincoln C, et al. Conducting tissues in congenitally corrected transposition with situs inversus. Br Heart J 1978;40:41–8.

32. Ma J, Bian C, Ying ZQ. Successful ablation of atrioventricular nodal reentrant tachycardia in a patient with coexistent congenitally corrected transposition of the great vessels and situs inversus. Intern Med 2014;53:1519–22.

33. Lev M. The architecture of the conduction system in congenital heart disease. II. Tetralogy of Fallot. AMA Arch Pathol 1959;67:572–87.

34. Dickinson DF, Wilkinson JL, Smith A, et al. Variations in the morphology of the ventricular septal defect and disposition of the atrioventricular conduction tissues in Tetralogy of Fallot. Thorac Cardiovasc Surg 1982;30:243–9.

35. Kurosawa H, Imai Y. Surgical anatomy of the atrioventricular conduction bundle in tetralogy of Fallot. New findings relevant to the position of the sutures. J Thorac Cardiovasc Surg 1988;95:586–91.

36. Becker AE, Connor M, Anderson RH. Tetralogy of Fallot: a morphometric and geometric study. Am J Cardiol 1975;35:402–12.

37. Hasegawa T. Studies on the conduction system in congenital malformations of the heart, especially of tetralogy of fallot. Jpn Heart J 1961;2:377–96.

38. Zeppenfeld K, Schalij MJ, Bartelings MM, et al. Catheter ablation of ventricular tachycardia after repair of congenital heart disease: electroanatomic identification of the critical right ventricular isthmus. Circulation 2007;116:2241–52.

39. Moore JP, Seki A, Shannon KM, et al. Characterization of anatomic ventricular tachycardia isthmus pathology after surgical repair of Tetralogy of Fallot. Circ Arrhythm Electrophysiol 2013;6:905–11.

40. Dickinson DF, Wilkinson JL, Smith A, et al. Atresia of the right atrioventricular orifice with atrioventricular concordance. Br Heart J 1979;42:9–14.

41. Dickinson DF, Wilkinson JL, Smith A, et al. Atrioventricular conduction tissues in univentricular hearts of left ventricular type with absent right atrioventricular connection ('tricuspid atresia'). Br Heart J 1979;42: 1–8.

42. Bharati S, Lev M. The conduction system in tricuspid atresia with and without regular (d-) transposition. Circulation 1977;56:423–9.

43. Guller B, DuShane JW, Titus JL. The atrioventricular conduction system in two cases of tricuspid atresia. Circulation 1969;40:217–26.

44. Serratto M, Pahlajani DB. Electrophysiologic studies in tricuspid atresia. Am J Cardiol 1978;42:983–6.

45. Abrams DJ, Earley MJ, Sporton SC, et al. Successful ablation of atrioventricular nodal reentry tachycardia following the atriopulmonary Fontan procedure. Europace 2006;8:907–10.

46. Frommeyer G, Milberg P, Eckardt L, et al. Slow pathway modulation in a patient with tricuspid valve atresia. Cardiol Young 2015;25:149–50.

47. Khairy P, Seslar SP, Triedman JK, et al. Ablation of atrioventricular nodal reentrant tachycardia in tricuspid atresia. J Cardiovasc Electrophysiol 2004;15:719–22.

48. Arana-Rueda E, Pedrote A, Sanchez-Brotons JA, et al. Ablation of atrioventricular nodal reentrant tachycardia in a patient with tricuspid atresia guided by electroanatomic mapping. Pacing Clin Electrophysiol 2012;35:e293–5.

49. Arana-Rueda E, Pedrote A, Duran-Guerrero JM, et al. Simplified approach for ablation of nodal reentrant tachycardia in a patient with tricuspid atresia and extracardiac Fontan palliation. Rev Esp Cardiol (Engl Ed) 2013;66:314–6.

50. Anderson RH, Arnold R, Thapar MK, et al. Cardiac specialized tissue in hearts with an apparently single ventricular chamber (double inlet left ventricle). Am J Cardiol 1974;33:95–106.

51. Bharati S, Lev M. The course of the conduction system in single ventricle with inverted (L-) loop and inverted (L-) transposition. Circulation 1975;51:723–30.

52. Becker AE, Wilkinson JL, Anderson RH. Atrioventricular conduction tissues in univentricular hearts of left ventricular type. Herz 1979;4:166–75.

53. Uemura H, Ho SY, Devine WA, et al. Atrial appendages and venoatrial connections in hearts from patients with visceral heterotaxy. Ann Thorac Surg 1995;60:561–9.

54. Smith A, Ho SY, Anderson RH, et al. The diverse cardiac morphology seen in hearts with isomerism of the atrial appendages with reference to the disposition of the specialised conduction system. Cardiol Young 2006;16:437–54.

55. Dickinson DF, Wilkinson JL, Anderson KR, et al. The cardiac conduction system in situs ambiguus. Circulation 1979;59:879–85.

56. Wren C, Macartney FJ, Deanfield JE. Cardiac rhythm in atrial isomerism. Am J Cardiol 1987;59:1156–8.

57. Ho SY, Cook A, Anderson RH, et al. Isomerism of the atrial appendages in the fetus. Pediatr Pathol 1991;11:589–608.

58. Wu MH, Wang JK, Lin JL, et al. Supraventricular tachycardia in patients with right atrial isomerism. J Am Coll Cardiol 1998;32:773–9.

59. Cheung YF, Cheng VY, Yung TC, et al. Cardiac rhythm and symptomatic arrhythmia in right atrial isomerism. Am Heart J 2002;144:159–64.

60. Bae EJ, Noh CI, Choi JY, et al. Twin AV node and induced supraventricular tachycardia in Fontan palliation patients. Pacing Clin Electrophysiol 2005;28:126–34.

61. Kato Y, Horigome H, Takahashi-Igari M, et al. Tachycardia associated with twin atrioventricular nodes in an infant with heterotaxy and interruption of inferior vena cava. Pacing Clin Electrophysiol 2012;35:e302–5.

62. Anderson RH, Smith A, Wilkinson JL. Right juxtaposition of the auricular appendages. Eur J Cardiol 1976;4:495–503.

63. Bharati S, Lev M. The course of the conduction system in dextrocardia. Circulation 1978;57:163–71.

64. Ho SY, Fagg N, Anderson RH, et al. Disposition of the atrioventricular conduction tissues in the heart with isomerism of the atrial appendages: its relation to congenital complete heart block. J Am Coll Cardiol 1992;20:904–10.

65. Ih S, Fukuda K, Okada R, et al. The location and course of the atrioventricular conduction system in common atrioventricular orifice and in its related anomalies with transposition of the great arteries—A histopathological study of six cases. Jpn Circ J 1983;47:1262–73.

66. Pohanka I, Vitek B. The conducting system of the heart in the syndrome of visceral symmetry. Folia Morphol (Praha) 1978;26:379–88.

67. Stolte M. The conduction system of the heart. In: Davies MJ, Anderson RH, Becker AE, editors. Clinical cardiology, vol. 6. London: Butterworths; 1983. p. 336. illustrations, $53.75 (approx.) ISBN: 0-407-00133-6:A43.

Bradyarrhythmias in Congenital Heart Disease

Steven K. Carlson, MD[a],*, Akash R. Patel, MD[b], Philip M. Chang, MD[c]

KEYWORDS

- Brady arrhythmia • Congenital heart disease • Conduction system defects • Atrioventricular block
- Sinus node dysfunction

KEY POINTS

- Brady arrhythmias are frequently encountered in adults with congenital heart disease (CHD), can occur in any form of CHD, and occur with increasing frequency with longer duration of follow-up.
- Bradyarrhythmias in CHD can be a result of congenital abnormalities of the conduction system, a consequence from postsurgical or postinterventional trauma to the conduction system, or the cumulative endpoint of a combination of both.
- Clinical sequelae of bradyarrhythmias can include symptomatic bradycardia, bradycardia-induced tachyarrhythmias, heart failure, and, in some cases, increased mortality.
- Treatment of bradyarrhythmias with permanent pacing in CHD patients can lead to long-term complications, such as ventricular dysfunction, lead complications, and vascular compromise.

INTRODUCTION

Arrhythmias account for the highest proportion of complications in adult patients living with congenital heart disease (CHD). Because of advancements in both surgical and medical care, CHD patients who previously would not have lived into adult life are now doing so at an exponential rate.[1] The incidence of arrhythmias also progressively increases with age and duration of follow-up, further escalating the burden of arrhythmias not only for individual patients but also for the entire adult congenital heart disease (ACHD) population.

Bradyarrhythmias represent one end of the spectrum of arrhythmia disorders that can affect patients with ACHD. Although different in cause, frequency, and management in comparison to tachyarrhythmias, bradyarrhythmias remain a source of tremendous morbidity and mortality and require close attention. The arrhythmias encountered in patients with ACHD are frequently the consequence of surgical interventions and hemodynamic derangements that can impair conduction system function by directly damaging the conduction tissue, altering cardiac chamber size and wall thickness, and causing myocardial fibrosis. However, some patients can be born with bradyarrhythmias or carry an anatomic substrate that predisposes them to their development over time, even in the absence of corrective or palliative intervention.

Bradyarrhythmias can result in significant clinical sequelae and often require treatment through permanent pacing. Of equal importance to understanding the mechanisms and clinical sequelae of these bradyarrhythmias in patients with ACHD is

Disclosure Statement: The authors have nothing to disclose.
a Clinical Cardiac Electrophysiology, Keck Hospital of USC, Keck School of Medicine of the University of Southern California, 1510 San Pablo Street, Suite 322, Los Angeles, CA 90033, USA; b Department of Pediatrics, UCSF Benioff Children's Hospital, UCSF School of Medicine, 1825 4th Street, San Francisco, CA 94158, USA; c USC Adult Congenital Heart Disease Care Program, Keck Hospital of USC, Keck School of Medicine of the University of Southern California, 1510 San Pablo Street, Suite 322, Los Angeles, CA 90033, USA
* Corresponding author.
E-mail address: steven.carlson@med.usc.edu

Card Electrophysiol Clin 9 (2017) 177–187
http://dx.doi.org/10.1016/j.ccep.2017.02.002
1877-9182/17/© 2017 Elsevier Inc. All rights reserved.

cardiacEP.theclinics.com

the complexity of managing the potential complications, morbidity, and mortality associated with long-term permanent pacing, which is often used very early in their lives. This section discusses the incidence and prevalence of bradyarrhythmias in the CHD population, their timing of occurrence with respect to specific disease entities and interventions, and their short- and long-term clinical sequelae.

THE SPECTRUM OF BRADYARRHYTHMIAS IN CONGENITAL HEART DISEASE

Bradyarrhythmias in CHD encompass both sinus and atrioventricular (AV) node dysfunction resulting in varying degrees of bradycardia. These 2 broad categories can be further grouped based on causes:

- Congenital abnormalities involving the conduction system
- Acquired bradyarrhythmias secondary to surgical or percutaneous intervention
- Combined/mixed cause involving CHD conditions with inherent abnormalities in the structure of the conduction system that may lead to progressive development of bradyarrhythmias or, when coupled with surgical interventions, carry a heightened risk of postsurgical conduction system impairment

Table 1 lists the most common CHD lesions and causes of sinus and AV node dysfunction, respectively, in patients with ACHD.

Unrepaired Congenital Heart Disease

Sinus and AV node impairment can be associated with specific forms of CHD where there is either inadequacy or lack of development of either structure in the malformed heart or abnormalities in structural formation that predispose them to progressive deterioration. In addition, the derangement in

structural formation can increase risk of damage during surgical or percutaneous interventions.

Congenital abnormalities in sinus node location and formation are generally rare aside from the case of heterotaxy syndrome and left juxtaposition of the atrial appendages. Greater variability in AV node and distal conduction system anatomy exists across a variety of defects.[2] AV discordance, deficiency in atrial and/or ventricular septal development, and abnormalities in ventricular looping create the potential for duplication or malalignment of conduction system structures that increase the risk of heart block. Depending on the specific defect or defects, either the sinus node, AV node, or both may be affected.

Heterotaxy syndromes

Heterotaxy syndromes can lead to significant abnormalities in sinus and AV node anatomy. In right atrial isomerism, or asplenia, there is the potential for duplication of conduction system structures. Asplenic patients may therefore present with 2 separate atrial rhythms or 2 distinct QRS complexes owing to duplicated sinus nodes, AV nodes, and infranodal systems. Furthermore, those with duplicated AV nodes and distal conduction systems may develop re-entrant tachyarrhythmias if a concomitant Mönckeberg sling is present.[3]

In contrast, left atrial isomerism, or polysplenia, is more commonly associated with the development of bradyarrhythmias. Owing to the mirror-imaged left sidedness in polysplenia, the usual right-sided conduction system structures may, in fact, be absent.

The incidence of sinus node dysfunction with polysplenia has been reported between 16% and 50% among young patients.[4,5] Of further importance is the observation that these patients can develop combined tachycardia-bradycardia syndrome, with 1 study demonstrating that 79%

Table 1
Common causes of sinus node and atrioventricular node dysfunction in congenital heart disease

	Sinus Node Dysfunction	AV Node Dysfunction
Congenital	Heterotaxy/polysplenia	Heterotaxy/polysplenia, ccTGA
Combined/mixed	Heterotaxy/polysplenia, left juxtaposition of atrial appendages	Heterotaxy/polysplenia, ccTGA, AVSD, tricuspid atresia
Acquired	Postsurgical: atriotomy, SVC/pulmonary vein/atrial repairs (SVASD), atrial switch operations (Mustard/Senning), Fontan variants	Postsurgical: VSD closure/tunneling, ventricular myotomy/myomectomy, subaortic membrane resection, Konno operation, valve replacement

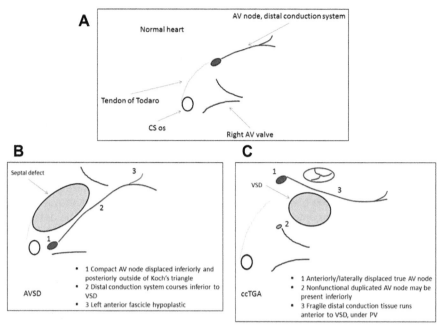

Fig. 1. AV node and distal conduction system structure and course in the normal heart (*A*), AVSD (*B*), and ccTGA (*C*). CS, coronary sinus; PV, pulmonary vein.

of patients who developed supraventricular tachycardia also had evidence of sinus node dysfunction.[4]

Heart block has been reported to occur in up to 34% of cases in polysplenia and usually develops within the first 5 years of life.[6,7] In an anatomic study of polysplenia patients, those with complete heart block (CHB) had identifiable AV nodes, but absence of a penetrating connection between the node and distal conduction system. Conversely, among those without heart block, a penetrating connection was present.[8]

Long-term follow-up of polysplenic patients is progressively growing. In a single-center experience, Gilljam and colleagues[9] reported on a cohort of 163 patients with left atrial isomerism followed over a 28-year period. Congenital CHB was present in 7% of patients. Both univariate and multivariate analyses showed congenital CHB to be significantly associated with earlier mortality. Only 1 of 11 patients with congenital CHB survived at the end of the follow-up period, and 80% of patients who received early pacing therapy died before further surgical interventions. The postnatal development of bradycardia secondary to progressive absence of atrial rhythms occurred in 16% and postsurgical heart block in patients with preoperative intact conduction occurred in 4 patients. By combining congenital and postnatally acquired bradyarrhythmias, 25% of the cohort experienced significant bradyarrhythmias requiring pacing support.

Atrioventricular septal defects

The anatomy of the AV node and distal conduction system is significantly distorted in patients with atrioventricular septal defects (AVSDs) (**Fig. 1**B). In AVSDs, the AV node is displaced to an inferior position outside of Koch triangle and anterior to the mouth of the coronary sinus. In addition, the distal conduction system runs along the lower ridge of the ventricular septum, which can predispose it to injury during surgical repair of associated ventricular septal defects (VSDs). The anterior fascicle of the left bundle is usually hypoplastic and resultant left-axis deviation is commonly seen on surface electrocardiogram (ECG). In a small study examining the rhythms of patients with AVSDs, it was found that most had intra-atrial conduction delay and 28% had suprahisian first-degree AV block.[10]

Bradyarrhythmia risk in patients with AVSDs largely stems from the baseline fragile architecture of the conduction system. Relatively recent appraisal of postsurgical heart block following corrective surgery for CHD revealed that AVSDs carry a significantly higher risk of postsurgical heart block with an odds ratio of 1.77 compared with other common VSD types.[11] This finding highlights the augmented risk of damage during surgery unique to this particular defect.

Congenitally corrected transposition of the great arteries

Patients with congenitally corrected transposition of the great arteries (ccTGA) can have congenital or progressive heart block and are also at higher risk of developing postoperative heart block owing to the significant anatomic distortion of the conduction system (see **Fig. 1**). Duplicated AV nodes have been described in ccTGA with a hypoplastic and nonfunctional node located more posteriorly along the right AV valve annulus and the functioning node located rightward and anteriorly. The functional AV node is located outside of Koch triangle and connects to the distal conduction system, which itself takes an unusual course, becoming elongated, running medially toward the septum, and then along the anterior rim of the pulmonary valve.[12] These anatomic abnormalities have a significant impact on the stability of the AV conduction system over time.

Heart block risk is seen throughout the lifetime of the ccTGA patient. Up to 10% of infants with ccTGA are born with CHB. The progressive risk of heart block in ccTGA patients has been estimated at 1% to 2% per person-year with an overall incidence ranging between 13% and 38% depending on the presence of associated defects.[13–15] The mean age of heart block occurrence was 18 years.[14] Pathologic studies in ccTGA patients with acquired heart block show fibrosis of the common bundle above the level of the His.[13]

Connelly and colleagues[15] followed 52 ccTGA patients greater than 18 year old, of which 39 patients survived during the study period. Nearly 60% of the deceased and half of survivors had pacemakers implanted. Although most patients who died had pacemakers, bradycardia-related sequelae were not reported as the cause of death. Among the 18 survivors who received pacemakers, 3 had congenital CHB, 6 developed progressive heart block requiring pacing, and the remaining patients developed postsurgical heart block. These findings suggest that bradycardia-associated mortality is not typically seen and is likely prevented with permanent pacing.

Other congenital heart disease defects

Other CHD defects with associated abnormalities in the conduction system include lesions with left juxtaposition of the atrial appendages and certain forms of single-ventricle defects. In left juxtaposed atrial appendages, the sinus node is displaced inferior and anterior to the crista terminalis.[16] Although this displacement may not necessarily alter sinus node function, the atypical location of the node may increase the risk of trauma and dysfunction following cardiac surgery.

Among patients with single-ventricle defects, those with tricuspid atresia and ventricular inversion have been found to have structural abnormalities of the conduction system. In tricuspid atresia, the atretic tricuspid valve is frequently a fibrous plate with associated displacement of the AV node to the floor of the right atrium. The AV node subsequently courses to a malformed central fibrous body before connecting to the His bundle on the left side of the ventricular septum. This derangement in course can lead to progressive fibrosis and heart block over time. Similar conduction system distortion as well as risk of developing heart block as described above in ccTGA patients also exists in single-ventricle defects with associated ventricular inversion and AV discordance.[17]

Repaired Congenital Heart Disease

Traumatic damage to the conduction system during surgical repair or palliation of CHD is the most common reason for the development of bradyarrhythmias in patients with ACHD. The incidence of these arrhythmias varies widely depending on the specific CHD lesion and type of surgery performed. Postsurgical conduction system impairment certainly is not unique to CHD patients. However, what is unique is the occurrence of postsurgical bradyarrhythmias much earlier in life. These early arrhythmias introduce tremendous challenges in permanent pacemaker management in these patients over a much longer lifespan than typically encountered for adult patients who require permanent pacing later in life.

Spanning all severity types of CHD, sinus node dysfunction can occur after atrial surgeries that may injure the sinus node, its blood supply, or its autonomic inputs. Damage to the AV node and distal conduction tissue secondary to surgical intervention occurs most commonly from surgical procedures aimed at closing VSDs or using VSDs as tunneling conduits. Operations that require surgical incision into or excision of some portion of the ventricular septum also carry an increased risk of AV nodal and distal conduction system damage. Heart block can also arise following surgical valve repair or replacement (see **Table 1**).

Postsurgical sinus node dysfunction

With regards to postsurgical sinus node dysfunction, several CHD defects and surgical procedures deserve special mention and discussion. These CHD defects and surgical procedures include atrial switch operations for the physiologic repair of D-transposition of the great arteries (D-TGA) and surgical procedures used for the repair of sinus venosus-type atrial septal defects (SVASDs). Patients with single-ventricle CHD and Fontan connections also carry a high risk of developing sinus node impairment.

The Mustard and Senning operations used for physiologic repair of D-TGA and double-switch repair for ccTGA are associated with a high risk of postoperative and progressive sinus node dysfunction owing to their extensive atrial dissection and manipulation to create intra-atrial baffles. Early postoperative sinus node dysfunction after the Mustard operation has been reported to be between 11% and 19% with only a fraction requiring permanent pacing.[18,19] A similar incidence has also been reported following the Senning operation.

In a meta-analysis of studies following patients who have undergone atrial switch operations, the Mustard operation appeared to be associated with a greater long-term risk of sinus node dysfunction with several reports noting a 5-year incidence of sinus node dysfunction between 35% and 64.4% versus 22% and 32.6% following the Senning.[20] Furthermore, risk of sinus node dysfunction appears to be related to duration of follow-up. In long-term follow-up studies, sinus rhythm was seen in only 77% of Mustard patients and 53% of Senning patients at 5 years, but only 40% of Mustard and Senning patients at 20 years following surgery.[18,21]

In SVASDs, particularly the superior vena cava (SVC) type of the defect with or without anomalous pulmonary venous connections, postsurgical sinus node dysfunction is a well-recognized complication. The incidence is quite variable and appears to be related to the surgical technique used to repair the defect. Stewart and colleagues[22] reported the highest incidence of sinus node dysfunction following a 2-patch repair approach, followed next by a single-patch approach, and no incidence among the small cohort of patients that underwent a Warden repair with SVC anastomosis to the right atrial appendage. Given the potential for diagnosing and treating SVASDs in pediatric and even late adult age groups, postsurgical sinus node dysfunction can theoretically occur at any age, depending on when surgical correction is undertaken.

Sinus node dysfunction is frequently encountered both acutely following staged single-ventricle palliation procedures and over longer duration follow-up of patients who have undergone Fontan completion. Incidence of early sinus node dysfunction following cavopulmonary shunts, Glenn anastomosis, or the hemi-Fontan operation has been reported between 6% and 15% with recovery often seen.[23]

Dysfunction occurring early after Fontan surgery is often transient and seen in 23% to 47%.[24] Risk varies to some degree based on whether a lateral tunnel or extracardiac Fontan is performed. Both are associated with substantially lower rates of sinus node dysfunction in comparison to the antiquated "classic" atriopulmonary Fontan. In one study, bradycardia at 30 days or later occurred in 18% of lateral tunnel Fontans in comparison to only 9% of extracardiac Fontans.[25] Alternatively, the type of surgical dissection required in proceeding from the Glenn to extracardiac Fontan may result in greater blood supply compromise to the sinus node in comparison to that required for a lateral tunnel approach.[26]

Although sinus node dysfunction in Fontan patients is thought to be most frequently due to direct surgical trauma, other factors contribute as well. Atrial remodeling is recognized to be a significant contributor to the development atrial tachyarrhythmias. Atrial wall thickening and fibrosis are certainly appreciated in Fontan patients over longer durations of follow-up.[27] These changes parallel the observation of the increasing incidence of bradyarrhythmias in Fontan patients over longer durations of follow-up.[28] Although direct correlation between remodeling and sinus node dysfunction has not been established, this is certainly a possible explanation for the progressive development of sinus node dysfunction in these patients. Furthermore, chronic or persistent atrial tachyarrhythmias are frequently associated with adverse atrial remodeling that begets more atrial arrhythmias and possibly concomitant sinus node dysfunction.

Postsurgical complete heart block

Postsurgical heart block most commonly occurs after repair of CHD defects where surgical intervention is performed in close proximity to the AV node and distal conduction system. This risk appears further compounded in defects with pre-existing, deranged, and fragile conduction system architecture. Not surprisingly, rates of AV conduction system injury following surgery are highest in patients undergoing repairs in ccTGA and AVSDs.

The KID (Kids' Inpatient Database) reported on the incidence of postsurgical heart block in roughly 16,000 patients undergoing VSD, AVSD, and tetralogy of Fallot (TOF) repairs.[2] The investigators found that, over a 10-year period, CHB occurred in 4.14% of VSD repairs, 7.66% of AVSD repairs, and 3.72% of TOF repairs. The overall development of postsurgical CHB remained unchanged over the surgical era despite decreases in surgical mortality over time, and age was not found to be a predictor based on logistic regression analysis.

In a recent multicenter study, Liberman and colleagues[29] reported a 1% overall incidence of advanced second- or third-degree AV block among patients who underwent greater than 100,000 surgical procedures for CHD repair. Surgical procedures that involved some component of VSD closure or baffling or surgical resection for the relief of outflow tract obstruction accounted for nearly 28% of the patients with postsurgical heart block. Mitral, tricuspid, and aortic valve operations accounted for another 24% of cases. The double-switch operation for ccTGA repair carried the highest risk of CHB and pacemaker implantation.

Most cases of postsurgical CHB are transient with 43% to 95% recovering conduction in the first 7 to 10 days[30] (**Fig. 2**). Therefore, it is generally agreed that patients with persistent CHB beyond 10 days should undergo permanent pacemaker implantation. Those who recover conduction may have different short- and long-term courses, including the potential for redevelopment of advanced conduction disease. Aziz and colleagues[31] noted that nearly 16% of patients who had recovered AV conduction after initially having postoperative CHB developed late CHB again. Those with redevelopment of CHB had substantially longer median durations of initial postoperative CHB before conduction recovery. Gross and colleagues[30] further cited additional variables that may potentially serve as risk factors for late redevelopment of high-grade block, or even sudden death, among long-term survivors with repaired CHD and history of postsurgical conduction impairment. These variables include the level of conduction impairment, the escape rhythm versus recovered rhythm QRS morphology, and recovery of conduction with residual bifascicular

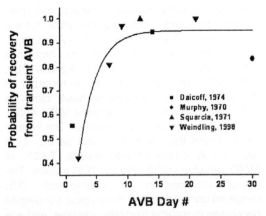

Fig. 2. Probability of recovery from transient postsurgical heart block (atrioventricular block, AVB). (*From* Gross GJ, Chiu CC, Hamilton RM, et al. Natural history of postoperative heart block in congenital heart disease: implications for pacing intervention. Heart Rhythm 2006;3(5):602; with permission.)

block. Alternatively, those with persistent heart block even beyond 14 days have been shown to recover AV conduction late in follow-up. Batra and colleagues[32] reported recovery in nearly 10% of patients at a median 41 days following surgery. Very late recovery, even out to 20 years (median 5.5 years) after initial surgery, was reported by Bruckheimer and colleagues[33] in 32% of patients with persistent postsurgical CHB.

The development of very late-onset heart block following a history of CHD surgery has also been reported. This presentation is highly variable, may not be the result of surgical AV node injury, and can occur even decades after surgery.[34] The timing of this presentation is likely influenced by the specific CHD substrate, surgical techniques used, the natural progression of AV node dysfunction in those forms of CHD, and long-term patient survival.

Heart block is also a recognized complication in percutaneous interventions. Catheter-based interventions are increasingly being used over surgical repair for atrial and VSDs. The development of CHB following transcatheter closure of atrial septal defects was found to be 1.12% compared with none among patients repaired surgically.[35] In a small cohort of patients with muscular VSDs, there was no incidence of heart block following percutaneous device closure.[36] However, a higher risk of heart block was seen following percutaneous closure of perimembranous VSDs. In a large series of patients who underwent percutaneous perimembranous VSD closure, periprocedural heart block occurred in nearly 2% of patients with an additional 1.5% of patients developing heart block within 30 days after the procedure as well.[37]

Transcatheter valve replacement is increasing in application and integration in the care of patients with ACHD. This expanding form of therapy must also be recognized as potentially carrying some risk of AV conduction system injury. Heart block generally is not encountered following percutaneous pulmonary valve insertion. Conversely, the risk of heart block following transcatheter aortic valve replacement (TAVR) has been reported around 10% at 1 year in the normal adult population.[38] It is unclear if similar or higher risk should be expected in CHD patients following TAVR.

CLINICAL SEQUELAE AND TREATMENT OF BRADYARRHYTHMIAS IN ADULT CONGENITAL HEART DISEASE

The short- and long-term clinical sequelae of bradyarrhythmias in both unrepaired and repaired CHD are highly variable. Consequences can include symptoms attributable to bradycardia, the development of concomitant tachyarrhythmias, and, in some cases, an increase in mortality. In addition, the long-term requirement for permanent ventricular pacing may lead to pacing-induced cardiomyopathy. Published and endorsed treatment guidelines provide a framework to guide the integration of permanent pacing in patients with ACHD with clinically significant bradyarrhythmias (**Table 2**).

By far the most common sequelae of bradyarrhythmias in CHD are symptoms attributable to bradycardia where slow heart rates are insufficient to meet metabolic needs either at rest or during exertion. Alternatively, patients may develop symptoms related to the loss of AV synchrony, which may cause or worsen existing valve dysfunction and impair cardiac output, thereby causing or worsening heart failure.

Table 2
Proposed recommendations for permanent pacing in adults with congenital heart disease extrapolated from published American College of Cardiology, the American Heart Association, Heart Rhythm Society, Pediatric And Congenital Electrophysiology Society guidelines and consensus statements

Class I	1. Permanent pacing is recommended for adults with CHD and symptomatic sinus node dysfunction, including documented sinus bradycardia or chronotropic incompetence that is intrinsic or secondary to required drug therapy. Devices that minimize ventricular pacing are preferred.
	2. Permanent pacing is recommended in adults with CHD and symptomatic bradycardia in conjunction with any degree of heart block or with ventricular arrhythmias presumed to be due to heart block.
	3. Permanent pacing is recommended in adults with congenital CHB and wide QRS escape rhythm, complex ventricular ectopy, or ventricular dysfunction.
	4. Permanent pacing is recommended for adults with CHD and postsurgical high-grade second- or third-degree heart block that is not expected to resolve.
	5. CRT is recommended for adults with biventricular CHD, reduced morphologic systemic LV function, wide left bundle branch block with QRS duration >150 ms, and evidence of mechanical dyssynchrony.
Class IIa	1. Permanent pacing is reasonable for adults with CHD and impaired hemodynamics, as assessed by noninvasive or invasive means, due to sinus bradycardia or loss of AV synchrony.
	2. Permanent pacing is reasonable for adults with CHD and sinus or junctional bradycardia for the prevention of recurrent intra-atrial reentrant tachycardia (IART). Devices with atrial antitachycardia pacing (ATP) function should be considered in this subpopulation of patients.
	3. Permanent pacing is reasonable in adults with congenital CHB and average daytime resting heart rate <50 bpm.
	4. Permanent pacing is reasonable for adults with complex CHD and an awake resting heart rate (sinus or junctional) <40 bpm or ventricular pauses >3 s. An ATP device may be considered if concomitant IART risk is present.
	5. CRT may be reasonable in patients with ACHD with reduced EF <35% and anticipated ventricular pacing requirement >40%.
Class IIb	1. Permanent pacing may be reasonable in adults with CHD of moderate complexity and an awake resting heart rate (sinus or junctional) <40 bpm or ventricular pauses >3 s. An ATP device may be considered if concomitant IART risk is present.
	2. Permanent pacing may be considered in adults with CHD, a history of transient postsurgical CHB, and residual bifascicular block.
	3. CRT may be reasonable in patients with ACHD with reduced EF >35% and anticipated ventricular pacing requirement >40%.
	4. CRT may be reasonable in patients with ACHD with univentricular or systemic morphologic RV substrates, evidence of reduced systemic ventricular function, mechanical dyssychrony, and wide QRS duration of at least 130 ms.
Class III	1. Pacing is not indicated in asymptomatic adults with CHD and bifascicular block with or without first-degree AV block in the absence of a history of transient CHB.
	2. Endocardial leads are generally avoided in adults with CHD and intracardiac shunts. Risk assessment regarding hemodynamic circumstances, concomitant anticoagulation, shunt closure before endocardial lead placement, or alternative approaches for lead access should be individualized.

Concomitant tachyarrhythmias and bradyarrhythmias are frequently encountered in patients with ACHD. Prevention of excessive bradycardia with permanent pacing can permit more aggressive antiarrhythmic treatment of tachyarrhythmias with less concern over medication-induced bradycardia. Furthermore, provision of a consistent atrial rhythm with pacing may also prevent or reduce ectopy that could otherwise trigger atrial tachyarrhythmias.

Adverse atrial remodeling likely contributes to both bradyarrhythmias and tachyarrhythmias in patients with ACHD. In some, these opposite arrhythmias may develop independent of each other, but more commonly, they arise from shared factors. Abnormal atrial hemodynamics combined with scar promotes the development of intra-atrial re-entrant tachyarrhythmias in the setting of pre-existing, chronic bradycardia. Conversely, chronic and persistent atrial tachyarrhythmias may beget adverse atrial remodeling that may secondarily result in sinus node dysfunction. In all of these scenarios, the implantation of permanent pacing devices with antitachycardia pacing may be of some benefit to address both bradyarrhythmias and tachyarrhythmias.

In some forms of CHD, chronic bradycardia or the requirement for permanent pacing increases long-term mortality. Persistent sinus node dysfunction after palliation in hypoplastic left heart syndrome is associated with increased mortality.[39] The requirement for permanent pacing after atrial switch operations was also found to be the only predictor of long-term mortality in patients with repaired D-TGA.[40] Finally, it has been well documented that postoperative CHB following CHD surgery that remains untreated results in almost universally poor outcomes with near 100% mortality.[30]

Cardiac resynchronization therapy (CRT) is presently recognized as a valuable tool in the treatment of patients with cardiomyopathies and significant electromechanical dyssynchrony.[41] This form of pacing therapy can treat and help prevent ventricular dysfunction related to chronic single-site ventricular pacing. As such, resynchronization when applied in appropriate settings has been demonstrated to facilitate improvements in dyssynchrony measures and systemic ventricular ejection fraction (EF).

In the context of CHD, there are no prospective randomized controlled studies of single-site ventricular pacing versus biventricular pacing. Similarly, resynchronization pacing as a principal treatment tool for the management of primary ventricular dysfunction related to CHD defects, including systemic morphologic right ventricles

or single ventricle/Fontan substrates with resultant congestive heart failure, has yielded very mixed results. However, insight into the potential deleterious effects of single-site ventricular pacing can be found within several retrospective studies evaluating the benefit of CRT with respect to improved left ventricular (LV) function after CRT upgrade.[42,43] When pooled, these studies demonstrated improvements in left ventricular ejection fraction (LVEF) with CRT on average between 6% and 11% with associated improvements in New York Heart Association functional class scores. However, present experience remains inadequate to derive more generalized recommendations for the application of CRT in CHD.[44] The strongest recommendations for CRT remain reserved for patients with cardiomyopathy and ECG evidence of mechanical dyssynchrony, particularly wide left bundle branch block and QRS durations in excess of 150 milliseconds. Current guidelines give class IIa and IIb recommendations for the upgrade to a CRT devices in CHD patients anticipated to require greater than 40% ventricular pacing and either LVEF less

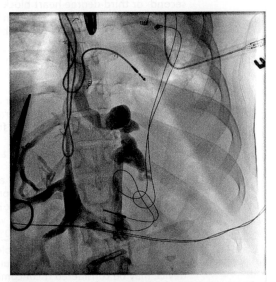

Fig. 3. Example of complexities in permanent pacing device management in patients with ACHD with history of early transvenous endocardial pacing. In this example, complete inferior vena cava (IVC) obstruction due to prolapsed transvenous pacing leads resulting in liver cirrhosis was discovered in a 24-year-old woman with original transvenous pacemaker implantation at 9 years. Complete extraction of the prolapsed leads was performed with angioplasty of the IVC to re-establish antegrade IVC flow. (*From* Carlson SK, Chang P, Doshi RN. Prolapse of pacemaker leads resulting in complete IVC obstruction in an adult congenital patient. Journal of Innovations in Cardiac Rhythm Management 2015; 2118; with permission.)

than 35% or greater than 35%, respectively[45] (see **Table 2**).

From a simplistic perspective, with presently available technology and techniques, the treatment of bradyarrhythmias with permanent pacing would seem to be relatively intuitive and effective. The application of permanent pacing affords the ability to provide chronotropic responsiveness, AV synchrony, and even multisite pacing for CRT. In comparison to the management of tachyarrhythmias, which can involve multiple options, the management of bradyarrhythmias can appear rather straightforward. However, it is important to recognize the implications of the permanency of pacing systems, along with their associated complications, lifelong care needs, required repeat interventions, and significant shortcomings.

Epicardial pacing systems are known to exhibit reduced system longevity, owing to known differences between endocardial versus epicardial pacing and the atypical system configurations that are frequently used when integrating permanent pacing in young CHD patients with either unconventional anatomy or small body sizes.[46] On the other hand, although transvenous endocardial pacing can be effectively achieved over long durations of time, transvenous lead implantation in younger and smaller patients can certainly be associated with a wide range of long-term complications, particularly as they grow into adulthood. These complications can include the need for reintervention for lead failure, lead fracture, infection, and venous obstruction[47] (**Fig. 3**).

Furthermore, surgical interventions for certain types of CHD may yield unconventional venous anatomy and narrowed passageways that should be approached by implanters who are knowledgeable and experienced in device implantation in

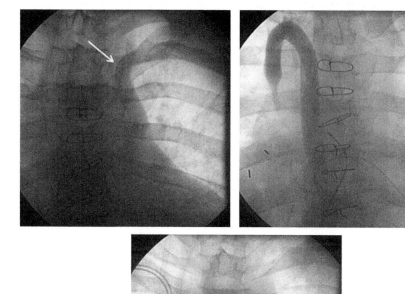

Fig. 4. Example of complexities in permanent pacing device management in patients with ACHD with prior surgical repair. In this example, SVC superior limb baffle occlusion was diagnosed in a 43-year-old man with D-TGA after atrial switch, advanced conduction disease, recurrent nonsustained ventricular tachycardia, and severely reduced systemic right ventricular function. Recanalization was achieved, and the superior limb was stented before right-sided implantable cardioverter-defibrillator implantation. Of note, a left SVC was present (*arrow*), but a bridging innominate vein was absent.

complex patients with ACHD (**Fig. 4**). Appropriate and close follow-up of permanent pacing systems, reasonable timing of conversion from epicardial to endocardial pacing, and careful monitoring for clinical sequelae and complications related to pacing leads must be integrated into the long-term care of patients with ACHD with permanent pacemakers.

SUMMARY

Bradyarrhythmias in patients with ACHD comprise a complex group of disorders with congenital and acquired origins, highly variable long-term sequelae, and highly complex treatment options. Untreated bradyarrhythmias can contribute substantially to morbidity and mortality in the ACHD population, whereas permanent pacing poses tremendous challenges in the long-term management of these patients. These aspects highlight the importance of early recognition of significant bradyarrhythmias and the careful and judicious use of permanent pacing for the treatment of this highly heterogeneous set of arrhythmias in an equally heterogeneous ACHD population.

REFERENCES

1. Warnes CA, Liberthson R, Danielson GK, et al. Task force 1: the changing profile of congenital heart disease in adult life. J Am Coll Cardiol 2001;37(5): 1170–5.
2. Anderson RH, Ho SY, Becker AE. The surgical anatomy of the conduction tissues. Thorax 1983;38(6): 408–20.
3. Khairy P, Fournier A, Dubuc M. Monckeberg's sling. Can J Cardiol 2003;19(6):717–8.
4. Miyazaki A, Sakaguchi H, Ohuchi H, et al. The incidence and characteristics of supraventricular tachycardia in left atrial isomerism: a high incidence of atrial fibrillation in young patients. Int J Cardiol 2013;166(2):375–80.
5. Momma K, Takao A, Shibata T. Characteristics and natural history of abnormal atrial rhythms in left isomerism. Am J Cardiol 1990;65(3):231–6.
6. Wren C, Macartney FJ, Deanfield JE. Cardiac rhythm in atrial isomerism. Am J Cardiol 1987; 59(12):1156–8.
7. Loomba RS, Willes RJ, Kovach JR, et al. Chronic arrhythmias in the setting of heterotaxy: differences between right and left isomerism. Congenit Heart Dis 2016;11(1):7–18.
8. Ho SY, Fagg N, Anderson RH, et al. Disposition of the atrioventricular conduction tissues in the heart with isomerism of the atrial appendages: its relation to congenital complete heart block. J Am Coll Cardiol 1992;20(4):904–10.
9. Gilljam T, McCrindle BW, Smallhorn JF, et al. Outcomes of left atrial isomerism over a 28-year period at a single institution. J Am Coll Cardiol 2000;36(3):908–16.
10. Fournier A, Young ML, Garcia OL, et al. Electrophysiologic cardiac function before and after surgery in children with atrioventricular canal. Am J Cardiol 1986;57(13):1137–41.
11. Anderson JB, Czosek RJ, Knilans TK, et al. Postoperative heart block in children with common forms of congenital heart disease: results from the KID Database. J Cardiovasc Electrophysiol 2012;23(12): 1349–54.
12. Anderson RH, Becker AE, Arnold R, et al. The conducting tissues in congenitally corrected transposition. Circulation 1974;50(5):911–23.
13. Daliento L, Corrado D, Buja G, et al. Rhythm and conduction disturbances in isolated, congenitally corrected transposition of the great arteries. Am J Cardiol 1986;58(3):314–8.
14. Huhta JC, Maloney JD, Ritter DG, et al. Complete atrioventricular block in patients with atrioventricular discordance. Circulation 1983;67(6):1374–7.
15. Connelly MS, Liu PP, Williams WG, et al. Congenitally corrected transposition of the great arteries in the adult: functional status and complications. J Am Coll Cardiol 1996;27(5):1238–43.
16. Ho SY, Monro JL, Anderson RH. Disposition of the sinus node in left-sided juxtaposition of the atrial appendages. Br Heart J 1979;41(2):129–32.
17. Bharati S, Lev M. The conduction system in tricuspid atresia with and without regular (d-) transposition. Circulation 1977;56(3):423–9.
18. Gelatt M, Hamilton RM, McCrindle BW, et al. Arrhythmia and mortality after the Mustard procedure: a 30-year single-center experience. J Am Coll Cardiol 1997;29(1):194–201.
19. Deanfield J, Camm J, Macartney F, et al. Arrhythmia and late mortality after Mustard and Senning operation for transposition of the great arteries. An eight-year prospective study. J Thorac Cardiovasc Surg 1988;96(4):569–76.
20. Khairy P, Landzberg MJ, Lambert J, et al. Long-term outcomes after the atrial switch for surgical correction of transposition: a meta-analysis comparing the Mustard and Senning procedures. Cardiol Young 2004;14(3):284–92.
21. Dos L, Teruel L, Ferreira IJ, et al. Late outcome of Senning and Mustard procedures for correction of transposition of the great arteries. Heart 2005; 91(5):652–6.
22. Stewart RD, Bailliard F, Kelle AM, et al. Evolving surgical strategy for sinus venosus atrial septal defect: effect on sinus node function and late venous obstruction. Ann Thorac Surg 2007;84(5):1651–5 [discussion: 1655].
23. Cohen MI, Bridges ND, Gaynor JW, et al. Modifications to the cavopulmonary anastomosis do not

eliminate early sinus node dysfunction. J Thorac Cardiovasc Surg 2000;120(5):891–900.

24. Cohen MI, Wernovsky G, Vetter VL, et al. Sinus node function after a systematically staged Fontan procedure. Circulation 1998;98(19 Suppl):II352–8 [discussion: II358–9].

25. Balaji S, Daga A, Bradley DJ, et al. An international multicenter study comparing arrhythmia prevalence between the intracardiac lateral tunnel and the extracardiac conduit type of Fontan operations. J Thorac Cardiovasc Surg 2014;148(2):576–81.

26. Rajanbabu BB, Gangopadhyay D. Sinus node dysfunction after extracardiac conduit and lateral tunnel Fontan operation: the importance of the type of prior superior cavopulmonary anastomosis. World J Pediatr Congenit Heart Surg 2016;7(2):210–5.

27. Wolf CM, Seslar SP, den Boer K, et al. Atrial remodeling after the Fontan operation. Am J Cardiol 2009; 104(12):1737–42.

28. Stamm C, Friehs I, Mayer JE Jr, et al. Long-term results of the lateral tunnel Fontan operation. J Thorac Cardiovasc Surg 2001;121(1):28–41.

29. Liberman L, Silver ES, Chai PJ, et al. Incidence and characteristics of heart block after heart surgery in pediatric patients: a multicenter study. J Thorac Cardiovasc Surg 2016;152(1):197–202.

30. Gross GJ, Chiu CC, Hamilton RM, et al. Natural history of postoperative heart block in congenital heart disease: implications for pacing intervention. Heart Rhythm 2006;3(5):601–4.

31. Aziz PF, Serwer GA, Bradley DJ, et al. Pattern of recovery for transient complete heart block after open heart surgery for congenital heart disease: duration alone predicts risk of late complete heart block. Pediatr Cardiol 2013;34(4):999–1005.

32. Batra AS, Wells WJ, Hinoki KW, et al. Late recovery of atrioventricular conduction after pacemaker implantation for complete heart block associated with surgery for congenital heart disease. J Thorac Cardiovasc Surg 2003;125(6):1291–3.

33. Bruckheimer E, Berul CI, Kopf GS, et al. Late recovery of surgically-induced atrioventricular block in patients with congenital heart disease. J Interv Card Electrophysiol 2002;6(2):191–5.

34. Fischbach PS, Frias PA, Strieper MJ, et al. Natural history and current therapy for complete heart block in children and patients with congenital heart disease. Congenit Heart Dis 2007;2(4): 224–34.

35. Wu MH, Chen HC, Wang JK, et al. Paradigm shift in the intervention for secundum atrial septal defect in an era of transcatheter closure: a national birth cohort study. Am Heart J 2015;170(6):1070–6.

36. Kanaan M, Ewert P, Berger F, et al. Follow-up of patients with interventional closure of ventricular septal defects with Amplatzer Duct Occluder II. Pediatr Cardiol 2015;36(2):379–85.

37. Bai Y, Xu XD, Li CY, et al. Complete atrioventricular block after percutaneous device closure of perimembranous ventricular septal defect: a single-center experience on 1046 cases. Heart Rhythm 2015;12(10):2132–40.

38. Leon MB, Smith CR, Mack MJ, et al. Transcatheter or surgical aortic-valve replacement in intermediate-risk patients. N Engl J Med 2016;374(17):1609–20.

39. Trivedi B, Smith PB, Barker PC, et al. Arrhythmias in patients with hypoplastic left heart syndrome. Am Heart J 2011;161(1):138–44.

40. Vejlstrup N, Sorensen K, Mattsson E, et al. Long-term outcome of Mustard/Senning correction for transposition of the great arteries in Sweden and Denmark. Circulation 2015;132(8):633–8.

41. European Heart Rhythm Association, European Society of Cardiology, Heart Rhythm Society, et al. 2012 EHRA/HRS expert consensus statement on cardiac resynchronization therapy in heart failure: implant and follow-up recommendations and management. Heart Rhythm 2012;9(9):1524–76.

42. Cecchin F, Frangini PA, Brown DW, et al. Cardiac resynchronization therapy (and multisite pacing) in pediatrics and congenital heart disease: five years experience in a single institution. J Cardiovasc Electrophysiol 2009;20(1):58–65.

43. Motonaga KS, Dubin AM. Cardiac resynchronization therapy for pediatric patients with heart failure and congenital heart disease: a reappraisal of results. Circulation 2014;129(18):1879–91.

44. Thambo JB, Dos Santos P, Bordachar P. Cardiac resynchronization therapy in patients with congenital heart disease. Arch Cardiovasc Dis 2011;104(6–7): 410–6.

45. Khairy P, Van Hare GF, Balaji S, et al. PACES/HRS expert consensus statement on the recognition and management of arrhythmias in adult congenital heart disease: developed in partnership between the Pediatric And Congenital Electrophysiology Society (PACES) and the Heart Rhythm Society (HRS). Endorsed by the governing bodies of PACES, HRS, the American College of Cardiology (ACC), the American Heart Association (AHA), the European Heart Rhythm Association (EHRA), the Canadian Heart Rhythm Society (CHRS), and the International Society for Adult Congenital Heart Disease (ISACHD). Heart Rhythm 2014;11(10):e102–65.

46. Radbill AE, Triedman JK, Berul CI, et al. System survival of nontransvenous implantable cardioverter-defibrillators compared to transvenous implantable cardioverter-defibrillators in pediatric and congenital heart disease patients. Heart Rhythm 2010;7(2): 193–8.

47. Carlson SK, Chang P, Doshi RN. Prolapse of pacemaker leads resulting in complete IVC obstruction in an adult congenital patient. The Journal of Innovations in Cardiac Rhythm Management 2015;6:2117–20.

Supraventricular Tachycardia in Adult Congenital Heart Disease
Mechanisms, Diagnosis, and Clinical Aspects

Christopher M. Janson, MD[a],*, Maully J. Shah, MBBS[b]

KEYWORDS

- Supraventricular tachycardia (SVT) • Adult congenital heart disease (ACHD) • Accessory pathway
- Atrioventricular reciprocating tachycardia (AVRT) • AV nodal reentrant tachycardia (AVNRT)
- Intra-atrial reentrant tachycardia (IART) • Atrial fibrillation

KEY POINTS

- Anatomic variants, postoperative conduction barriers, and hemodynamic derangements all contribute to a unique electrophysiologic milieu that is ripe for the development of supraventricular tachycardia (SVT) in the adult congenital heart disease (ACHD) patient.
- Slow pathway modification for atrioventricular (AV) nodal reentrant tachycardia in ACHD patients should be guided by knowledge of the variations in AV node and His bundle location expected in specific lesions.
- Atrioventricular reciprocating tachycardia (AVRT) is common in Ebstein's anomaly, due to the high prevalence of accessory pathways. The presence of multiple pathways and difficulty localizing the true AV groove can make ablation challenging.
- Intra-atrial reentrant tachycardia (IART) is the most common form of SVT in the ACHD population. Clinicians must maintain a high index of suspicion for IART because slowed conduction around large circuits can result in relatively slow SVT.
- Management of all forms of SVT in the ACHD patient must take into account underlying substrate, existing conduction disease, hemodynamic status, and issues of intravascular and intracardiac access.

INTRODUCTION

Supraventricular arrhythmias represent a major source of morbidity in adults with congenital heart disease (ACHD). The prevalence of atrial arrhythmias is estimated to be 15% in the ACHD population, with a cumulative life-time risk of approximately 50% for 20-year-olds.[1] Factors predisposing to the high incidence of arrhythmias include anatomic considerations, such as

Disclosure Statement: The authors have nothing to disclose.
[a] Division of Cardiology, The Children's Hospital at Montefiore, Albert Einstein College of Medicine, 3415 Bainbridge Avenue, R1, Bronx, NY 10467, USA; [b] Division of Cardiology, The Children's Hospital of Philadelphia, Perelman School of Medicine at the University of Pennsylvania, 34th & Civic Center Boulevard, Philadelphia, PA 19104, USA
* Corresponding author.
E-mail address: cjanson@montefiore.org

cardiacEP.theclinics.com

accessory pathways (APs) and atrioventricular (AV) nodal abnormalities; postoperative factors, such as scarring and suture lines; and hemodynamic derangements, including elevated atrial pressure and chronic hypoxemia. Intrinsic myocardial abnormalities and genetic factors may also play a role.[2,3]

GENERAL MECHANISMS OF SUPRAVENTRICULAR TACHYCARDIA

As in the general population, the primary mechanisms of supraventricular tachycardia (SVT) in ACHD patients include reentry, increased automaticity, and triggered activity. Macroreentry circuits include AP-mediated AV reciprocating tachycardia (AVRT), AV nodal reentrant tachycardia (AVNRT), and intra-atrial reentrant tachycardia (IART), which includes typical atrial flutter. Tachycardia mediated by twin AV nodes is a rare form of AVRT unique to patients with specific forms of complex congenital heart disease (CHD). Atrial fibrillation (AF) can be considered a form of microreentry tachycardia. Focal tachycardias, including atrial and junctional tachycardias (JTs), may show features of increased automaticity, triggered activity, or rarely microreentry. Each of these tachycardia mechanisms is discussed in detail, with a focus on mechanism, diagnosis, and clinical aspects specific to the ACHD population.

CHALLENGES IN THE DIAGNOSIS AND MANAGEMENT OF SUPRAVENTRICULAR TACHYCARDIA IN ADULTS WITH CONGENITAL HEART DISEASE

The ACHD patient with SVT presents several unique challenges, with regard to both diagnosis and management. Intrinsic electrophysiologic abnormalities can complicate interpretation of electrocardiogram (ECG) tracings. In the simplest example, SVT in a repaired tetralogy of Fallot (TOF) patient will likely present as a wide QRS tachycardia due to pre-existing right bundle branch block (RBBB) (**Fig. 1**). A more subtle example is IART in a Fontan patient, in whom a large circuit around scarred atrial tissue may generate a slow tachycardia with 1-to-1 AV conduction and very low amplitude P-waves (**Fig. 2**). Acute management of SVT in the ACHD patient should take into account residual lesions and abnormal hemodynamics, which may make tachycardia less tolerable. Medications for chronic management are likewise selected with attention to ventricular function and potential for bradycardia due to coexisting sinus or AV nodal conduction disease. Evaluation of a new arrhythmia in a repaired CHD patient should include a comprehensive functional assessment because new hemodynamic derangements can be a precipitating factor.[2,4] Finally, when ablation is indicated, additional challenges arise, including unusual

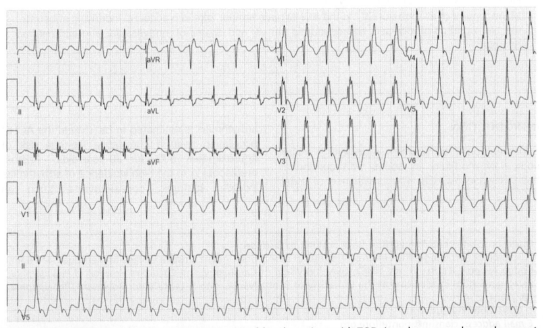

Fig. 1. 12-lead ECG demonstrating SVT in a 21-year-old male patient with TOF s/p pulmonary valve replacement. Pre-existing RBBB leads to a wide QRS morphology in SVT.

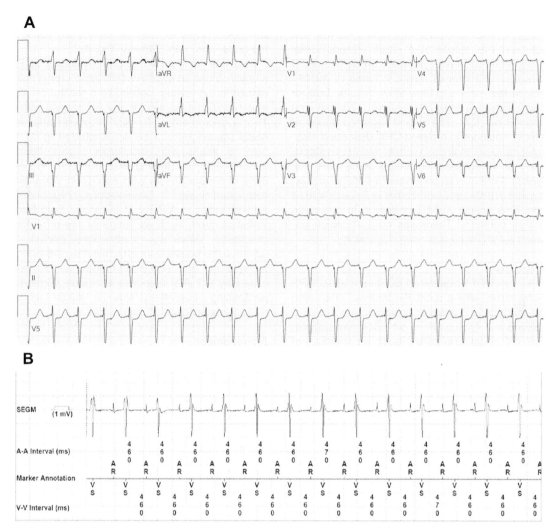

Fig. 2. (*A*) 12-lead ECG demonstrating IART in a 36-year-old female patient with tricuspid atresia, most recently s/p Fontan revision with an extracardiac conduit, as well as Maze procedure. Low amplitude P-waves can be appreciated in the limb leads. (*B*) Pacemaker interrogation confirms an atrial tachycardia with cycle length 460 ms and 1:1 conduction.

conduction anatomy and difficulty accessing vessels and intracardiac chambers due to prior procedures. For example, in a 2004 study of ablation in subjects with CHD, 24% of subjects had limited catheter access due to prior interventions, precluding mapping and ablation in 4 cases.[5] In the following sections, these issues will be addressed in more depth in the context of each specific tachycardia.

Atrioventricular Nodal Reentrant Tachycardia

Although AVNRT accounts for less than 8% of clinical SVT in adults with repaired CHD, it is estimated to occur in the CHD population with a similar frequency to the general population, in which it represents the most common paroxysmal

SVT mechanism in otherwise healthy adults.[4,6] AVNRT may be encountered in CHD patients as an additional tachycardia mechanism during invasive treatment of a different clinical arrhythmia. In a recent series of AVNRT ablations in CHD subjects, one-third were a secondary tachycardia induced at electrophysiology (EP) study.[7]

Pathophysiology

The substrate for AVNRT consists of 2 functionally discrete atrial inputs to the AV node: the fast pathway, which exhibits shorter conduction time and a longer effective refractory period (ERP), and the slow pathway, which displays longer conduction time but a shorter ERP.[8,9] The most common form of AVNRT is typical (slow-fast) AVNRT, with antegrade conduction across the slow pathway, and retrograde activation via the fast pathway; this results in a short ventriculoatrial (VA) interval ($\leq$70 ms), manifest on surface ECG as a short RP interval. Atypical forms of AVNRT include fast-slow and slow-slow circuits, both of which exhibit a long VA interval (>70 ms) and long RP on ECG. The largest reported series of AVNRT ablations in repaired CHD described electrophysiologic findings in a heterogeneous population of 49 subjects (including some children). Typical AVNRT was observed in 63% of cases, atypical in 28%, and both forms in 8% (compared with 90% typical AVNRT observed in otherwise healthy adults).[7,8] There was no association between AVNRT type and anatomic lesion.[7]

Diagnosis

Typical AVNRT presents on ECG as a usual QRS tachycardia, with a short RP interval, often with the retrograde P-wave obscured within the QRS (pseudo r').[9] Observations on ECG may suggest dual AV nodal physiology, such as initiation of tachycardia following a premature atrial contraction (PAC) with marked lengthening of the AV interval (jump), or with a 2-for-1 response, in which there is simultaneous conduction via fast and

slow pathways (**Fig. 3**). Rarely, AVNRT may occur with VA dissociation due to conduction block in the upper common pathway (**Fig. 4**).[10]

Evidence for dual AV nodal physiology at EP study includes an atrial-His (AH) jump during atrial extrastimulus testing, defined as a greater than or equal to 50 ms increase in the AH interval with a 10 ms decrement in S1-S2.[8] Although dual AV nodal physiology can be demonstrated in up to 85% of adults with structurally normal hearts and AVNRT, this finding was observed in only 38% of CHD subjects with AVNRT in the aforementioned study.[7,11] Observations in support of a mechanism of AVNRT at EP study have been well-described, such as failure of His-refractory premature ventricular contractions (PVCs) to advance the subsequent atrial electrogram during tachycardia, and entrainment from the RV followed by a V-A-V response and long corrected postpacing interval–tachycardia cycle length (TCL) (greater than 110 ms).[12,13]

Management

Catheter ablation has been established to be a safe and effective means of treatment of AVNRT. Slow pathway (SP) modification can be challenging in the setting of repaired ACHD for several

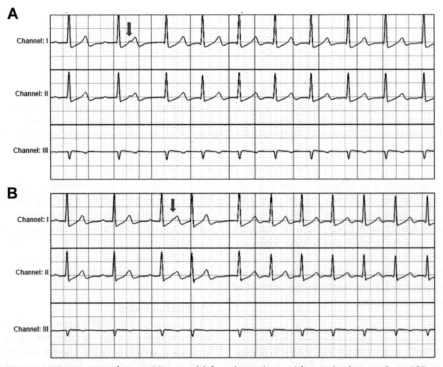

Fig. 3. (*A*) Event monitor tracing from a 23-year-old female patient with repaired secundum ASD and palpitations. A PAC (*solid arrow*) conducts with a long AV interval (jump), initiating a narrow QRS tachycardia. (*B*) Another tracing from the same patient shows a PAC (*solid arrow*), with a 2-for-1 response, initiating tachycardia. These tracings suggest a mechanism of typical AVNRT.

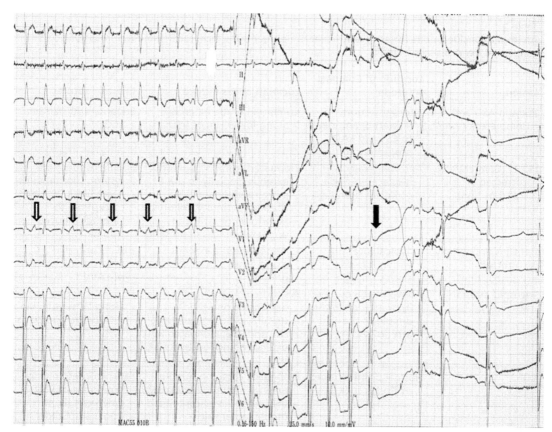

Fig. 4. ECG showing SVT at 130 bpm in a 20-year-old patient with heterotaxy syndrome (polysplenia type), dextrocardia, complete common AV canal, single right ventricle, pulmonary stenosis and bilateral SVC s/p extracardiac Fontan. Note that there appears to be ventricular-atrial dissociation during tachycardia (P-waves marked by *open arrows*). The QRS morphology during tachycardia is similar to that in sinus rhythm, ruling out ventricular tachycardia. The underlying mechanism is, therefore, either AVNRT with upper common pathway block or junctional tachycardia. An EP study is necessary to delineate the precise mechanism. Tachycardia terminates with adenosine after a QRS complex (*solid arrow*).

reasons. First, the compact AV node and His may be displaced from Koch's triangle in certain congenital lesions, such as AV canal defects (posterior displacement) and AV discordance or levo-transposition of the great arteries (L-TGA) (anterolateral displacement) (**Table 1**).[14] Also, fluoroscopic landmarks and catheter position may be altered by atrial enlargement, annular displacement, and coronary sinus (CS) abnormalities.[7] Access to the SP region may require transbaffle puncture in the case of Fontan and Mustard or Senning repairs. Finally, the implications of AV nodal injury can be profound in patients with underlying hemodynamic derangements, so medical management may be preferable in such cases.[7]

Despite these concerns, reported results of AVNRT ablation in repaired CHD have shown high success rates. In their recent series, Upadhyay and colleagues[7] described techniques and outcomes of SP modification for a wide variety of lesions. For conditions with atrial situs solitus, D-looped ventricles, and biventricular circulation, the site of successful SP modification was most often in the conventional locale in the lower third of Koch's triangle anterior to the CS os. This observation was true for TOF (n = 5), Ebstein's anomaly (n = 3), and several miscellaneous lesions, such as aortic stenosis, pulmonary stenosis, secundum atrial septal defect (ASD), and subpulmonary ventricular septal defect (VSD), with single cases described for each.[7] Usual locale for SP modification was also found in subjects with dextro-transposition (D-TGA) status post (s/p) atrial switch (n = 5), although this site was located on the pulmonary venous side of the baffle, necessitating transbaffle access. One exception was a subject with a repaired transitional AV canal, in whom ablation was performed inferior to the CS os, taking into account the expected posterior deviation of the compact node in this lesion. Another

Table 1
Anatomic considerations for atrioventricular nodal reentrant tachycardia ablation in specific congenital heart disease lesions

Lesion	Location of Compact AV Node	Location of His Bundle	Clinical Features
Primum ASD and complete AV canal	Inferoposteriorly displaced; anterior to CS os in RAO projection	Common bundle extends along lower rim of VSD	Superior QRS axis on ECG
{S,L,L} (Congenitally corrected transposition)	Anterolaterally displaced outside of Koch's triangle	Elongated common bundle extends medially to site of mitral-pulmonary valve fibrous continuity; follows anterior edge of PV, or upper rim of VSD (if present)	Fragile conduction system; spontaneous heart block 2%/year; susceptible to catheter-induced trauma
{I,D,D} (Congenitally corrected transposition)	In typical location within left-sided Koch's triangle	Common bundle extends along lower rim of VSD if present	HBE recorded at anteromedial aspect of LAVV
Tricuspid atresia	Above the CS os, and in or inferior to the dimple of the atretic TV	A short common bundle descends along the LV septum, dividing early into LBB and RBB; elongated RBB extends along lower rim of VSD	HBE can be recorded along LV septum via retrograde approach
TOF	Normal position (apex of Koch's triangle)	Elongated common bundle extends along lower rim of VSD, with deviation toward the LV septal side	HBE recorded in usual position, but VSD patch can blunt signal amplitude
D-TGA {S,D,D}	Normal position (apex of Koch's triangle)	Common bundle extends along lower rim of VSD if present	In Mustard or Senning repairs, HBE can be recorded via retrograde approach in NCC of AoV or flexed toward TV

Abbreviations: AoV, aortic valve; LAVV, left atrioventricular valve; LBB, left bundle branch; NCC, non-coronary cusp; PV, pulmonary valve; RAO, right anterior oblique; RBB, right bundle branch.
Data from Mullin M, Van Praagh R, Walsh E. Development and anatomy of the cardiac conducting system. In: Walsh EP, Saul JP, Triedman JK, editors. Cardiac arrhythmias in children and young adults with congenital heart disease. Philadelphia: Lippincott Williams & Wilkins; 2001. p. 3–22.

exception was a subject with a left-sided superior vena cava (LSVC) to CS, in whom the site of successful ablation was at the roof of the CS os. Other subjects with venous anomalies, including 3 other cases of LSVC to CS, underwent successful SP modification in the usual locale.[7]

SP modification in congenitally corrected transposition has been a subject of interest, given the abnormal anatomic location and fragile nature of the conduction system in L-looped ventricles. In a study that included 7 subjects with {S,L,L} anatomy, 6 of 7 subjects had a single His potential recorded in an anteroseptal position along the right-sided mitral annulus, and 1 subject had an additional His potential in a more posterior location (twin AV nodes). Excluding the subject with twin AV nodes, the site of successful SP modification was in the right posterior septum in 2, in the right midseptum in 3 (following attempts in the posterior septum), and in the left posterior septum in 1 via trans-septal approach (following right-sided attempts).[15] Other reports of SP modification in {S,L,L} have described successful ablation in the right posterior septum[7] and right anterior septum[16] in individual cases. SP modification in patients with {I,D,D} anatomy is expected to be more conventional, given D-looped ventricular anatomy, albeit in a left-sided Koch's triangle. There are only a few described cases in the literature: 2 with successful ablation in the midseptum of the left-sided right atrium (following attempts in the posterior septum),[15] 1 with successful ablation in the posterior septum of the left-sided right atrium,[7] and 1 with unsuccessful SP elimination after ablation on both sides of the septum with transient AV block on the final attempt with cryoablation.[7]

Ablation for AVNRT in patients with single ventricle anatomy is complex and not well-described. The anatomic location of specialized conduction tissue is variable, depending on ventricular morphology, looping, and associated AV canal defects or heterotaxy.[14] Access to the SP region depends on the location of surgical baffles relative to the nodal region, with antegrade transvenous, transbaffle, and retrograde routes all described.[7] Traditional landmarks can be absent or difficult to identify, including challenges to CS cannulation.[7] Upadhyay and colleagues[7] described their general approach to SP modification in this group of subjects, including a preference for inferior ablation sites far from the His, as well as using cryoablation over radiofrequency (RF) ablation. They reported ablation success in 8 out of 10 attempted cases, with cryoablation used in 6, RF in 3, and both in 1 case; 1 failure was complicated by first-degree AV block with cryoablation. They also cautioned a conservative approach in this population, given the profound consequences of AV block in patients with a univentricular circulation.[7] Thus, although ablation is reasonable in single ventricle patients with symptomatic AVNRT refractory to medications, a more conservative approach may be appropriate in cases of pharmacologically well-controlled tachycardia or incidentally discovered AVNRT during invasive evaluation of a different clinical arrhythmia.

Accessory-Pathway Mediated Tachycardia

Pathophysiology

AVRT mediated by an AP is an important consideration in the ACHD patient with SVT, although it accounts for less than 8% of SVT in this population.[4] APs are sites of persistent electrical continuity between the atrium and ventricle along the AV valves, due to defects in the annulus fibrosus.[17] Antegrade conduction across APs manifests as pre-excitation on surface ECG, known as Wolff-Parkinson-White (WPW) syndrome. APs with exclusive retrograde conduction are concealed, with a normal surface ECG in sinus rhythm. APs create substrate for orthodromic AVRT (ORT), in which the circuit consists of antegrade AV nodal conduction and retrograde AP conduction, as well as antidromic AVRT, with antegrade AP conduction and retrograde nodal conduction.[17]

APs are strongly associated with specific forms of CHD. The prevalence of WPW syndrome is 9% in Ebstein's anomaly and 1.4% in L-TGA (which itself is often associated with an Ebsteinoid left-sided tricuspid valve [TV]) compared with 0.15% in the general population.[18] The developmental abnormality of Ebstein's, including failure of delamination and subsequent apical displacement of the septal leaflet of the TV, creates substrate for persistent AV muscular connections along the tricuspid annulus.[19,20] APs have been reported to occur in approximately 25% of patients with Ebstein's, often along the posterior and septal aspect of the tricuspid annulus.[19,21]

In other forms of CHD, the prevalence of APs is similar to that of the general population. Due to both the natural history of AVRT, with presentation in childhood, and the unnatural history in the present era, with ECG screening identifying asymptomatic WPW syndrome patients, many patients with APs will be identified and treated before adulthood, although exceptions still exist.

Similar to those in structurally normal hearts, APs in CHD generally demonstrate nondecremental conduction and adenosine insensitivity. However, there are rare variants that exhibit slow and decremental conduction. For example, one type of slowly conducting, decremental AP, usually located in the right posteroseptum, is responsible for a specific form of SVT, known as the permanent form of junctional reciprocating tachycardia (PJRT). Due to the decremental nature of this AP, tachycardia can initiate with sinus beats, often creating incessant SVT and potential for tachycardia-induced cardiomyopathy, with usual presentation at a young age.[22] A second type of decremental AP is the Mahaim fiber, which is typically an atriofascicular fiber, originating in the lateral right atrium and inserting into the distal right bundle, although AV variants and even left-sided fibers have also been described. Mahaim fibers exhibit decremental antegrade conduction, with absent retrograde conduction in most (**Fig. 5**).[23] Additional rare AP variants include nodofascicular pathways and nodoventricular pathways, which can participate in reentry tachycardia, and fasciculoventricular pathways, which do not participate in SVT.[4]

Diagnosis

The diagnosis of a manifest AP is made with a 12-lead ECG, which shows a short PR interval and widened QRS, with slurring of its upstroke (delta wave) (**Fig. 6**). Caution should be taken in the diagnosis of WPW syndrome in certain CHD lesions due to the occasional observation of pseudo–pre-excitation, in which there is the appearance of a delta wave, without a true accessory AV connection (**Fig. 7**).[24] Pseudo–pre-excitation has been described with highest prevalence in

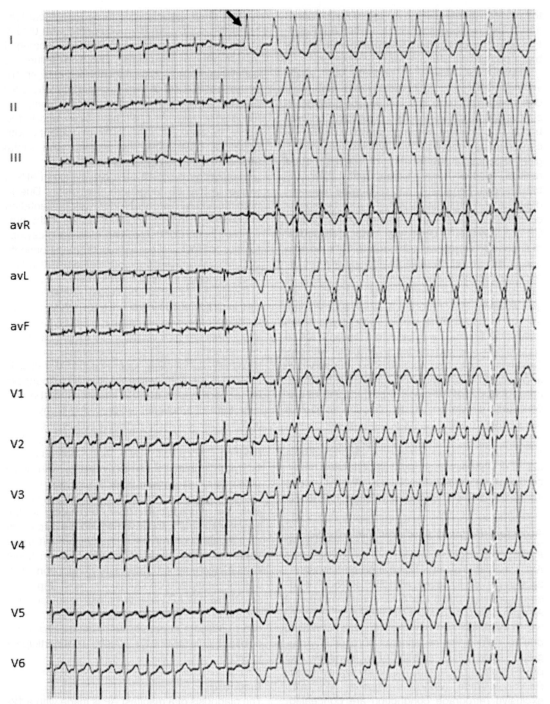

I

II

III

avR

avL

avF

V1

V2

V3

V4

V5

V6

Fig. 5. 12-lead rhythm strip showing atrial pacing with progressive lengthening of the AV interval and with non–pre-excited QRS complexes. The last atrial paced beat results in AV conduction with a pre-excited QRS (*arrow*), which is associated with retrograde conduction over the right bundle, His bundle, and AV node, and induction of antidromic tachycardia. Antegrade conduction occurs over a right-sided atriofascicular fiber, and retrograde conduction occurs via the right bundle, His bundle, and AV node axis. The resultant ECG produces a typical left bundle branch block pattern and superior frontal plane QRS axis.

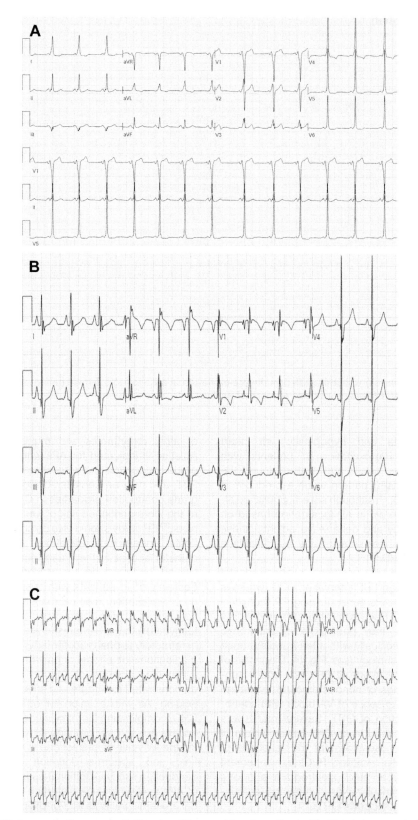

Fig. 6. (*A*) ECG demonstrating pre-excitation in a 21-year-old male patient with Ebstein's anomaly. (*B*) ECG from an 18-year-old with Ebstein's demonstrating normal sinus rhythm, right atrial enlargement, right ventricular conduction delay and absence of pre-excitation. (*C*) ECG of the same 18-year-old patient showing SVT at 185 beats per minute with a long RP interval and RBBB (EP study confirmed presence of an AP with antegrade and retrograde conduction).

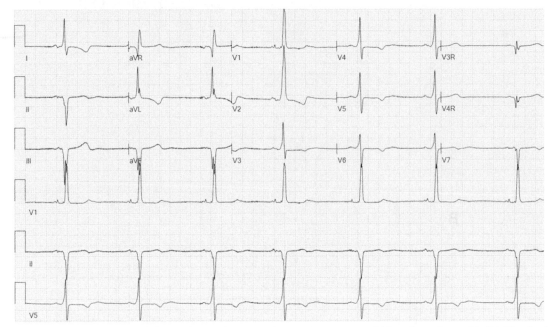

Fig. 7. ECG showing sinus rhythm with pseudo–pre-excitation in a 22-year-old female patient with {S,L,L}, mitral atresia, and DORV. EP study confirmed absence of an AP.

tricuspid atresia and hypoplastic left heart syndrome.[24,25] Pre-excitation in patients with Ebstein's is often subtle and a study found the absence of a RBBB pattern to be a predictor of an AP (see **Fig. 6**).[26] Although several published algorithms exist to aid in AP localization based on QRS morphology and delta wave polarity, these algorithms have been shown to be less reliable in the setting of CHD.[27–29]

ORT mediated by a traditional nondecremental AP results in a short RP interval on ECG, whereas nondecremental APs generate long RP tachycardias, as in PJRT. Because Mahaim fibers conduct antegrade only, they participate in antidromic tachycardia, specifically with a left bundle branch block QRS morphology (see **Fig. 5**). Diagnosis of a concealed AP is made at EP study and is supported by findings of nondecremental, eccentric VA conduction, absence of VA block with adenosine, and induction of ORT. Several maneuvers have been described to confirm a mechanism of ORT, including assessment of the response of tachycardia to His-refractory PVCs (advancement of the subsequent atrial electrogram supports ORT) and to ventricular overdrive pacing (entrainment with fusion supports ORT).[12,13]

Management
In patients with CHD and WPW syndrome, EP study is generally recommended even in the absence of symptoms due to the high incidence of atrial arrhythmias and multiple pathways.[30] Ablation is indicated for APs with high-risk antegrade conduction characteristics and for inducible SVT, and may be considered regardless of antegrade conduction properties in CHD patients due to the aforementioned risk of future atrial arrhythmias.[30] EP study should also be considered for patients undergoing operations that may limit catheter access in the future, and AP ablation is viewed by many to be standard of care for Ebstein's.[3,4] In patients with suspected ORT but no pre-excitation, medical management is an option, with catheter ablation preferred in cases of tachycardia that is hemodynamically embarrassing or refractory to pharmacotherapy, or in the event of medication side effects or patient preference.

Catheter ablation of APs in CHD has been demonstrated to be safe and effective, albeit challenging. As with ablation for other substrates in CHD, complicating factors include limited vascular access due to prior procedures, difficulty accessing the AV valve of interest due to intracardiac baffles, and abnormal location of normal AV conduction tissue. Additional issues in the ablation of APs in CHD include distortion of landmarks by CS anatomic variants and/or difficulty cannulating the CS. Chamber enlargement can affect catheter stability and myocardial hypertrophy can affect delivery of energy and lesion depth.[2,18] Multiple APs are more commonly observed in CHD than in structurally normal hearts.[31]

Many of the series describing AP ablation in subjects with CHD include both children and adults but the observations remain relevant to a discussion of APs in ACHD. In a 2004 series that included 110 APs in 70 subjects with CHD (n = 27 with Ebstein's), 66 APs were manifest, 36 were concealed, and 8 were Mahaim fibers.[5] Twenty percent of subjects had multiple APs, compared with 5% to 10% generally reported for subjects with structurally normal hearts.[5,31,32] Most were right-sided APs (65%), whereas a 45% to 55% distribution of right-sided and left-sided APs has been reported for subjects without structural heart disease.[33] Acute success was 70% for right-sided APs and 82% for left-sided APs, with a recurrence rate of 24% and a complication rate of 5.5% (2 major, 3 minor).[5] Interpretation of these results should take into account the older era of ablation included (1990–2002).

Electrophysiologic findings and ablation techniques for APs in ACHD patients are best described in the Ebstein's population, owing to the high prevalence of APs in this condition. Ablation in this population is challenging, with lower acute success rates and higher recurrence rates reported compared with the general population.[34,35] A recent multicenter study of adults with Ebstein's reported an 80% acute success rate for AP ablation, with 40% recurrence.[35] Because most APs in Ebstein's are associated with the TV, the intrinsic difficulties of right-sided ablation are a factor. However, several additional elements complicate the ablation of APs in Ebstein's. First, these cases can be electrophysiologically complex, with a high incidence of multiple APs, including AP variants such as Mahaim fibers, and the frequent finding of additional non-AP–mediated tachycardia mechanisms. In recent adult series of AP ablation in Ebstein's, more than 1 AP was observed in 35% to 50% of subjects, with decremental properties in 6% to 9% of APs.[19,36] In an earlier pediatric study of Ebstein's subjects at EP study, 52% had a single AP, and 29% had multiple APs, with approximately 6% of APs characterized as Mahaim fibers.[34] Challenges of mapping include right atrial and TV annular enlargement, which can interfere with catheter stability; long sheaths and deflectable sheaths can facilitate catheter stability and contact.[35,36] A major difficulty lies in identifying appropriate ablation targets along the true tricuspid annulus, where ventricular signals may be low amplitude and/or fractionated. Techniques for defining the true AV ring include right coronary angiography or introduction of a multielectrode microcatheter into the right coronary artery, although this latter technology is no longer available.[37] Angiography of the right atrium and right ventricle also helps to identify the true annular plane, and allows visualization of the extent of atrialized right ventricle, an important consideration for signal analysis.[19,36,38] In a recent study of 32 right-sided APs in 22 adult Ebstein's subjects, 50% had fractioned ventricular electrograms at the site of success.[36] APs with fractionated ventricular electrograms corresponded anatomically to sites of atrialized RV, and were associated with higher atrial to ventricular signal ratios than controls.[36] Because the multiple components within these fractioned electrograms can complicate differentiation of atrial and ventricular signals during activation mapping, the investigators recommend the delivery of extrastimuli at the AP refractory period to separate atrial and ventricular components.[36] A final challenge in this population is the frequent occurrence of broad APs, with a study reporting 26% prevalence of such APs, defined by the site of early activation and ablation success measuring greater than 1 cm in width.[19]

Twin Atrioventricular Nodes

A rare form of AVRT in patients with CHD occurs in the setting of duplication of the specialized conduction system or so-called twin AV nodes. Suspicion for this uncommon form of tachycardia should be raised in patients with complex lesions, particularly when AV discordance and AV canal defects coexist, or in the setting of heterotaxy syndrome.[14]

Pathophysiology

Histologic studies have documented the presence of 2 distinct compact AV nodes, His bundles, and bundle branches in several lesions (**Box 1**).[39] The classic description by Mönckeberg includes an

---

Box 1
Lesions in which twin atrioventricular nodes have been observed histologically

- {S,L,L} TGA
- {I,D,D} TGA
- {I,L,L} Double outlet right ventricle (DORV)
- {S,L,L} DORV
- Heterotaxy with asplenia
- Heterotaxy with polysplenia

Data from Epstein MR, Saul JP, Weindling SN, et al. Atrioventricular reciprocating tachycardia involving twin atrioventricular nodes in patients with complex congenital heart disease. J Cardiovasc Electrophysiol 2001;12(6):671–9.

anterior and posterior node, with a connecting fiber between the distal portions of the anterior and posterior bundle branches; this specialized connection at the ventricular level, or so-called Mönckeberg sling, completes the potential reentry circuit.[14]

Diagnosis

The observation on ECG in sinus rhythm of 2 distinct non–pre-excited QRS morphologies with differing QRS axis suggests the existence of twin AV nodes (**Fig. 8**). The QRS pattern may provide a clue to the anatomic location of the associated AV node, especially when taking the underlying congenital defect into account. For example, in a patient with {S,L,L} and unbalanced complete atrioventricular canal, a superior QRS axis reflects conduction via the posteriorly displaced AV node seen in AV canal defects; whereas a normal axis with qR pattern in leads V1 or aVR reflects conduction across the anteriorly displaced AV node typical of L-looped ventricles.[39]

ECGs during tachycardia will show 1 stable QRS morphology, and tachycardia episodes may

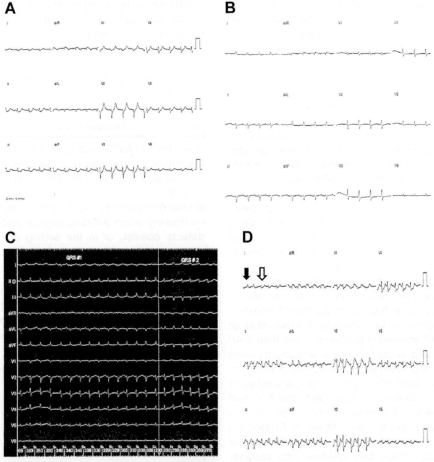

Fig. 8. (*A*) 21-year-old patient with heterotaxy syndrome (asplenia type), malaligned common AV canal, right ventricle to aorta, pulmonary atresia and total anomalous pulmonary venous connection to a vertical vein, s/p lateral tunnel Fontan procedure. ECG (25 mm/s, 10 mm/mV) shows normal sinus rhythm with a rightward frontal QRS axis and R/S transition in the precordial leads in lead V6 (QRS morphology #1). (*B*) ECG in the same patient shows normal sinus rhythm with a superiorly directed frontal QRS axis and R/S transition in the precordial leads in V3 (QRS morphology #2). (*C*) Decremental atrial pacing during EP study in the same patient shows a shift in antegrade conduction from the anterior/superior AV conduction bundle (QRS morphology #1) to the posterior/inferior AV conduction bundle (QRS morphology #2). (*D*) ECG showing SVT in the same patient. Adenosine administration results in a change in QRS morphology from #2 (*solid arrow*) to #1 (*open arrow*), suggesting a shift in antegrade conduction via the posterior-inferior AV conduction bundle to the second AV conduction bundle, which is located in a more anterior-superior position.

exclusively demonstrate 1 QRS pattern if only 1 of the nodes conducts retrograde. Adenosine will successfully treat tachycardia, and both PR and RP prolongation may be observed before termination.[39]

Epstein and colleagues[39] described several findings at EP study that support the diagnosis, including the following:

1. Two discrete His bundle electrograms (HBEs) recorded at anatomically separate sites
2. Two non–pre-excited QRS morphologies, with QRS morphology dependent on the site of atrial depolarization, whether spontaneous or stimulated (ie, preferential conduction across 1 atrioventricular node-HBE); each activation pattern is associated with 1 of the 2 HBE signals with a normal HV interval (the HBE can still be recorded at the alternate site but with an obscured or short HV interval)
3. Decremental AV conduction, with no change in HV interval or QRS morphology; for a given site of atrial depolarization, once the ERP of the primary AVN for that site has been reached, there is a shift to the alternate QRS morphology (and associated HBE) (provided the ERP of the alternate node is shorter), without any preceding fusion of the 2 QRS patterns (see **Fig. 8**).

Fusion of the 2 QRS patterns was only observed in the rare instance of fused activation from 2 separate atrial sites. This absence of fusion, in addition to AV and VA block during adenosine administration, favors the absence of an AP. Finally, there must be decremental, retrograde conduction over at least 1 of the AV nodes in order for AVRT to occur. Interestingly, in their series, Epstein and colleagues[39] did not observe an AH (or AV) jump for any of the studied cases of twin AV nodes. For some cases of tachycardia, they demonstrated that PVCs timed to His bundle refractoriness advanced the subsequent atrial electrogram, confirming the presence of an additional VA connection.[39]

Management

Epstein and colleagues[39] described ablative treatment of 3 cases of AVRT secondary to twin AV nodes. Their technique described first determining which node forms the antegrade limb and which forms the retrograde limb of the circuit. In each case, ablation was directed at the AV node responsible for the retrograde limb of the circuit. They also considered antegrade conduction properties of the nodes, preferentially targeting the weaker of the 2, as well as potential for future dysfunction, in the case of anteriorly displaced nodes in L-looped ventricles. RF energy was applied during atrial-paced

rhythm at either the site of the recorded HBE of the target node or at the site of earliest atrial activation mapped during tachycardia. Junctional acceleration of the targeted node was observed at the correct site in 2 of 3 cases, with success in all 3 ultimately demonstrated by an abrupt change to the alternate AV conduction pattern. Ablation successfully eliminated retrograde conduction and inducible tachycardia, although antegrade conduction via the targeted node could still be demonstrated in 2 cases.

Intra-atrial Reentry Tachycardia

IART, involving macro-reentry within atrial muscle, represents the most frequent form of SVT in the ACHD population.[3]

Pathophysiology

The requirements for intra-atrial reentry include distinct corridors of conduction, with different refractory periods, separated by a nonconductive anatomic barrier, with a zone of slow conduction in between. The suture lines, scars, patches, and baffles from prior operations, as well as annular and atrial enlargement from volume loading lesions, together with natural conduction barriers (eg, the crista terminalis and AV valve and caval orifices), provide ideal substrates for such circuits.[40–42] Atrial remodeling secondary to chronic hemodynamic stress also modifies myocardial conduction properties and contributes to creation of these circuits.[43,44] IART includes typical and atypical atrial flutter but the category encompasses several additional potential circuits due to the unique anatomic and electrophysiologic milieu in each ACHD patient.

The prevalence of atrial tachycardia in the ACHD population is estimated to be 15%, with a lifetime risk of up to 50%.[1] Conditions with abnormal hemodynamics and extensive atrial incisions, such as D-TGA following Mustard or Senning atrial switch procedures and single ventricles with older style atriopulmonary Fontan procedures, are associated with the highest rates of IART.[3] However, atrial tachycardias occur in up to one-third of repaired-TOF patients, and are frequently seen following simple ASD repair as well.[3] Sinus node dysfunction is a risk factor for IART (so-called tachycardia-bradycardia syndrome).[45] Of note, surgical modifications have been introduced with the goal of reducing this arrhythmia burden. The modern techniques of lateral tunnel and extracardiac conduits for the Fontan operation, which minimize right atrial dilation, have been associated with lower rates of IART.[3]

As in the adult with a structurally normal heart, typical flutter in the ACHD patient involves counterclockwise propagation of a wavefront around the tricuspid annulus, with a critical zone of slow conduction in the cavotricuspid isthmus (CTI). Likewise, atypical atrial flutter refers to a CTI-dependent circuit with clockwise propagation.

The term IART includes nonisthmus-dependent circuits in the atrium, with wavefronts propagating around atriotomy incisions and other scars.[40] With atrial rates in the 150 to 250 beats per minute range, IART is generally slower compared with typical atrial flutter. This slower atrial rate can translate to 1:1 conduction, with rapid ventricular rates and resultant hemodynamic instability.[3] IART typically involves right atrial tissue, although this tissue may be sequestered by baffles to the pulmonary venous atrium, and left atrial circuits have been described as well.

Specific patterns of IART circuits have been observed in relation to the anatomic and surgical substrate. For example, in repaired ASD and TOF, the tachycardia circuit will often involve the CTI but with a so-called dual-loop configuration, in which a second, outer loop traverses the atriotomy incision.[46–48] IART following Mustard or Senning operations also typically involves the CTI, part of which is usually confined to the pulmonary venous atrium, necessitating transbaffle or retrograde access for ablation.[38,49] In single ventricle patients with older atriopulmonary Fontan baffles, there are often multiple IART circuits, which can occur in any part of the enlarged right atrium.[38]

Diagnosis

The diagnosis of IART on ECG can be rendered difficult due to low amplitude P-waves. IART with 2:1 AV conduction may masquerade as sinus tachycardia if P-waves are buried within the QRS complex or T-wave (**Fig. 9**).[3] The classic sawtooth atrial flutter waves may not be present with CTI-dependent flutter in ACHD patients. The clinician should maintain a high index of suspicion for IART when approaching an ACHD patient with even mild tachycardia. Abrupt onset and fixed cycle length are useful diagnostic features when analyzing tracings from telemetry, Holter monitoring, or device interrogation. Finally, changes in R-R intervals due to modulations in AV conduction, either spontaneous or provoked with vagal maneuvers, can reveal otherwise hidden P-waves[3].

At EP study, features of a reentry mechanism will be apparent, including tachycardia initiation and termination with programmed stimulation and overdrive pacing. Voltage mapping in sinus rhythm is useful to identify sites of scar and patch (low voltage sites), around which conduction isthmuses can propagate tachycardia circuits. Activation mapping in tachycardia will reveal an early-meets-late propagation pattern. Entrainment maneuvers are used to ascertain sites within the tachycardia circuit. Careful attention must be paid to the surface P-wave morphology and intracardiac activation pattern while mapping IART because multiple circuits often coexist and transition to a different tachycardia can occur.

Management

Acute management of IART in the ACHD patient must take into account hemodynamic stability during tachycardia, as well as thromboembolic risk profile, both of which relate to underlying severity of CHD. Standard methods for acute termination apply, including direct current synchronized electrical cardioversion, pharmacologic cardioversion, and pace-termination. Alternate pad positions may be required, as in cases of cardiac malposition such as dextrocardia; anteroposterior positions have been recommended if there is severe atrial enlargement.[2,4]

Regarding thromboprophylaxis, standard guidelines should be followed in cases of simple, nonvalvular lesions. Recommendations are more conservative for patients with CHD of moderate or severe complexity, due to the higher risk of intracardiac thrombus. For example, recent guidelines recommend 3 weeks of anticoagulation or transesophageal echocardiography (TEE) before cardioversion, regardless of tachycardia duration, in patients with stable IART and CHD of moderate or severe complexity (class IIa).[2] Furthermore, for lesions at highest risk of thromboembolism, such as Fontan circulations, TEE before cardioversion has been suggested, even after a period of therapeutic anticoagulation.[2] Guidelines for long-term anticoagulation in the ACHD population have recently been published.[2]

Although acute termination of IART is generally successful, prevention of further episodes and maintenance of sinus rhythm is the greater challenge.[3] Although a rate control strategy is a reasonable option for simple CHD lesions, rhythm control is preferred for moderate to severe CHD, in part due to the hemodynamic consequences of impaired AV synchrony.[2] For chronic medical management, selection of an anti-arrhythmic agent must consider underlying sinus or AV nodal dysfunction, ventricular dysfunction, and potential for proarrhythmia. Class I drugs are generally not recommended in ACHD patients with coronary artery disease, or with systemic or subpulmonary ventricular dysfunction, due to proarrhythmic

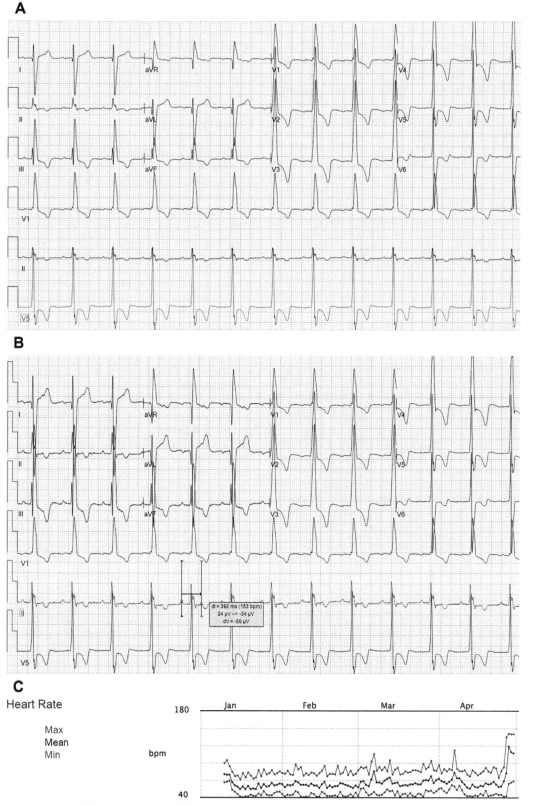

Fig. 9. (*A*) 12-lead ECG demonstrating IART with 2:1 conduction in a 43-year-old male patient s/p Mustard procedure for D-TGA (also s/p pacemaker due to sinus node dysfunction). Every other P-wave is obscured by the T-wave and the tracing could easily be mistaken for sinus tachycardia. (*B*) Same ECG with the limb lead gain at twice normal. The P-waves are now more obvious, and atrial tachycardia with cycle length of 392 ms is evident. (*C*) Rate histograms from pacemaker interrogation mark the onset of IART with abrupt increase in the monitored heart rate.

concerns.[2] Amiodarone has reasonable efficacy but its use is limited by long-term systemic side effects; it can be considered a first-line agent for maintenance of sinus rhythm in ACHD patients with ventricular dysfunction.[2] Adjunctive therapy with an AV nodal blocking agent may be prudent in patients with normal AV conduction to prevent a rapid ventricular response, which has been associated with sudden cardiac death, particularly in patients with single ventricles or systemic right ventricles.[2,50,51] The recently published joint Pediatric and Congenital Electrophysiology Society and Heart Rhythm Society (PACES/HRS) expert consensus statement includes an algorithm to further guide the selection of agents for rhythm control in the ACHD population with moderate to severe disease severity.[2] For patients with simple forms of CHD, standard adult management guidelines may be followed.[52]

Pacemaker implantation is a potential adjunctive therapy, especially in the setting of sinus node dysfunction, because atrial pacing has been shown to decrease frequency of IART episodes.[4,53,54] Anti-tachycardia pacing is a useful device feature, with options for manual in-office overdrive pacing and automated algorithms for tachycardia detection and therapy.[55]

Catheter ablation is preferred over chronic pharmacologic management for patients with frequent, symptomatic IART.[2] Isthmuses of tissue critical to maintenance of tachycardia are targeted, and linear lesions are placed to transect these paths and create lines of conduction block. Acute success rates ranging from 76% to 96% have been published; however, recurrence rates are as high as 40%.[38] Several recent technologies have contributed to improved procedural success. Data from advanced imaging modalities can be integrated with electroanatomic maps, as with the superimposition of fluoroscopic, angiographic, or other images onto the anatomic shell registered by the catheter.[38] Intracardiac echo has the additional benefit of allowing visualization of the catheter-myocardium interface to ensure adequate contact during ablation.[38] Irrigated-tip catheters are used to increase lesion depth, especially in the face of hypertrophied atrial tissue and low-flow sites that limit power delivery with temperature-controlled RF catheters.[38] Although technology has improved IART ablation outcomes, preprocedural planning remains of utmost importance. Careful review of operative notes and imaging studies allows for hypothesis generation regarding potential circuits, understanding of potential access issues, and knowledge of probable location of normal conduction tissue.[38]

Atrial Fibrillation

AF is an important consideration in ACHD patients, with an increasing incidence as this population ages.

Pathophysiology

AF occurs with highest incidence in patients with unoperated or palliated CHD, unrepaired or late-repaired ASD, and those with residual left-sided lesions following complete repair.[56] As in structurally normal hearts, chronic left atrial volume and pressure overload are factors.[56] In a multicenter study of TOF subjects, AF was noted to be more common than IART in subjects older than 55 years, and AF was associated with left-sided disease, including left atrial dilation and reduced LV ejection fraction.[57] The electrophysiologic substrate for the development of AF includes areas of slow conduction, dispersion of atrial refractoriness, as well as premature beats, all of which are promoted by the atrial scarring and dilation that often follow CHD repair.[58] It has been observed that patients with repaired CHD develop AF at a younger age compared with those without CHD. A recent multicenter study of 199 CHD subjects with AF reported a mean age of onset of 49 years. Subjects with complex anatomy, including D-TGA s/p atrial switch and single ventricle lesions, presented even earlier, at a mean age of 35 and 29 years, respectively.[58] In contrast, AF presents with increasing frequency during the fifth decade in the general population.[59,60]

In one-third of this recent CHD cohort, AF coexisted with organized atrial tachycardia mechanisms, such as IART, and the regular atrial tachycardia preceded the development of AF in most (65%).[58] Regular atrial tachycardia has been observed to result in electrophysiologic remodeling of the atria, which can then promote development of AF. Some investigators have hypothesized that catheter ablation of regular atrial tachycardias may delay or prevent the later onset of AF.[58] In this same cohort, progression from paroxysmal to persistent AF was observed in 26% of subjects, within a relatively short time (mean 3 years).[58]

Diagnosis

AF typically presents as an irregularly irregular narrow QRS tachycardia without distinct P-waves (**Fig. 10**). In ACHD patients, pre-existing QRS abnormalities may result in a wide QRS tachycardia during AF. Because ventricular pre-excitation occurs with a higher than average frequency in the ACHD population (especially Ebstein's), consideration should be given to the possibility of pre-excited AF, which may degenerate into VF with

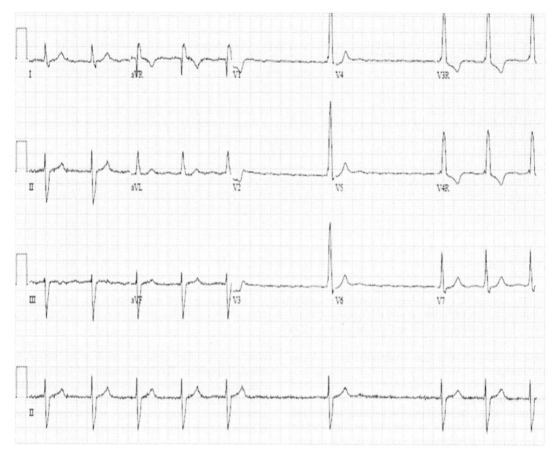

Fig. 10. ECG showing AF in a 40-year-old s/p Mustard procedure for D-TGA. There are no visible P-waves and the ventricular rate is irregular.

rapid AP conduction. Pre-excited AF displays narrow and wide QRS complexes, reflecting degrees of fusion between AV nodal and AP activation (**Fig. 11**). The P-waves of ACHD patients may be low amplitude and poorly defined at baseline, which can complicate interpretation of AF tracings. Furthermore, organized atrial tachycardias often coexist in patients with AF, and transition from an organized to a disorganized rhythm has been observed to occur on the same rhythm strip.[58] In patients with pacemakers, AF may be diagnosed by review of stored high-rate events, which will show rapid, irregular atrial activity with variable electrograms.

Management

Acute management of AF parallels that of IART with regard to decisions about cardioversion and anticoagulation. Chronic rhythm control strategies include anti-arrhythmic medication, surgical Maze procedures, and catheter ablation. As with IART, pharmacologic management of AF should be guided by consideration of coexisting conduction disease, ventricular function, lesion complexity,

and risk of proarrhythmia.[2] In the absence of specific guidelines for the management of AF in the ACHD population, recommendations for the general adult population may be considered.[2,52] For patients with AF undergoing cardiac surgery, a left atrial Cox-Maze III should be considered.[2] There are few studies on catheter ablation of AF in the ACHD population. In a recent single-center study including 36 adult subjects with repaired CHD (61% ASD), pulmonary vein isolation was successful in 42% at 300 days and 27% at 4 years; this compared with respective success rates of 53% and 36% in controls without CHD.[61] As the ACHD population grows and the incidence of AF increases, expertise in catheter ablation in this setting is expected to increase. Finally, AV nodal ablation with postablation pacing should be viewed as a last resort, particularly in complex ACHD patients in whom chronic ventricular pacing may worsen hemodynamic status.[2]

Focal Atrial Tachycardia

Although intra-atrial reentry represents the most common form of atrial tachycardia in ACHD

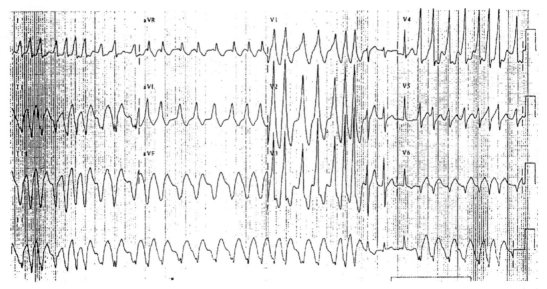

Fig. 11. 12-lead ECG of a 20-year-old patient presenting to the emergency room with palpitations. An irregularly irregular rhythm with narrow and wide QRS complexes is seen, consistent with pre-excited AF. Subsequent diagnosis of WPW syndrome and Ebstein's anomaly is made.

patients, tachycardia can emanate from a focal atrial origin.

Pathophysiology

In focal atrial tachycardia, activation originates from a point source in the atrium, spreading centrifugally to depolarize the rest of the atrium. The most common mechanism underlying focal atrial tachycardia in adults with structurally normal hearts is increased automaticity. This condition is usually indicated by the term ectopic atrial tachycardia (EAT). The foci of abnormal automaticity in EAT tend to occur in characteristic anatomic locations, such as the crista terminalis, tricuspid annulus, right atrial appendage, and pulmonary veins.[62–65] Although EAT can occur in ACHD patients, the more common form of focal atrial tachycardia in the ACHD population is nonautomatic focal atrial tachycardia (NAFAT). In a cohort of 216 children and ACHD subjects undergoing ablation for atrial tachycardia, 8% of subjects (n = 17) were determined to have a tachycardia mechanism of NAFAT.[66] In another study of 62 atrial tachycardias in 43 ACHD subjects, 16% of tachycardias had a focal atrial origin.[67] Focal atrial tachycardia may coexist with additional atrial tachycardia mechanisms in the ACHD population.[66,67]

Triggered activity and microreentry have been postulated to play a role in the generation of NAFAT. Some investigators have hypothesized that chronic atrial stretch can lead to triggered activity. Foci responsible for NAFAT have been observed to localize to areas with abnormal

conduction, often adjacent to scar or surgically created barriers. The observation of fractionated electrograms at these sites supports the notion that conduction abnormalities play a role.[67] NAFAT more commonly maps to the right atrium; in cases of left atrial foci, the sites of origin cluster in proximity to the pulmonary veins.[66] Some investigators have hypothesized that the proximity to natural or unnatural conduction barriers implies a microreentry mechanism.[66] Additional evidence for microreentry is the observation of continuous electrical activity at the site of successful ablation for some foci.[67]

Diagnosis

A diagnosis of EAT may be suspected from the clinical presentation, with features of warm-up and cool-down behavior, as well as sensitivity to catecholamines. Surface ECG may show a long RP tachycardia, with a distinct, nonsinus P-wave morphology. Algorithms to ascertain the site of origin of the focus based on P-wave axis have been published, although they may not be applicable to the adult with repaired CHD.[68,69] At EP study, activation mapping will demonstrate focal origin with radial propagation of the wavefront. Tachycardia induction may require isoproterenol; programmed electrical stimulation will not typically induce or terminate EAT.

NAFAT is more difficult to diagnose by noninvasive means and often masquerades as IART in the ACHD population.[66] In the study of NAFAT by Seslar and colleagues,[66] 11 of 17 cases of NAFAT were initially labeled as atrial flutter based on ECG;

all 11 subjects had CHD, and 7 had single ventricle lesions. NAFAT can only be definitively differentiated from IART with invasive EP testing; NAFAT will exhibit a focal source of activation, in contrast to the circulating wavefront of IART. Adenosine administration may aid in the differentiation of NAFAT and IART because NAFAT is more likely to terminate with adenosine.[66,70] NAFAT can also resemble EAT clinically and electrocardiographically; therefore, only EP testing can make the diagnosis. At EP study, NAFAT can be initiated and terminated with pacing. Focal atrial tachycardia can also present with AF. de Groot and colleagues[67] described 2 subjects in whom the surface ECG demonstrated AF, whereas the intracardiac activation map revealed a focal source of activation. In each of these cases, they hypothesized a single tachycardia focus with fibrillatory conduction.

Management

In focal atrial tachycardia, regardless of underlying mechanism, catheter ablation targets the site of earliest atrial activation. In their ACHD cohort, de Groot and colleagues[67] observed abnormal electrograms at the sites of ablation success, describing both low-amplitude fractionated potentials and continuous electrical activity. They reported tachycardia termination in all cases with ablation directed at the site of earliest atrial activation. In some cases, they also described encircling the area of fractionated potentials at these sites with additional lesions, as a means of source isolation.[67]

Junctional Tachycardia

Focal JT is an uncommon form of SVT in the ACHD population.

Pathophysiology

Focal JT results from disordered impulse generation originating in the region of the AV junction, with hypothesized foci in the transitional cells, compact AV node, or His bundle.[71] Focal JT presents as a rapid, often irregular, tachycardia, with narrow QRS (or QRS matching that of sinus rhythm), and with possible VA dissociation.[71] Both increased automaticity and triggered activity have been proposed as underlying mechanisms.

A form of focal JT commonly occurs immediately following surgery for CHD; in this scenario, the term junctional ectopic tachycardia (JET) is used. The incidence of JET following congenital heart surgery has been reported to range from 5.0% to 15.3%, occurring most frequently in neonates and children, with adults more rarely affected.[72,73] JET has typically been attributed to

mechanical injury to the conduction system, either directly via sutures or indirectly via stretch and edema. More recently, however, ischemia and reperfusion injury have been proposed as alternative mechanisms.[72,74] In support of this, Moak and colleagues[72] observed higher rates of JET after repair of conotruncal and single ventricle lesions (many without associated VSD repair), compared with simple VSD repair. Predictors of JET included surgical time and postoperative use of inotropes. JET usually occurs within 24 hours of surgery and runs a self-limited course; however, the combination of tachycardia and AV dyssynchrony can significantly impair cardiac output, and JET has been associated with increased postoperative morbidity and mortality.[72,74]

Focal JT has also been described in adults, in paroxysmal and incessant forms, unrelated to structural heart disease or recent cardiac surgery. In an early report of RF ablation for focal JT, 2 of 11 subjects in the series had repaired CHD.[75] A more recent series described late postoperative focal JT in a group of subjects with CHD.[76] Interestingly, 10 of 12 subjects had complex single ventricle heart disease palliated by the Fontan procedure, of whom 8 had an associated AV canal defect and 7 had associated heterotaxy. Moreover, 8 of 10 Fontan subjects with late focal JT also had a history of immediate postoperative JET. In 5 of these cases, the JET was described as atypical in that it behaved paroxysmally, did not respond to cooling, and either terminated with adenosine or slowed in response to calcium channel blockers. These observations led the investigators to speculate that intrinsic abnormalities of the specialized conduction tissue in certain lesions predispose to both atypical acute postoperative JET and late focal JT.[76]

Diagnosis

Electrocardiographic features of focal JT include a rapid, often irregular, narrow QRS tachycardia, with VA dissociation. However, 1:1 VA conduction during tachycardia may occur. In patients with pre-existing bundle branch block, tachycardia is wide complex, with the QRS matching that of sinus rhythm. Rate-related aberration has also been described, especially when tachycardia starts suddenly after a pause, further confounding the diagnosis.[71]

Features of both automatic and triggered mechanisms are evident at EP study. Spontaneous tachycardia initiation with isoproterenol has been described (favoring increased automaticity), although initiation with overdrive pacing and termination with adenosine have also been observed (favoring triggered activity). In most descriptions of JT in adults, extrastimulus testing does not have a role in tachycardia induction or termination, making a reentry mechanism unlikely.[71]

Proof that the atrium is a bystander of the tachycardia includes spontaneous VA dissociation, VA dissociation during adenosine administration, and variable VA conduction without change in the TCL.[76] In cases of 1:1 VA conduction, JT can be differentiated from AVNRT by the response to His-refractory PACs.[77] Initiation with extrastimulus testing after reaching a critical AH interval also favors AVNRT. Differentiation from AVRT using a concealed nodofascicular pathway can be made by assessing the response to His-refractory PVCs.[71]

In their series of focal JT in ACHD subjects, Bae and colleagues[76] reported a few electrophysiologic differences compared with the typical description of focal JT in adults. First, they observed evidence for a reentry mechanism in 5 of 11 cases studied, with induction by programmed stimulation and/or termination by overdrive pacing or extrastimuli (of note, a case with reentry features had a concealed nodofascicular AP, which confounds interpretation). Interestingly, all cases of focal JT were adenosine-sensitive. Finally, VA intervals during tachycardia were significantly longer than previously described for focal JT. They reported intervals from QRS onset to earliest atrial activation ranging from 120 to 208 ms, compared with a range of 77 to 100 ms reported by Hamdan and colleagues[71] The long VA interval during JT led Bae and colleagues[76] to surmise a tachycardia origin at the AV node or His, in contrast to the supposition by Hamdan and colleagues[71] that the short VA interval implied JT origin above the level of the node in the perinodal atrium. With only limited data on focal JT in adults with repaired CHD it is difficult to draw conclusions from these observed differences, but observation of a long VA during JT may affect ablation site (see later discussion).

Management

Acute treatment of postoperative JET is well-described, and includes strategies to decrease circulating catecholamines (sedation, weaning inotropes), cooling, anti-arrhythmic medication (amiodarone or procainamide), and/or atrial pacing to restore AV synchrony.[78] Because JET runs a self-limited course, chronic treatment is not usually necessary.

Treatment of late focal JT in ACHD patients includes antiarrhythmic medications and catheter ablation. Bae and colleagues[76] described reasonable success with class III medications (sotalol and amiodarone). Catheter ablation for focal JT

involves targeting the site of earliest retrograde atrial activation during tachycardia.[71,75] However, as Bae and colleagues[76] surmise, this approach may not be applicable for JT with a long VA interval if the site of origin is distal to the perinodal atrium. When retrograde conduction cannot be mapped, an ablation strategy has been described in which lesions are placed initially in the posterior septum, followed by sequentially higher attempts.[71] A 5% to 10% incidence of complete heart block has been reported for JT ablation in adults with normal anatomy.[71,75] When considering JT ablation in the adult with CHD, the clinician must take into account the abnormal anatomic substrate, and the high hemodynamic cost of iatrogenic AV block.

REFERENCES

1. Bouchardy J, Therrien J, Pilote L, et al. Atrial arrhythmias in adults with congenital heart disease. Circulation 2009;120(17):1679–86.
2. Khairy P, Van Hare GF, Balaji S, et al. PACES/HRS expert consensus statement on the recognition and management of arrhythmias in adult congenital heart disease: developed in partnership between the Pediatric and Congenital Electrophysiology Society (PACES) and the Heart Rhythm Society (HRS). Endorsed by the governing bodies of PACES, HRS, the American College of Cardiology (ACC), the American Heart Association (AHA), the European Heart Rhythm Association (EHRA), the Canadian Heart Rhythm Society (CHRS), and the International Society for Adult Congenital Heart Disease (ISACHD). Heart Rhythm 2014; 11(10):e102–65.
3. Walsh EP, Cecchin F. Arrhythmias in adult patients with congenital heart disease. Circulation 2007; 115(4):534–45.
4. Page RL, Joglar JA, Caldwell MA, et al. 2015 ACC/AHA/HRS guideline for the management of adult patients with supraventricular tachycardia: a report of the American College of Cardiology/American Heart Association task force on clinical practice guidelines and the Heart Rhythm Society. J Am Coll Cardiol 2016;67(13):e27–115.
5. Chetaille P, Walsh EP, Triedman JK. Outcomes of radiofrequency catheter ablation of atrioventricular reciprocating tachycardia in patients with congenital heart disease. Heart Rhythm 2004;1(2):168–73.
6. Koyak Z, Kroon B, de Groot JR, et al. Efficacy of antiarrhythmic drugs in adults with congenital heart disease and supraventricular tachycardias. Am J Cardiol 2013;112(9):1461–7.
7. Upadhyay S, Marie Valente A, Triedman JK, et al. Catheter ablation for atrioventricular nodal reentrant tachycardia in patients with congenital heart disease. Heart Rhythm 2016;13(6):1228–37.

8. Kwaku KF, Josephson ME. Typical AVNRT–an update on mechanisms and therapy. Card Electrophysiol Rev 2002;6(4):414–21.

9. Katritsis DG, Camm AJ. Atrioventricular nodal reentrant tachycardia. Circulation 2010;122(8):831–40.

10. Wellens HJ, Wesdorp JC, Duren DR, et al. Second degree block during reciprocal atrioventricular nodal tachycardia. Circulation 1976;53(4):595–9.

11. Zimmerman FJ. Atrioventricular node reentry tachycardia. In: Walsh EP, Saul JP, Triedman JK, editors. Cardiac arrhythmias in children and young adults with congenital heart disease. Philadelphia: Lippincott Williams & Wilkins; 2001. p. 161–72.

12. Veenhuyzen GD, Quinn FR, Wilton SB, et al. Diagnostic pacing maneuvers for supraventricular tachycardia: part 1. Pacing Clin Electrophysiol 2011;34(6):767–82.

13. Veenhuyzen GD, Quinn FR, Wilton SB, et al. Diagnostic pacing maneuvers for supraventricular tachycardias: part 2. Pacing Clin Electrophysiol 2012; 35(6):757–69.

14. Mullin M, Van Praagh R, Walsh E. Development and anatomy of the cardiac conducting system. In: Walsh EP, Saul JP, Triedman JK, editors. Cardiac arrhythmias in children and young adults with congenital heart disease. Philadelphia: Lippincott Williams & Wilkins; 2001. p. 3–22.

15. Liao Z, Chang Y, Ma J, et al. Atrioventricular node reentrant tachycardia in patients with congenitally corrected transposition of the great arteries and results of radiofrequency catheter ablation. Circ Arrhythm Electrophysiol 2012;5(6):1143–8.

16. Tada H, Nogami A, Naito S, et al. Selected slow pathway ablation in a patient with corrected transposition of the great arteries and atrioventricular nodal reentrant tachycardia. J Cardiovasc Electrophysiol 1998;9(4):436–40.

17. Blaufox AD, Saul JP. Accessory-pathway-mediated tachycardias. In: Walsh EP, Saul JP, Triedman JK, editors. Cardiac arrhythmias in children and young adults with congenital heart disease. Philadelphia: Lippincott Williams & Wilkins; 2001. p. 173–99.

18. Saul JP. Ablation of accessory pathways. In: Walsh EP, Saul JP, Triedman JK, editors. Cardiac arrhythmias in children and young adults with congenital heart disease. Philadelphia: Lippincott Williams & Wilkins; 2001. p. 393–425.

19. Wei W, Zhan X, Xue Y, et al. Features of accessory pathways in adult Ebstein's anomaly. Europace 2014;16(11):1619–25.

20. Frescura C, Angelini A, Daliento L, et al. Morphological aspects of Ebstein's anomaly in adults. Thorac Cardiovasc Surg 2000;48(4):203–8.

21. Van Hare GF, Lesh MD, Stanger P. Radiofrequency catheter ablation of supraventricular arrhythmias in patients with congenital heart disease: results and technical considerations. J Am Coll Cardiol 1993; 22(3):883–90.

22. Kang KT, Potts JE, Radbill AE, et al. Permanent junctional reciprocating tachycardia in children: a multicenter experience. Heart Rhythm 2014;11(8): 1426–32.

23. Bohora S, Dora SK, Namboodiri N, et al. Electrophysiology study and radiofrequency catheter ablation of atriofascicular tracts with decremental properties (Mahaim fibre) at the tricuspid annulus. Europace 2008;10(12):1428–33.

24. Carlson AM, Turek JW, Law IH, et al. Pseudo-preexcitation is prevalent among patients with repaired complex congenital heart disease. Pediatr Cardiol 2015;36(1):8–13.

25. Zellers TM, Porter CB, Driscoll DJ. Pseudo-preexcitation in tricuspid atresia. Tex Heart Inst J 1991; 18(2):124–6.

26. Iturralde P, Nava S, Salica G, et al. Electrocardiographic characteristics of patients with Ebstein's anomaly before and after ablation of an accessory atrioventricular pathway. J Cardiovasc Electrophysiol 2006;17(12):1332–6.

27. Bar-Cohen Y, Khairy P, Morwood J, et al. Inaccuracy of Wolff-Parkinson-white accessory pathway localization algorithms in children and patients with congenital heart defects. J Cardiovasc Electrophysiol 2006;17(7):712–6.

28. Arruda MS, McClelland JH, Wang X, et al. Development and validation of an ECG algorithm for identifying accessory pathway ablation site in Wolff-Parkinson-White syndrome. J Cardiovasc Electrophysiol 1998;9(1):2–12.

29. Fitzpatrick AP, Gonzales RP, Lesh MD, et al. New algorithm for the localization of accessory atrioventricular connections using a baseline electrocardiogram. J Am Coll Cardiol 1994;23(1):107–16.

30. Pediatric and Congenital Electrophysiology Society (PACES), Heart Rhythm Society (HRS), American College of Cardiology Foundation (ACCF), et al. PACES/HRS expert consensus statement on the management of the asymptomatic young patient with a Wolff-Parkinson-white (WPW, ventricular pre-excitation) electrocardiographic pattern: developed in partnership between the Pediatric and Congenital Electrophysiology Society (PACES) and the Heart Rhythm Society (HRS). Endorsed by the governing bodies of PACES, HRS, the American College of Cardiology Foundation (ACCF), the American Heart Association (AHA), the American Academy of Pediatrics (AAP), and the Canadian Heart Rhythm Society (CHRS). Heart Rhythm 2012;9(6):1006–24.

31. Zachariah JP, Walsh EP, Triedman JK, et al. Multiple accessory pathways in the young: the impact of structural heart disease. Am Heart J 2013;165(1): 87–92.

32. Weng KP, Wolff GS, Young ML. Multiple accessory pathways in pediatric patients with Wolff-Parkinson-White syndrome. Am J Cardiol 2003;91(10):1178–83.

33. Kugler JD, Danford DA, Houston K, et al. Radiofrequency catheter ablation for paroxysmal supraventricular tachycardia in children and adolescents without structural heart disease. Pediatric EP society, radiofrequency catheter ablation registry. Am J Cardiol 1997;80(11):1438–43.

34. Reich JD, Auld D, Hulse E, et al. The pediatric radiofrequency ablation Registry's experience with Ebstein's anomaly. Pediatric Electrophysiology Society. J Cardiovasc Electrophysiol 1998;9(12):1370–7.

35. Roten L, Lukac P, Groot DE, et al. Catheter ablation of arrhythmias in ebstein's anomaly: a multicenter study. J Cardiovasc Electrophysiol 2011;22(12):1391–6.

36. Guo XG, Liu XU, Zhou GB, et al. Frequency of fractionated ventricular activation and atrial/ventricular electrogram amplitude ratio at successful ablation target of accessory pathways in patients with Ebstein's anomaly. J Cardiovasc Electrophysiol 2015;26(4):404–11.

37. Shah MJ, Jones TK, Cecchin F. Improved localization of right-sided accessory pathways with microcatheter-assisted right coronary artery mapping in children. J Cardiovasc Electrophysiol 2004; 15(11):1238–43.

38. Sherwin ED, Triedman JK, Walsh EP. Update on interventional electrophysiology in congenital heart disease: evolving solutions for complex hearts. Circ Arrhythm Electrophysiol 2013;6(5):1032–40.

39. Epstein MR, Saul JP, Weindling SN, et al. Atrioventricular reciprocating tachycardia involving twin atrioventricular nodes in patients with complex congenital heart disease. J Cardiovasc Electrophysiol 2001;12(6):671–9.

40. Collins KK, Love BA, Walsh EP, et al. Location of acutely successful radiofrequency catheter ablation of intraatrial reentrant tachycardia in patients with congenital heart disease. Am J Cardiol 2000;86(9): 969–74.

41. Love BA, Collins KK, Walsh EP, et al. Electroanatomic characterization of conduction barriers in sinus/atrially paced rhythm and association with intra-atrial reentrant tachycardia circuits following congenital heart disease surgery. J Cardiovasc Electrophysiol 2001;12(1):17–25.

42. Lindsay I, Moore JP. Cardiac arrhythmias in adults with congenital heart disease: scope, specific problems, and management. Curr Treat Options Cardiovasc Med 2015;17(12):56.

43. Wolf CM, Seslar SP, den Boer K, et al. Atrial remodeling after the Fontan operation. Am J Cardiol 2009; 104(12):1737–42.

44. Morton JB, Sanders P, Vohra JK, et al. Effect of chronic right atrial stretch on atrial electrical remodeling in patients with an atrial septal defect. Circulation 2003;107(13):1775–82.

45. Fishberger SB, Wernovsky G, Gentles TL, et al. Factors that influence the development of atrial flutter after the Fontan operation. J Thorac Cardiovasc Surg 1997;113(1):80–6.

46. Mah DY, Alexander ME, Cecchin F, et al. The electroanatomic mechanisms of atrial tachycardia in patients with Tetralogy of Fallot and double outlet right ventricle. J Cardiovasc Electrophysiol 2011; 22(9):1013–7.

47. de Groot NM, Lukac P, Schalij MJ, et al. Long-term outcome of ablative therapy of post-operative atrial tachyarrhythmias in patients with Tetralogy of Fallot: a European multi-centre study. Europace 2012; 14(4):522–7.

48. Akar JG, Kok LC, Haines DE, et al. Coexistence of type I atrial flutter and intra-atrial re-entrant tachycardia in patients with surgically corrected congenital heart disease. J Am Coll Cardiol 2001; 38(2):377–84.

49. Correa R, Walsh EP, Alexander ME, et al. Transbaffle mapping and ablation for atrial tachycardias after mustard, senning, or Fontan operations. J Am Heart Assoc 2013;2(5):e000325.

50. Khairy P, Fernandes SM, Mayer JE Jr, et al. Long-term survival, modes of death, and predictors of mortality in patients with Fontan surgery. Circulation 2008;117(1):85–92.

51. Khairy P, Harris L, Landzberg MJ, et al. Sudden death and defibrillators in transposition of the great arteries with intra-atrial baffles: a multicenter study. Circ Arrhythm Electrophysiol 2008;1(4):250–7.

52. January CT, Wann LS, Alpert JS, et al. 2014 AHA/ACC/HRS guideline for the management of patients with atrial fibrillation: a report of the American College of Cardiology/American Heart Association task force on practice guidelines and the Heart Rhythm Society. Circulation 2014;130(23):e199–267.

53. Silka MJ, Manwill JR, Kron J, et al. Bradycardia-mediated tachyarrhythmias in congenital heart disease and responses to chronic pacing at physiologic rates. Am J Cardiol 1990;65(7):488–93.

54. Ragonese P, Drago F, Guccione P, et al. Permanent overdrive atrial pacing in the chronic management of recurrent postoperative atrial reentrant tachycardia in patients with complex congenital heart disease. Pacing Clin Electrophysiol 1997;20(12 Pt 1):2917–23.

55. Stephenson EA, Casavant D, Tuzi J, et al. Efficacy of atrial antitachycardia pacing using the Medtronic AT500 pacemaker in patients with congenital heart disease. Am J Cardiol 2003;92(7):871–6.

56. Kirsh JA, Walsh EP, Triedman JK. Prevalence of and risk factors for atrial fibrillation and intra-atrial reentrant tachycardia among patients with congenital heart disease. Am J Cardiol 2002;90(3):338–40.

57. Khairy P, Aboulhosn J, Gurvitz MZ, et al. Arrhythmia burden in adults with surgically repaired Tetralogy of Fallot: a multi-institutional study. Circulation 2010; 122(9):868–75.

58. Teuwen CP, Ramdjan TT, Gotte M, et al. Time course of atrial fibrillation in patients with congenital heart defects. Circ Arrhythm Electrophysiol 2015;8(5): 1065–72.

59. Kannel WB, Abbott RD, Savage DD, et al. Epidemiologic features of chronic atrial fibrillation: the Framingham study. N Engl J Med 1982;306(17): 1018–22.

60. Heeringa J, van der Kuip DA, Hofman A, et al. Prevalence, incidence and lifetime risk of atrial fibrillation: the Rotterdam study. Eur Heart J 2006;27(8): 949–53.

61. Philip F, Muhammad KI, Agarwal S, et al. Pulmonary vein isolation for the treatment of drug-refractory atrial fibrillation in adults with congenital heart disease. Congenit Heart Dis 2012;7(4):392–9.

62. Kalman JM, Olgin JE, Karch MR, et al. "Cristal tachycardias": origin of right atrial tachycardias from the crista terminalis identified by intracardiac echocardiography. J Am Coll Cardiol 1998;31(2):451–9.

63. Zhang T, Li XB, Wang YL, et al. Focal atrial tachycardia arising from the right atrial appendage: electrophysiologic and electrocardiographic characteristics and catheter ablation. Int J Clin Pract 2009;63(3):417–24.

64. Kistler PM, Sanders P, Fynn SP, et al. Electrophysiological and electrocardiographic characteristics of focal atrial tachycardia originating from the pulmonary veins: acute and long-term outcomes of radiofrequency ablation. Circulation 2003;108(16): 1968–75.

65. Morton JB, Sanders P, Das A, et al. Focal atrial tachycardia arising from the tricuspid annulus: electrophysiologic and electrocardiographic characteristics. J Cardiovasc Electrophysiol 2001;12(6): 653–9.

66. Seslar SP, Alexander ME, Berul CI, et al. Ablation of nonautomatic focal atrial tachycardia in children and adults with congenital heart disease. J Cardiovasc Electrophysiol 2006;17(4):359–65.

67. de Groot NM, Zeppenfeld K, Wijffels MC, et al. Ablation of focal atrial arrhythmia in patients with congenital heart defects after surgery: role of circumscribed areas with heterogeneous conduction. Heart Rhythm 2006;3(5):526–35.

68. Kistler PM, Roberts-Thomson KC, Haqqani HM, et al. P-wave morphology in focal atrial tachycardia: development of an algorithm to predict the anatomic site of origin. J Am Coll Cardiol 2006;48(5):1010–7.

69. Tang CW, Scheinman MM, Van Hare GF, et al. Use of P wave configuration during atrial tachycardia to predict site of origin. J Am Coll Cardiol 1995;26(5): 1315–24.

70. Markowitz SM, Stein KM, Mittal S, et al. Differential effects of adenosine on focal and macroreentrant atrial tachycardia. J Cardiovasc Electrophysiol 1999;10(4):489–502.

71. Hamdan MH, Badhwar N, Scheinman MM. Role of invasive electrophysiologic testing in the evaluation and management of adult patients with focal junctional tachycardia. Card Electrophysiol Rev 2002;6(4):431–5.

72. Moak JP, Arias P, Kaltman JR, et al. Postoperative junctional ectopic tachycardia: risk factors for occurrence in the modern surgical era. Pacing Clin Electrophysiol 2013;36(9):1156–68.

73. Mildh L, Hiippala A, Rautiainen P, et al. Junctional ectopic tachycardia after surgery for congenital heart disease: incidence, risk factors and outcome. Eur J Cardiothorac Surg 2011;39(1):75–80.

74. Tharakan JA, Sukulal K. Post cardiac surgery junctional ectopic tachycardia: a 'Hit and Run' tachyarrhythmia as yet unchecked. Ann Pediatr Cardiol 2014;7(1):25–8.

75. Hamdan M, Van Hare GF, Fisher W, et al. Selective catheter ablation of the tachycardia focus in patients with nonreentrant junctional tachycardia. Am J Cardiol 1996;78(11):1292–7.

76. Bae EJ, Noh CI, Choi JY, et al. Late occurrence of adenosine-sensitive focal junctional tachycardia in complex congenital heart disease. J Interv Card Electrophysiol 2005;12(2):115–22.

77. Padanilam BJ, Manfredi JA, Steinberg LA, et al. Differentiating junctional tachycardia and atrioventricular node re-entry tachycardia based on response to atrial extrastimulus pacing. J Am Coll Cardiol 2008;52(21):1711–7.

78. Walsh EP, Saul JP, Sholler GF, et al. Evaluation of a staged treatment protocol for rapid automatic junctional tachycardia after operation for congenital heart disease. J Am Coll Cardiol 1997;29(5): 1046–53.

Ventricular Arrhythmias in Adult Congenital Heart Disease
Mechanisms, Diagnosis, and Clinical Aspects

Gnalini Sathananthan, MBBS, BSc (Med), FRACP,
Louise Harris, MD, FRCPC, Krishnakumar Nair, MBBS, MD, DM*

KEYWORDS

- Ventricular tachycardia • Ventricular arrhythmias • Congenital heart disease

KEY POINTS

- Ventricular arrhythmias are not infrequently seen in patients with congenital heart disease beyond the second decade of life.
- The frequency of ventricular arrhythmias depends on the complexity of the congenital defect, whether it has been repaired or not, and the type and timing of initial repair.
- The mechanism and type of ventricular arrhythmia varies depending on the congenital defect.
- Risk stratification for sudden death in patients with congenital heart disease remains challenging and is an area that will continue to evolve.

INTRODUCTION

The proportion of adult patients with congenital heart disease (CHD) has continued to increase over the last few decades due to the evolution in surgical techniques, improved intensive care and anesthetic medicine, and overall experience with the disease process involved.

Ventricular arrhythmias are rare in the first and second decade of life. Atrial arrhythmias are more common and better described than ventricular arrhythmias in the CHD population. It is not unusual for CHD patients to develop arrhythmias in adulthood, which often become an important aspect of their ongoing long-term care. The risk of ventricular arrhythmia increases after the second decade of life but largely depend on several factors, including the complexity of the congenital defect, whether it is repaired or unrepaired, the type of repair performed, and the age at which the repair was performed.

Ventricular arrhythmias are thought to be the predominant cause of sudden cardiac death in adult CHD patients and, therefore, physicians' understanding, diagnosis, and appropriate management of ventricular arrhythmias remains crucial to the long-term survival of these patients. Sudden cardiac death is the leading cause of death in the adult CHD population, alongside heart failure. Contemporary figures report up to 23% of deaths in adult CHD patients are due to sudden cardiac death, and these figures have interestingly remained largely unchanged when compared with older studies.[1–3]

The Pediatric and Congenital Electrophysiology Society–Heart Rhythm Society (PACES/HRS) expert consensus statement on the recognition and management of arrhythmias in adult congenital heart disease gives guidance on risk stratification and management of ventricular arrhythmias in CHD patients. However it is worth noting that

There are no commercial or financial conflicts of interest or funding for any of the authors.
Department of Cardiology, Peter Munk Cardiac Centre, University Health Network, University of Toronto, 585 University Avenue, Toronto, ON M5G 2N2, Canada
* Corresponding author.
E-mail address: Krishnakumar.Nair@uhn.ca

Card Electrophysiol Clin 9 (2017) 213–223
http://dx.doi.org/10.1016/j.ccep.2017.02.004

many of the recommendations are based on expert consensus in the absence of large randomized controlled trials. Secondary prevention guidelines for implantable cardioverter defibrillator (ICD) insertion are clearly defined, with a class I (level B) recommendation for adults with CHD who have had sustained ventricular tachycardia (VT) or resuscitated cardiac arrest in the absence of reversible causes.[4] A recent study found that 14% of CHD subjects who had an ICD received an appropriate shock, and the frequency was similar between those who had received an ICD for primary or secondary prevention. Forty-five percent of these patients, however, suffered significant complications in the form of inappropriate shocks, inappropriate anti-tachycardia pacing, infections requiring extraction, lead complications, and pneumothorax.[5] Therefore, it remains vital to develop firm guidelines for primary prevention ICD implantation in CHD.

PATHOPHYSIOLOGY OF VENTRICULAR ARRHYTHMIAS

Ventricular arrhythmias are, in general, a result of abnormal electrophysiological changes at the cellular level or abnormal changes at the myocardial level leading to abnormal cellular properties.[6,7] Abnormal transmembrane properties at the cellular level can result in areas of conduction block and, therefore, provoke ventricular arrhythmias.[6] An abnormal architectural arrangement of myocardial fibers as a result of intercellular fibrosis or interrupted intercellular connections may create areas of slow conduction or unidirectional block, which, in turn, results in anisotropic re-entry.[8]

Monomorphic VT is a broad complex tachycardia with a QRS morphology that is usually identical from beat to beat, indicating repetitive ventricular activation using a consistent substrate. Scar-related re-entry is the most common cause of sustained monomorphic VT in patients with structural heart disease, such as myocardial infarction, cardiomyopathy, and surgical incisions, in which the scar tissue delays electrical propagation, facilitating the initiation of reentry.[8] This form of VT is not uncommon in CHD and is the most common mechanism for VT in tetralogy of Fallot (TOF).

Focal VT, on the other hand, has 1 site of earliest ventricular activation, with the spread of activation away from this site in all directions. The mechanisms underlying focal VT can either be automaticity, triggered activity, or microreentry.[6,9] Automaticity refers to spontaneous depolarization during phase 4 of the action potential, which may give rise to ventricular arrhythmias.[10] Accelerated idioventricular rhythms as seen in acute ischemia or reperfusion are thought to be due to this mechanism. It has also been seen in cases of acute myocarditis.[11–13] Triggered activity can occur in the presence of early or delayed after-depolarizations. Outflow tract VT, which typically occurs in those without structural heart disease, can occur as a result of triggered activity due to delayed after-depolarizations. It can often present as a monomorphic VT or with frequent premature ventricular complexes. Meanwhile, early after-depolarizations are thought to be the mechanism behind ventricular arrhythmias in long QT syndrome.[10] It has also been suggested in the mechanism of ventricular arrhythmias in hypertrophied and postinfarction ventricular myocardium. Microreentry, on the other hand, refers to small re-entrant circuits that give the appearance of focal activation. This may occur if conduction is particularly slow, such that it allows for recovery of excitability in neighboring tissue, thus enabling localized re-entry.[14]

Polymorphic VT has QRS complexes that vary in morphology from beat to beat. It can be due to a functional re-entry, which is not determined by anatomic boundaries but occurs as a result of dynamic heterogeneities. The location and size of these circuits can vary but are often small and unstable. As a consequence, there may not necessarily be a structural target for ablation. It is often, however, initiated by premature beats from 1 or a few foci, and these can be ablated if they occur with sufficient frequency to be located. Polymorphic VT tends to be hemodynamically unstable and can often only be tolerated for a few seconds before resulting in sudden cardiac death. Polymorphic VT can terminate spontaneously but also has the potential to deteriorate into VF.[15]

ELECTROCARDIOGRAPHIC DIAGNOSIS OF VENTRICULAR TACHYCARDIA

The diagnosis of a broad complex tachycardia on electrocardiogram (ECG) can often be a challenge. The arrhythmia can either be of ventricular or supraventricular origin, and making this distinction is crucial to the immediate and long-term management of the patient. VT is, however, the most common diagnosis in this setting and accounts for up to 80% of broad complex tachycardias.[16]

Individuals with pre-existing structural heart disease such as CHD will invariably have abnormal baseline ECGs, which may make diagnosing VT even more challenging. A broad complex tachycardia could be VT; supraventricular tachycardia (SVT) with a bundle branch block (either pre-existing or rate related); or pre-excited tachycardia, including antidromic tachycardia (eg, Wolff-Parkinson-White [WPW] syndrome, in which the baseline QRS is pre-excited). There are multiple published criteria to distinguish VT from SVT with aberrancy but these have not been validated in CHD. The presence of atrioventricular (AV) disassociation, capture beats, and fusions beats may be helpful in distinguishing VT from SVT with aberrancy. Discriminating between VT and SVT with aberrancy based on morphology may be difficult in those with a pre-existing bundle branch block, as is often the case in patients with CHD. A QRS morphology during VT that is different from that at baseline but not a typical bundle branch block is likely to be VT, rather than SVT. VT due to bundle branch re-entry is, however, a situation in which VT can produce a similar QRS morphology to that at baseline.[17]

VENTRICULAR ARRHYTHMIAS IN TETRALOGY OF FALLOT
Pathophysiology and Mechanisms for Ventricular Arrhythmias

Late-onset ventricular arrhythmias are well-recognized in the TOF population. The incidence of clinically sustained VT and sudden death is estimated to be 11.9% and 8.3%, respectively, 35 years after corrective surgery in TOF patients.[18] The timing of initial surgical repair in TOF and the type of repair plays an important part in an individuals' risk of developing ventricular arrhythmias in adulthood. Late repair in TOF, defined as after the first decade of life, is associated with poor right ventricular remodeling and there is a clear progression of biventricular hypertrophy and fibrosis in this population; however, this was less than that with unrepaired TOF.[19] This is thought to be due to long-standing cyanosis and high right ventricular pressures in the latter.

Total repair in TOF entails closure of the ventricular septal defect (VSD) and relief of the right ventricular outflow tract (RVOT) obstruction. Earlier repairs were performed via a vertical ventriculotomy in the free wall of the RVOT. Transverse incisions were later introduced in the hope of better preserving ventricular function and outflow tract contractility. Ventriculotomies were later superseded altogether by the transatrial-transpulmonary approach.[20,21] The latter approach avoids a ventricular incision and results in a reduction in the incidence of life-threatening ventricular arrhythmias as a consequence of less scarring, without an apparent increase in the incidence of supraventricular arrhythmias.[22]

The VSD is typically closed with a circular patch with a sufficient margin to avoid damaging the conduction system, which traverses inferior to the VSD. An RVOT or transannular patch is often used to augment the restrictive RVOT or to relieve the stenosis of the pulmonary orifice. This patch is often made from either synthetic material or composed of pericardium, either autologous or preserved.

Monomorphic VT secondary to a macroreentrant circuit is the most common cause of ventricular arrhythmia in the TOF population. Surgical incisions, patch material, and the valve annuli can result in areas of dense fibrosis that can act as regions of conduction block, with intervening isthmuses of myocardial bundles in between that contain re-entry circuits for VT.[21] VT in TOF typically has a left bundle branch pattern on ECG and an inferior frontal plane axis (**Fig. 1**).[23,24] Polymorphic VT and ventricular fibrillation (VF) are less common in this form of CHD.

Electrophysiology studies (EPs) in TOF patients have helped identify 4 discrete anatomic isthmuses as substrates for VT in this population.[25] (This will be discussed elsewhere in the issue.)

Risk Factors for Ventricular Arrhythmias and Sudden Cardiac Death

The use of transannular patches during surgery is thought to be associated with ventricular arrhythmias and sudden death in TOF patients.[20]

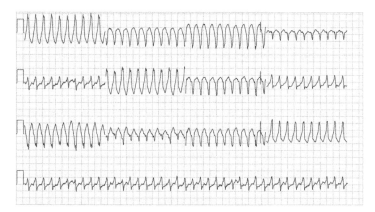

Fig. 1. VT in a patient with TOF physiology. The 12-lead ECG shows a broad QRS tachycardia with left bundle branch block morphology.

Event-free survival for those with a transannular patch was 27.6% at 25 years, versus 78.5% for those without a transannular patch. As a result, there has been a trend to avoid the use of transannular patches whenever possible. There has subsequently been a decrease in the use transannular patches from 89% to 64% over recent years.[26]

Free pulmonary regurgitation is common following transannular patch repair of the RVOT. It is often well-tolerated for many years, though it can eventually lead to chronic volume overload in the form of right ventricular dilatation and dysfunction. Pulmonary regurgitation was found to be the main underlying hemodynamic lesion for patients with VT and sudden death.[18] Indexed end-systolic and end-diastolic volumes were found to be significantly higher in patients with inducible sustained VT.[27] However, the optimal timing of pulmonary valve replacement (PVR) in asymptomatic patients with previous repaired TOF remains a contentious issue. Although most centers tend to be quite conservative, studies have shown that patients with a right ventricle (RV) end-diastolic volume less than 170 mL/m2 combined with an RV end-systolic volume less than 90 mL/m2 had favorable outcomes on RV remodeling following surgery.[28] This coincides with current practice based on the 2009 Canadian Cardiovascular Society Consensus Conference on the management of patients with Congenital Heart Disease.[29] Despite this, PVR alone has not been shown to reduce the risk of VT or sudden death.[30]

A QRS duration 180 ms or longer on ECG, or a QRS duration that increases at a rate of more than 3 ms per year has been found to be a strong predictor of VT and sudden death in TOF patients when used in conjunction other clinical parameters.[25,31,32] Increased QRS duration was found to correlate with chronic RV volume overload in TOF patients. This suggests an important mechanoelectrical interaction contributing to VT in TOF patients.[33] PVR in TOF patients was found to result in stabilization of the QRS duration on ECG when compared with those who did not undergo PVR.[34] Interestingly, although a reduction in RV volume has been noted following PVR, a reduction in the QRS duration was not seen.[24] The QRS prolongation, therefore, may be explained by changes restricted to the RVOT, as well as a conduction delay in 1 of the anatomic isthmuses.[35] In addition, a very broad QRS in operated TOF may also reflect delayed left ventricular activation.[36]

Despite extensive knowledge to date about VT in TOF and appreciation of the causative substrates, risk stratification for sudden death in this population still remains challenging. Several variables are at play, rather than any individual variable. A transannular RVOT patch, severe pulmonary regurgitation, RV dilatation, tricuspid regurgitation, and a QRS greater than or equal to 180 ms are strongly associated with ventricular arrhythmias and sudden death.[18]

Programmed ventricular stimulation has been found to be useful for risk stratification of patients with repaired TOF. Factors associated with inducible sustained VT include

- Prior palliative surgery
- Nonsustained VT
- Being greater than 18 years of age when tested
- Palpitations
- Frequent or complex ventricular ectopy
- Cardiothoracic ratio of 0.6 or more on chest radiograph.

Inducible VT by programmed ventricular stimulation was found to be a risk factor for sudden cardiac death or clinically sustained VT. An EP study was however found to be most beneficial for patients with intermediate risk based on noninvasive risk stratification, including a history of palpitations or syncope, older age at repair, transannular patch, QRS greater than or equal to 180 ms, or nonsustained VT.[37,38] Programmed ventricular stimulation yields insufficiently high positive predictive values so that an EP study cannot be recommended as a routine screening test in asymptomatic patients. TOF patients of intermediate risk will likely have the greatest benefit from an EP study.[39]

TRANSPOSITION OF THE GREAT ARTERIES
Pathophysiology and Mechanisms for Ventricular Arrhythmias

Before the 1980s, dextrotransposition of the great arteries (D-TGAs) was repaired via an atrial switch procedure using a baffle within the atria to divert blood to the appropriate ventricle. This was performed via a right atriotomy approach. The baffle was created using either autologous tissue, which was termed the Senning procedure, or using synthetic material that was termed the Mustard procedure. The atrial switch repair restores physiologic cardiac function but maintains a subpulmonic left ventricle and a systemic RV. A RV with long-standing exposure to systemic pressures inevitably develops dysfunction over time and is prone to the development of both atrial and ventricular arrhythmias. After the 1980s, most patients with D-TGA have undergone an arterial switch operation in which the great arteries are repositioned to create ventriculoarterial concordance, along with concurrent transfer of the coronaries.

This surgery has revolutionized the outlook for patients born with D-TGA. Although long-term outcomes continue to be observed, this surgical option has great promise with a potential for reduction in arrhythmias and systemic ventricular dysfunction.[40]

Most adult patients with D-TGA encountered today, however, will have previously undergone an atrial switch repair because this had been the repair of choice for several decades. Both Brady arrhythmias and atrial arrhythmias are common in this population, and have been well-documented.[41,42] The incidence of sudden death in the atrial switch population has been reported from 2% to 15%.[41,43,44]

Ventricular arrhythmias have been documented as the leading cause of sudden death in those who have had prior atrial switch repair. Polymorphic VT or VF was the terminal rhythm most often documented in cases of sudden death (**Fig. 2**). Monomorphic VT, though present, was found to be less common in this group and has been reported at 0.5% per year.[41,43] Atrial arrhythmias with rapid ventricular response rates can trigger ischemia and secondary ventricular arrhythmias with VT or VF as the final common endpoint. Indeed, the presence of symptoms and documented atrial flutter or fibrillation is the best predictor of sudden death in D-TGA.[41]

Risk Factors for Ventricular Arrhythmias and Sudden Cardiac Death

The mechanisms for ventricular arrhythmias late after atrial switch repair in simple D-TGA are primarily thought to be due to systemic ventricular dysfunction, chronic hemodynamic changes, and the subsequent mechanoelectrical interactions. Polymorphic VT and VF in atrial switch patients occur in the setting of a diffusely abnormal myocardium secondary to chronic pressure and volume loading on a systemic RV.[45] The mechanisms for VT in unrepaired levotransposition of the TGA (L-TGA) are similar to that in atrial switch repair patients because these patients also have a systemic RV. The RV is not accustomed to high systemic pressures and inevitably develops dysfunction over time.

The risk of sudden death in patients with D-TGA and atrial switch surgery has a 3-fold higher incidence compared with those with TOF. Despite this, risk stratifying this population is less well-delineated.[43] This is more so the case when it comes to L-TGA because the incidence of sudden cardiac death in this population has not been well-reported.

Risk factors for VT and sudden cardiac death in observational studies of patients following atrial switch repair include QRS duration 140 ms or longer, older age at time of repair,

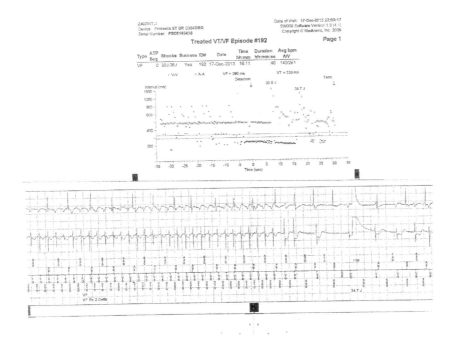

Fig. 2. Device tracings of a shock for VT in a patient with Mustard repair. Upper and lower panels show an interval plot and an electrogram plot, respectively. VT (with more ventricular signals and atrial signals) in the VF zone with 1 failed defibrillator shock (seen only in the interval plot), secondary termination, and a second defibrillator shock are shown.

and systemic ventricular dysfunction.[46,47] Significant systemic ventricular dysfunction is a marker of poor outcomes and this can also be extrapolated from extensive data on the systemic left ventricle. Current guidelines for a patient with a nonischemic cardiomyopathy provide a class I (level A) recommendation for a primary prevention ICD for those with a systemic left ventricular ejection fraction less than 35% and NYHA class II or III symptoms.[48] A normal subpulmonary RV ejection fraction in the patient with D-TGA has been reported between 43% and 65% in various studies and, therefore, using a threshold of 35% for a systemic RV has inherent limitations.[49,50] Those who received a primary prevention ICD with a systemic RV ejection fraction less than 35% had low rates of appropriate shocks at 0.5% per year compared with 6% per year for those who received a secondary prevention ICD following atrial switch surgery.[51]

The relationship between supraventricular arrhythmias and sudden death still remains a contentious issue in the atrial switch population. Although some studies do not show a significant relationship, others have implicated that supraventricular arrhythmias may play an important role in sudden cardiac death in atrial switch patients. Atrial switch repair patients with ICDs who received appropriate shocks for VT have been noted to have preceding or coexisting supraventricular arrhythmias, implying that either may precipitate or perpetuate the other. Beta-blockers were the only variable that seemed to moderate outcome by either limiting 1:1 conduction in intra-atrial reentrant tachycardia or moderating ischemia because of the mismatch of a right coronary artery supplying a systemic ventricle.[46,51,52]

EP studies have been used to risk stratify patients; however, various studies have found that inducible VT on EP study correlated poorly with clinical VT.[23,53] Thus, the mechanism for VT after atrial switch repair is multifactorial and is yet to be completely elucidated.

THE SINGLE VENTRICLE
Pathophysiology and Mechanisms for Ventricular Arrhythmias

Individuals with complex CHD in which biventricular repair is not feasible often undergo staged surgical procedures to create the Fontan circulation. This anatomic arrangement supports a univentricular physiology. There have been several modifications to the Fontan procedure over time, with the oldest method being the atriopulmonary Fontan. This was later superseded by

the lateral tunnel Fontan and, subsequently, the extracardiac Fontan.

The atriopulmonary Fontan involves an anastomosis between the right atrial appendage and main pulmonary artery. The lateral tunnel was later introduced in an attempt to ameliorate some of the adverse consequences of the atriopulmonary Fontan, which can lead to significant right atrial dilatation. The lateral tunnel uses a baffle within the right atrium to direct inferior vena caval blood to the right pulmonary artery. Both the atriopulmonary Fontan and lateral tunnel Fontan are performed via a right atriotomy approach. The extracardiac Fontan is the more recent modification and avoids the atrium altogether by using a synthetic, often polytetrafluoroethylene extracardiac conduit between the disconnected inferior vena cava and the right pulmonary artery to create total cavopulmonary anastamosis.[54]

Fontan patients have the highest mortality rates among patients with CHD.[55] Recent studies have shown the overall 10-year, 20-year, and 30-year survival after the Fontan operation as 74%, 61%, and 43%, respectively. Operations carried out before 1991, use of pre-operative diuretics, asplenia, and lack of preoperative sinus rhythm were all factors associated with decreased overall survival.[56]

One series found that death in the Fontan population predominantly occurred perioperatively (68%), followed by sudden death (9%), thromboembolism (8%), heart failure (7%), and sepsis (3%). Sudden death was presumed to be largely arrhythmic in origin.[57] Similar causes for late death were reported at the Mayo Clinic in Rochester.[58]

Atrial arrhythmias are more common in the atriopulmonary Fontan population compared with the lateral tunnel Fontan and the extracardiac Fontan groups, although long-term follow-up of the latter group is limited.[58,59] The incidence of atrial arrhythmias, however, remains similar between the lateral tunnel and extracardiac Fontan population.[60] Ventricular arrhythmias, on the other hand, have been poorly studied in this population. The incidence of complex ventricular ectopy on routine Holter monitoring in Fontan subjects was noted to be relatively common (25%). Interestingly, in another study, 2 subjects who had sudden cardiac events did not have nonsustained VT on Holter monitoring. This study detected sinus node dysfunction in nearly 20% of Fontan subjects, which frequently led to pacemaker implantation.[61,62]

Risk Factors for Ventricular Arrhythmias and Sudden Cardiac Death

There is currently a paucity of data on ventricular arrhythmias and risk stratification of sudden death in this population. Patients with single ventricles represent a very small proportion of CHD patients (<2%) who have received an ICD.[63] Although the link between atrial arrhythmias and sudden cardiac death has not been well-established, it is well-recognized that atrial arrhythmias are poorly tolerated in this population, resulting in increased Fontan pressures and, thereby, decreasing cardiac output. Additionally, sinus node dysfunction is not uncommon in this population.

EBSTEIN ANOMALY
Pathophysiology and Mechanisms for Ventricular Arrhythmias

Ebstein anomaly is a malformation of the tricuspid valve resulting from abnormal attachments of the leaflets and apical displacement of the functional annulus. The patient will often have tricuspid regurgitation, the severity of which will be determined by the extent of abnormality of the tricuspid valve. Progressive RV dilatation and dysfunction develop over time.[64]

VT has been found to be inducible on EP studies in a minority of patients with unrepaired Ebstein and has been incidentally detected during investigations for SVT. These were predominantly monomorphic VTs with a left bundle branch block QRS morphology.[65] The clinical significance of inducible VT on EP study, however, is unknown in this population. The cause of VT in unrepaired Ebstein is likely to be long-standing RV volume overload. Another mechanism for SCD in the patient with Ebstein anomaly can be seen in the presence of an accessory pathway where rapid conduction during atrial fibrillation can trigger VF and subsequent death.[65] Rapidly conducting or multiple AV accessory pathways are an important substrate for sudden cardiac death.[66] Up to 36% of patients with Ebstein anomaly will have 1 or more accessory pathways, also known as Wolff Parkinson-White syndrome.

Patients with Ebstein who survive infancy generally do very well, reaching adolescence or adulthood before surgical repair may need to be considered. The first and most commonly used surgical repair of the tricuspid valve in Ebstein was the creation of a monocuspid valve using the anterior leaflet of the tricuspid valve. The repair also consists of plication of the free wall of the atrialized portion of the RV, posterior tricuspid annuloplasty, and right reduction atrioplasty. Various other techniques are in practice today that use the same surgical principles. The newest and most promising technique is the Cone repair. RV plication is preferred in contrast to RV resection because the latter can result in full-thickness

scar and increase the likelihood of ventricular arrhythmias.[67]

One series reported VT in up to 7% of subjects following Ebstein repair in the immediate postoperative period. Subjects who demonstrated perioperative VT or VF were found to be at increased risk of sudden death during long-term follow-up.[68]

Risk Factors for Ventricular Arrhythmias and Sudden Cardiac Death

Unrepaired Ebstein anomaly poses a large hemodynamic burden on the right heart and this can, in turn, place an individual at risk of arrhythmias. The development of atrial arrhythmias and right heart failure are well-established in the unrepaired Ebstein population. The incidence of ventricular arrhythmias in this group, however, remains unknown. To date, there is also little known of the long-term risk of VT after Ebstein repair.

Sudden death is uncommon in Ebstein anomaly, though was found to be the most common mechanism of death in an observational trial. This included both repaired and unrepaired Ebstein. Interestingly, none of the subjects in this series had WPW syndrome.[2] Multiple accessory pathways, short pre-existing RR intervals during atrial fibrillation, and a history of both reciprocating tachycardia and atrial fibrillation are the major risk factors for an increased risk of VF in WPW syndrome.[69]

Ebstein anomaly is also associated with left heart disease in up to 40% of patients. This includes left ventricular noncompaction, mitral valve prolapse, bicuspid aortic valve, and VSDs, which provide other potential sources of ventricular arrhythmias.[70] Ebstein anomaly currently only constitutes 0.02% of all patients who have received an ICD and, thus, data remain limited.[4]

EISENMENGER SYNDROME
Pathophysiology and Mechanisms for Ventricular Arrhythmias

Eisenmenger syndrome refers to pulmonary vascular disease and cyanosis, secondary to reversed or bidirectional shunts, or in a single ventricle through a large defect between the systemic and pulmonary circulation at the ventricular, atrial, or aortopulmonary levels.[71] Patients with Eisenmenger syndrome have a poor prognosis, with a 15-year survival of 77%.[72] 18% of sudden cardiac deaths in individuals with CHD were seen in patients with Eisenmenger syndrome. These were presumed to be arrhythmic because no alternate cause could be identified on postmortem studies.[71]

Risk Factors for Ventricular Arrhythmias and Sudden Cardiac Death

Worsening symptoms, age, ventricular dysfunction, and noncardiac surgery were associated with a poor prognosis.[73] Impaired systemic and subpulmonic ventricular dysfunction were found to be associated with sudden cardiac death.[71]

AORTIC COARCTATION
Pathophysiology and Mechanisms for Ventricular Arrhythmias

Aortic coarctation is part of a diffuse arteriopathy, with a propensity to aneurysm formation and dissection remote from the coarctation site.[74] Ten percent of patients with aortic coarctation also have cerebral aneurysms detected on MRI.[75] Sudden death was found to be the most common mode of death in aortic coarctation.[2] Premature coronary disease, residual hypertension, cerebral aneurysmal rupture, aortic aneurysm and dissection are all potential underlying causes of early mortality in this population. Profound hypertrophy was mentioned in most of the fatalities.[43]

Risk Factors for Ventricular Arrhythmias and Sudden Cardiac Death

Risk stratification in this population is difficult because this condition has several extracardiac manifestations that contribute to an individual's risk of sudden death. It has yet to be delineated how frequently ventricular arrhythmias contribute to this.

VENTRICULAR SEPTAL DEFECTS

Early studies from the 1950s and 60s noted a high prevalence of serious arrhythmias and sudden death in those with VSDs at long-term follow up. Anecdotally, the authors have observed that patients operated in an earlier era with suboptimal bypass who have ventricular dysfunction are at risk for ventricular arrhythmias. This is unlikely to be seen in the contemporary cohort of VSD-repaired patients.[76]

SUMMARY

The incidence of ventricular arrhythmias in CHD varies depending on the diagnosis, type of repair, and timing of repair. Much of the current literature surrounds ventricular arrhythmias in TOF, despite there being a significantly higher incidence reported in patients following atrial switch repair. Monomorphic VT with a left bundle branch morphology is most commonly described in TOF, as well as Ebstein anomaly; whereas polymorphic VT and VF is best described in patients following atrial switch repair. There is currently a lack of data on ventricular arrhythmias in Fontan patients but there is an expectation that this will change over time. Atrial arrhythmias are, however, well-established as predictors of ventricular arrhythmias and sudden cardiac death in D-TGA, Ebstein anomaly, and Fontan patients.

Sudden cardiac death is well-recognized in those with Eisenmenger syndrome, which is predominantly thought to be due to ventricular arrhythmias. This has been largely derived from postmortem studies. Sudden death is noted not infrequently in those with aortic coarctation but this is a diffuse arteriopathy with extracardiac manifestations that make it difficult to attribute this solely to ventricular arrhythmias.

Understanding of ventricular arrhythmias and sudden death in CHD continues to grow and so too will the ability to better stratify the risk these patients in the future.

REFERENCES

1. Engelings CC, Helma PC, Abdul-Khaliq H, et al. Cause of death in adults with congenital heart disease - an analysis of the German National Register for congenital heart defects. Int J Cardiol 2016; 211:31–6.
2. Oechslin EN, Harrison DA, Connelly MS, et al. Mode of death in adults with congenital heart disease. Am J Cardiol 2000;86(10):1111–6.
3. Verheugt CL, Uiterwaal CS, van der Velde ET, et al. Mortality in adult congenital heart disease. Eur Heart J 2010;31:1220–9.
4. Khairy P, Van Hare GF, Balaji S, et al. PACES/HRS expert consensus statement on the recognition and management of arrhythmias in adult congenital heart disease: developed in partnership between the Pediatric and Congenital Electrophysiology Society (PACES) and the Heart Rhythm Society (HRS). Endorsed by the governing bodies of PACES, HRS, the American College of Cardiology (ACC), the American Heart Association (AHA), the European Heart Rhythm Association (EHRA), the Canadian Heart Rhythm Society (CHRS), and the International Society for Adult Congenital Heart Disease (ISACHD). Heart Rhythm 2014;11:e102–65.
5. Santharam S, Hudsmith L, Thorne S, et al. Long term follow up of implantable cardioverter-defibrillators in adult congenital heart disease patients: indications and outcomes. Europace 2017;19(3):407–13.
6. Pye MP, Cobbe SM. Mechanisms of ventricular arrhythmias in cardiac failure and hypertrophy. Cardiovasc Res 1992;26:740–50.

7. Bigger JT, Dresdale RJ, Heissenbuttel RH, et al. Ventricular arrhythmias in ischemic heart disease: mechanism, prevalence, significance, and management. Prog Cardiovasc Dis 1977;19(4):255–300.

8. Gaztanaga L, Marchlinski FE, Betensky BP. Mechanisms of cardiac arrhythmias. Rev Esp Cardiol 2012;65:174–85.

9. Pogwizd SM, Hoyt RH, Saffitz JE, et al. Reentrant and focal mechanisms underlying ventricular tachycardia in the human heart. Circulation 1992;86:1872–87.

10. Markowitz SM, Lerman BB. Mechanisms of focal ventricular tachycardia in humans. Heart Rhythm 2009;6:S81–5.

11. Grimm W. Accelerated idioventricular rhythm. Card Electrophysiol Rev 2001;5:328–31.

12. Tai YT, Lau CP, Fong PC, et al. Incessant automatic ventricular tachycardia complicating acute coxsackie B myocarditis. Cardiology 1992;80:339–44.

13. Zeppenfeld K, Blom NA, Bootsma M, et al. Incessant ventricular tachycardia in fulminant lymphocytic myocarditis: evidence for origin in the Purkinje system and successful treatment with ablation. Heart Rhythm 2007;4:88–91.

14. Qin D, Zhang ZH, Caref EB, et al. Cellular and ionic basis of arrhythmias in postinfarction remodeled ventricular myocardium. Circ Res 1996;79:461–73.

15. Stevenson WG. Ventricular scars and ventricular tachycardia. Trans Am Clin Climatol Assoc 2009;120:403–12.

16. Miller JM, Hsia HH, Rothman SA, et al. Ventricular tachycardia versus supraventricular tachycardia with aberration: electrocardiographic distinctions. In: Zipes D, Jalife J, editors. Cardiac electrophysiology: from cell to bedside. 3rd edition. Philadelphia: Sanders WB; 2000. p. 696–705.

17. Hadid C. Sustained ventricular tachycardia in structural heart disease. Cardiol J 2015;22:12–24.

18. Gatzoulis MA, Balaji S, Webber SA, et al. Risk factors for arrhythmia and sudden cardiac death later after repair of Tetralogy of Fallot: a multicentre trial. Lancet 2000;356:975–81.

19. Pradegan N, Vida VL, Geva T, et al. Myocardial histopathology in late repaired and unrepaired adults with Tetralogy of Fallot. Cardiovasc Pathol 2016;25:225–31.

20. Khairy P, Stevenson WG. Catheter ablation in Tetralogy of Fallot. Heart Rhythm 2009;6(7):1069–74.

21. Zeppenfield K, Jongbloed M, Schalij MJ. Cardiac electrophysiology. From cell to bedside. Ventricular arrhythmias in congenital heart disease. 6th edition. Philadelphia: Elsevier Saunders; 2014. p. 1009–18.

22. Dietl CA, Cazzaniga ME, Dubner SJ, et al. Life threatening arrhythmias and RV dysfunction after surgical repair of Tetralogy of Fallot. Comparison between transventricular and transatrial approaches. Circulation 1994;90:II7–12.

23. Khairy P, Harris L, Landzberg MJ, et al. Implantable cardioverter defibrillators in TOF. Circulation 2008;117:363–70.

24. Cheung EW, Wong WH, Cheung YF. Metaanalysis of pulmonary valve replacement after operative repair of Tetralogy of Fallot. Am J Cardiol 2000;106:552–7.

25. Zeppenfield K, Schaliji MJ, Bartelings MM, et al. Catheter ablation of ventricular tachycardia after repair of congenital heart disease: electroanatomic identification of the critical right ventricular isthmus. Circulation 2007;116(20):2241–52.

26. Luitjen LW, van den Bosch E, Duppen N, et al. Long term outcomes of transatrial-transpulmonary repair of Tetralogy of Fallot. Eur J Cardiothorac Surg 2015;47:527–34.

27. Marie PY, Marcon F, Brunotte F, et al. Right ventricular overload and induced sustained ventricular tachycardia in operatively 'repaired' Tetralogy of Fallot. Am J Cardiol 1992;69(8):785–9.

28. Alvarez-Fuente M, Garrido-Lestache E, Fernandez-Pineda L, et al. Timing of pulmonary valve replacement: how much can the right ventricle dilate before it loses its remodelling potential? Pediatr Cardiol 2016;37(3):601–5.

29. Silversides CK, Marelli A, Beauchesne L, et al. Canadian Cardiovascular Society 2009 Consensus Conference on the management of adults with congenital heart disease: executive summary. Can J Cardiol 2010;26(3):143–50.

30. Harrild DM, Berul CI, Cecchin F, et al. Pulmonary valve replacement in Tetralogy of Fallot. Impact on survival and ventricular tachycardia. Circulation 2009;119:445–51.

31. Valenre AM, Gauvreau K, Assenza GE, et al. Contemporary predictors of death and sustained ventricular tachycardia in patients with repaired Tetralogy of Fallot enrolled in the INDICATOR cohort. Heart 2014;100(3):247–53.

32. Muller J, Hager A, Diller GP, et al. Peak oxygen uptake, ventilatory efficiency and QRS-duration predict event free survival in patients late after surgical repair of Tetralogy of Fallot. Int J Cardiol 2015;196:158–64.

33. Gatzoullis M, Till JA, Somerville J, et al. Mechanoelectrical interaction in Tetralogy of Fallot. QRS prolongation relates to right ventricular size and predicts malignant ventricular arrhythmias and sudden death. Circulation 1995;92(2):231–7.

34. Therrien J, Siu SC, Harris L, et al. Impact of pulmonary valve replacement on arrhythmia propensity later after repair of Tetralogy of Fallot. Circulation 2001;103(20):2489–94.

35. Uebing A, Gibson DG, Babu-Narayan SV, et al. Right ventricular mechanics and QRS duration in patients with repaired Tetralogy of Fallot: implications of infundibular disease. Circulation 2007;116:1532–9.

36. Nanthakumar K, Masse S, Silversides CK, et al. Intraoperative high-density global mapping in adult repaired Tetralogy of Fallot. Altered left ventricular and right ventricular activation and implications for resynchronization strategies. J Am Coll Cardiol 2010; 55:2409–22.

37. Khairy P, Landzberg MJ, Gatzoulis MA, et al. Value of programmed ventricular stimulation after Tetralogy of Fallot repair: a multicenter study. Circulation 2004;109(16):1994–2000.

38. Khairy P, Dore A, Poirer N, et al. Risk stratification in surgically repaired Tetralogy of Fallot. Expert Rev Cardiovasc Ther 2009;7(7):755–62.

39. Khairy P. Programmed ventricular stimulation for risk stratification in patients with Tetralogy of Fallot: a Bayesian perspective. Nat Clin Pract Cardiovasc Med 2007;4(6):292–3.

40. Khairy P, Clair M, Fernandes SM, et al. Cardiovascular outcomes after the arterial switch operation for D-Transposition of the great arteries. Circulation 2013; 127:331–9.

41. Kammeraad JA, van Deurzen CH, Sreeram N, et al. Predictors of sudden cardiac death after Mustard or Senning repair for transposition of the great arteries. J Am Coll Cardiol 2004;44(5):1095–102.

42. El Said G, Rosenberg HS, Mullins CE, et al. Dysrythmias after Mustard's operation for transposition of the great arteries. Am J Cardiol 1972;30(5):526–32.

43. Silka MJ, Hardy BG, Menashe VD, et al. A population-based prospective evaluation of risk of sudden cardiac death after operation for common congenital heart defects. J Am Coll Cardiol 1998;32:245–51.

44. Gelatt M, Hamilton RM, McCrindle BW, et al. Arrhythmia and mortality after the Mustard procedure: a 30-year single-center experience. J Am Coll Cardiol 1997;29:194–201.

45. Sherwin ED, Triedman JK, Walsh EP. Update on interventional electrophsyiology in congenital heart disease. Evolving solutions for complex hearts. Circulation 2013;6:1032–40.

46. Schwerzmann M, Salehian O, Harris L, et al. Ventricular arrhythmias and sudden death in adults after a Mustard operation for transposition of the great arteries. Eur Heart J 2009;30:1873–9.

47. Cuypers JA, Eindhoven JA, Slager MA, et al. The natural and unnatural history of the Mustard procedure: long term outcome up to 40 years. Eur Heart J 2014;35:1666–74.

48. Epstein AE, DiMarco JP, Ellenbogen KA, et al. ACC/AHA/HRS 2008 guidelines for device based therapy of cardiac rhythm abnormalities: executive summary. J Am Coll Cardiol 2008;117:2820–40.

49. Kovalova S, Necas J, Vespalec J. What is a 'normal' right ventricle? Eur J Echocardiogr 2006;7:293–7.

50. Khairy P. Ventricular arrhythmias and sudden cardiac death in adults with congenital heart disease. Heart 2016;102:1703–9.

51. Khairy P, Harris L, Landzberg MJ, et al. Sudden death and defibrillators in transposition of the great arteries with intra atrial baffles. A multicenter study. Circ Arrhythm Electrophysiol 2008;1:250–7.

52. Birnie D, Tometzki A, Curzio J, et al. Outcomes of transposition of the great arteries in the era of atrial inflow correction. Heart 1998;80:170–3.

53. Backhoff D, Muller M, Ruschewski W, et al. ICD therapy for primary prevention of sudden cardiac death after Mustard repair for d-transposition of the great arteries. Clin Res Cardiol 2014;103:891–901.

54. Gersony WM. Fontan operation after 3 decades: what we have learned. Circulation 2008;117:13–5.

55. Khairy P, Fernandes SM, Mayer JE, et al. Long-term survival, modes of death and predictors of mortality in patients with Fontan surgery. Circulation 2008; 117(1):85–92.

56. Pundi KN, Johnson JN, Dearani JA, et al. 40-year follow-up after the Fontan operation. Long term outcomes of 1,052 patients. J Am Coll Cardiol 2015; 66(15):1700–10.

57. Mair DD, Puga FJ, Danielson GK. The Fontan procedure for tricuspid atresia: early and late results of a 25 year experience with 216 patients. J Am Coll Cardiol 2001;37(3):933–9.

58. D'Udekem Y, Iyengar AJ, Galati JC, et al. Redefining expectations of long-term survival after the Fontan procedure. Twenty-five years of follow up from the entire population of Australia and New Zealand. Circulation 2014;130(11 Suppl 1):S32–8.

59. Stephenson EA, Lu M, Berul CI, et al. Arrhythmias in a contemporary fontan cohort. J Am Coll Cardiol 2010;56:890–6.

60. Balaji S, Daga A, Bradley DJ, et al. An international multicenter study comparing arrhythmia prevalence between the intracardiac lateral tunnel and the extracardiac conduit type of Fontan operations. J Thorac Cardiovasc Surg 2014;148:576–81.

61. Czosek RJ, Anderson J, Khoury PR, et al. Utility of ambulatory monitoring in patients with congenital heart disease. J Am Coll Cardiol 2013;111:723–30.

62. Walsh EP. Sudden death in adult congenital heart disease: risk stratification in 2014. Heart Rhythm 2014;11:1735–42.

63. Vehmeijer JT, Brouwer TF, Limpens J, et al. Implantable cardioverter-defibrillators in adults with congenital heart disease: a systematic review and meta-analysis. Eur Heart J 2016;37:1439–48.

64. Attenhofer Jost CH, Connolly HM, Dearani JA, et al. Ebstein's anomaly. Circulation 2007;115:277–85.

65. Smith WM, Gallagher JJ, Kerr CR, et al. The electrophysiologic basis and management of symptomatic recurrent tachycardia in patients with ebstein's anomaly of the tricuspid valve. Am J Cardiol 1982; 49:1223–34.

66. Zachariah JP, Walsh EP, Triedman JK, et al. Multiple accessory pathways in the young: the impact

of structural heart disease. Am Heart J 2013;165: 87–92.

67. Dearani JA, Said SM, Burkhart HM, et al. Strategies for tricuspid re-repair in Ebstein malformation using the Cone technique. Ann Thorac Surg 2013;96: 202–10.

68. Oh JK, Holmes DR, Hayes DL, et al. Cardiac arrhythmias in patients with surgical repair of Ebstein's anomaly. J Am Coll Cardiol 1985;6(6):1351–7.

69. Klein GJ, Bashore TM, Sellers TD. Ventricular fibrillation in Wolff-Parkinson-White syndrome. N Engl J Med 1979;301:1080–5.

70. Attenhofer Jost CH, Connolly HM, O'Leary PW, et al. Left heart lesions in patients with Ebstein anomaly. Mayo Clin Proc 2005;80(3):361–8.

71. Koyak Z, Harris L, de Groot JR, et al. Sudden cardiac death in adult congenital heart disease. Circulation 2012;126:1944–54.

72. Saha A, Balakrishnan KG, Jasiwal PK, et al. Prognosis for patients with Eisenmenger syndrome of various aetiology. Int J Cardiol 1994;45:199–207.

73. Daliento L, Somerville J, Presbitero P, et al. Eisenmenger syndrome – factors relating to deterioration and death. Eur Heart J 1998;19:1845–55.

74. Warnes CA. Bicuspid aortic valve and coarctation: two villains part of a diffuse problem. Heart 2003; 89:965–6.

75. Connolly HM, Huston J, Brown RD, et al. Intracranial aneurysms in patients with coarctation of the aorta: a prospective magnetic resonance angiographic study of 100 patients. Mayo Clin Proc 2003;78: 1491–9.

76. Kidd L, Driscoll DJ, Gersony WM, et al. Second natural history study of congenital heart defects. Results of treatment of patients with ventricular septal defects. Circulation 1993;87:38–51.

Sudden Cardiac Death in Adult Congenital Heart Disease

Pablo Ávila, MD[a], Marie-A. Chaix, MD, MS[b],
Blandine Mondésert, MD[b], Paul Khairy, MD, PhD[b],*

KEYWORDS

- Congenital heart disease • Implantable cardioverter-defibrillator • Risk stratification
- Sudden cardiac death • Ventricular tachycardia

KEY POINTS

- Sudden cardiac death (SCD) is a leading cause of mortality in adults with congenital heart disease.
- SCD is predominantly due to malignant arrhythmias but other causes include myocardial infarction, heart failure, thromboemboli, and aneurysm rupture.
- Cardiac arrest survivors and patients with hemodynamically unstable ventricular tachycardia with no clearly identified reversible cause generally benefit from implantable cardioverter-defibrillator (ICD) therapy.
- Risk stratification for primary prevention ICDs remains challenging in this population of patients.
- Factors associated with SCD are relatively well defined in patients with tetralogy of Fallot, in contrast to those with systemic right ventricles or univentricular hearts.

INTRODUCTION

Remarkable medical and surgical breakthroughs in the care of children born with heart defects have resulted in a striking improvement in survival, particularly in younger age strata and in those with severe forms of congenital heart disease (CHD).[1] Consequently, most children now survive to adulthood, leading to a shift in population demographics with adults making up two-thirds of the entire CHD population.[2] Epidemiologic studies estimate that there are at least 3 million adults with CHD in North America and Europe.[3] Moreover, the prevalence of complex CHD in adults is steadily increasing.[2] Despite these medical achievements, patients with CHD cannot be considered cured even with successful repairs. They face a variety of long-term complications, including a broad spectrum of cardiac arrhythmias, and higher mortality compared with the general population.[4]

In this context, sudden cardiac death (SCD) is a leading cause of mortality. These catastrophic events often occur in otherwise relatively stable patients, typically in the third or fourth decade of life.[4–12] Identification of subjects deemed at high risk for SCD is a real challenge for the treating physician. These difficulties are reflected in a

Funding Sources: Dr P. Khairy is supported by a Research Chair in Electrophysiology and Adult Congenital Heart.
Conflict of Interest Disclosure: Dr B. Mondésert reports receiving consulting fees and grant support from Boston Scientific. The other authors report no conflicts.
[a] Department of Cardiology, Instituto de Investigación Sanitaria, Hospital Gregorio Marañón, Universidad Complutense, Madrid, Spain; [b] Adult Congenital Heart Center, Montreal Heart Institute, Université de Montréal, 5000 Belanger Street East, Montreal H1T 1C8, Canada
* Corresponding author.
E-mail address: paul.khairy@umontreal.ca

Card Electrophysiol Clin 9 (2017) 225–234
http://dx.doi.org/10.1016/j.ccep.2017.02.003
1877-9182/17/© 2017 Elsevier Inc. All rights reserved.

consensus document developed in partnership between the Pediatric and Congenital Electrophysiology Society and the Heart Rhythm Society, in which evidence-based recommendations were proposed.[13] This article focuses on mechanisms and risk factors for SCD in the adult with CHD and summarizes current recommendations regarding preventive strategies.

SCOPE OF THE PROBLEM

SCD is defined as death due to a cardiovascular cause that occurs within 1 hour of the onset of symptoms, or unwitnessed death in the absence of an obvious extracardiac condition as the proximate cause of death. The first reports that raised concerns about SCD following surgical repair of CHD were published more than 35 years ago.[14] The topic has since grown in interest, as reflected by numerous subsequent studies.

Contemporary studies on causes of late mortality in adults with CHD suggest that, after heart failure, SCD is the second most common cause of mortality, accounting for approximately 20% of all deaths (**Table 1**).[4–12] Trends indicate that the proportion of SCDs is on the decline.[11,12] Although the incidence of SCD in the CHD population at large is relatively low (<0.1% per year), identified subgroups at higher risk include tetralogy of Fallot, systemic right ventricle (ie, complete transposition of the great arteries [TGAs] with atrial switch or congenitally corrected TGA), left-sided outflow obstructive lesions (ie, aortic or subaortic stenosis, aortic coarctation), and Eisenmenger syndrome.[5,7,9,10] Furthermore, factors associated with SCD seem to differ among

specific defects, suggesting that risk stratification is best performed on a lesion-by-lesion basis.[15]

MECHANISMS OF SUDDEN CARDIAC DEATH

Arrhythmias account for approximately 80% of all SCDs in the CHD population. Ventricular arrhythmias, both monomorphic and polymorphic (**Figs. 1 and 2**), are the most common events. However, atrial tachyarrhythmias with rapid (eg, 1:1) atrioventricular (AV) conduction degenerating into ventricular fibrillation (VF) have also been described, as have bradyarrhythmic deaths due to AV block. It is also important to bear in mind that other pathologic conditions, such as thromboembolism, myocardial infarction, aortic dissection, and aneurysm rupture, account for up to 20% of SCDs.[13] In contrast to other forms of heart disease that afflict young adults (eg, hypertrophic cardiomyopathy and arrhythmogenic right ventricular cardiomyopathy), exercise and physical activity have not been associated with SCD in adults with CHD,[16] with few exceptions such as TGA with atrial switch surgery.[17] Overall, less than 10% of SCDs in adults with CHD occur during exercise.[8,18] Most adults with CHD should be encouraged to exercise regularly, although the nature and intensity of exercise training should be tailored following a comprehensive evaluation.[16,19]

SECONDARY PREVENTION OF SUDDEN CARDIAC DEATH

There are no randomized trials for secondary prevention implantable cardioverter-defibrillators (ICDs) in subjects with CHD. In general, ICDs are

Table 1
Sudden cardiac death in adults with congenital heart disease

Authors	Years	Subjects	Deaths	SCD
Oeschlin et al,[6] 2000	1981–1996	2609	197	26%
Silka et al,[5] 1998	1958–1996	3589	176	23%
Verheugt et al,[7] 2010	2001–2009	6933	197	19%
Zomer et al,[8] 2012	2001–2010	8595	231	22%
Gallego et al,[9] 2012	1990–2010	936	50	44%
Koyak et al,[10] 2012	1970–2011	25,790	1189	19%
Diller et al,[4] 2015	1991–2013	6969	524	7%
Engelings et al,[11] 2016	2001–2015	2596	239	23%
Raissadati et al,[12] 2016	1953–2009	10,964	721	21%
Total or average	—	63,936	3524	19%

Adapted from Khairy P, Van Hare GF, Balaji S, et al. PACES/HRS expert consensus statement on the recognition and management of arrhythmias in adult congenital heart disease: Developed in partnership between the Pediatric and Congenital Electrophysiology Society (PACES) and the Heart Rhythm Society (HRS). Endorsed by the governing bodies of PACES, HRS, the American College of Cardiology (ACC), the American Heart Association (AHA), the European Heart Rhythm Association (EHRA), the Canadian Heart Rhythm Society (CHRS), and the International Society for Adult Congenital Heart Disease (ISACHD). Heart Rhythm 2014;11(10):e132; with permission.

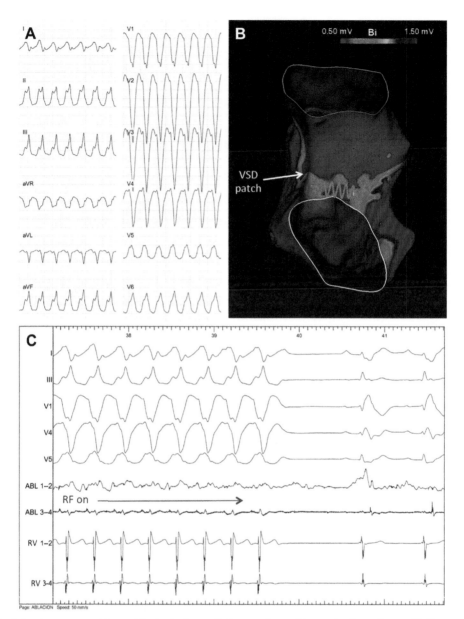

Fig. 1. Sustained monomorphic ventricular tachycardia in a patient with repaired tetralogy of Fallot status after pulmonary valve replacement. The electrocardiogram depicts ventricular tachycardia with a left bundle branch block morphology and inferior QRS axis (*A*). The critical isthmus was between the ventricular septal defect patch (*arrow*) and pulmonary annulus (*B*). Ablation at this site interrupted the tachycardia and produced bidirectional conduction block (*C*).

indicated in survivors of cardiac arrest due to VF or hemodynamically unstable ventricular tachycardia (VT) after ruling out reversible causes (**Table 2**). A high rate of appropriate ICD shocks has been observed during follow-up in this group of patients.[13,20] Catheter ablation has emerged as a useful tool to reduce episodes of VT or ICD shocks. However, as for other structural diseases, it should not be considered a substitute for an ICD but, rather, as complementary therapy. The subgroup of patients with successful ablation of VT isthmuses, demonstrated bidirectional conduction block across them, and preserved ventricular function seem to be at low risk of VT recurrence and SCD.[21,22] Yet, complete bidirectional block is not achievable in all patients and it may be difficult to assess in some cases. Moreover, catheter ablation does not address polymorphic VT, which

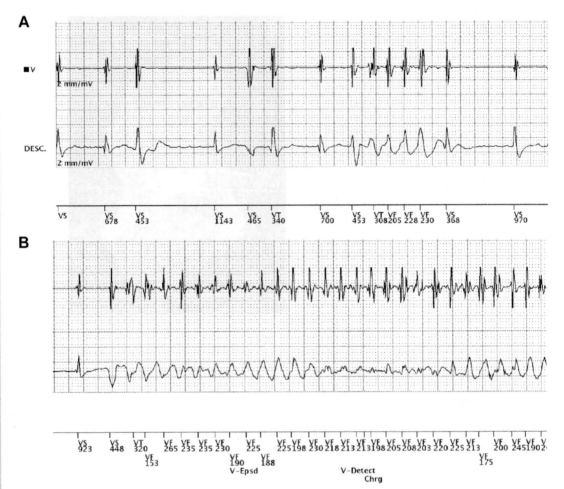

Fig. 2. Recorded tracings from a patient with non-Eisenmenger chronic cyanosis and severe systemic ventricular dysfunction with a secondary prevention implantable cardioverter-defibrillator following resuscitated cardiac arrest. Episodes of nonsustained (*A*) and sustained polymorphic ventricular tachycardia degenerating into ventricular fibrillation (*B*) are depicted. Monomorphic ventricular tachycardia was never recorded.

is also of concern, particularly in patients with severe systemic ventricular dysfunction, extensive hypertrophy, diffuse fibrosis, or myocardial ischemia.[23]

PRIMARY PREVENTION OF SUDDEN CARDIAC DEATH
Challenges in Risk Stratification

Risk stratification for SCD is, no doubt, among the most challenging issues encountered by the CHD specialist. Objectives are to predict which patients are likely to die suddenly and to prevent these catastrophic events. To date, the ICD is the only therapy demonstrated to effectively prevent SCD. Key factors involved in guiding decisions to implant an ICD must be carefully considered. These include objectively estimating risk for SCD, effectiveness of the ICD in

preventing the event, competing causes of death, and morbidity and mortality associated with the device.[23] The greatest benefit may be anticipated for young patients (ie, with a higher number of potential years of life saved) with a high probability of SCD due to ventricular arrhythmias and a low likelihood of dying from other causes. In addition, economic considerations associated with ICD therapy must be factored into the equation when establishing the threshold at which benefits exceed risks.[23]

Transvenous ICDs are associated with inherent challenges in the CHD population. Access to the cardiac chambers of interest may not be possible due to narrowed or obstructed venous pathways, conduits, or baffles; or because the venous system bypasses the heart (eg, total cavopulmonary connection Fontan). Implant-related complications are more frequent in patients with CHD

Table 2
Implantable cardioverter-defibrillator indications in adults with congenital heart disease

COR	LOE	Recommendation
Secondary Prevention		
I	B	ICD therapy is indicated in adults with CHD who are survivors of cardiac arrest due to VF or hemodynamically unstable VT after evaluation to define the cause of the event and exclude any completely reversible etiologic factors.
I	B	ICD therapy is indicated in adults with CHD and spontaneous sustained VT who have undergone hemodynamic and electrophysiologic evaluation.
	C	Catheter ablation or surgery may offer a reasonable alternative or adjunct to ICD therapy in carefully selected patients.
Primary Prevention		
I	B	ICD therapy is indicated in adults with CHD and a systemic LVEF ≤35%, biventricular physiology, and NYHA class II or III symptoms.
IIa	B	ICD therapy is reasonable in selected adults with tetralogy of Fallot and multiple risk factors for SCD, such as LV systolic or diastolic dysfunction, nonsustained VT, QRS duration ≥180 ms, extensive RV scarring, or inducible sustained VT at electrophysiologic study.
IIb	C	ICD therapy may be reasonable in adults with a single or systemic right ventricular ejection fraction <35%, particularly in the presence of additional risk factors such as complex ventricular arrhythmias, unexplained syncope, NYHA functional class II or III symptoms, QRS duration ≥140 ms, or severe systemic AV valve regurgitation.
IIb	B	ICD therapy may be considered in adults with CHD and syncope of unknown origin with hemodynamically significant sustained VT or fibrillation inducible at electrophysiologic study.
IIb	C	ICD therapy may be considered for adults with syncope and moderate or complex CHD in whom there is a high clinical suspicion of ventricular arrhythmia and in whom thorough invasive and noninvasive investigations have failed to define a cause.
IIb	C	ICD therapy may be considered in adults with CHD and a systemic ventricular ejection fraction <35% in the absence of overt symptoms (NYHA class I) or other known risk factors.

Abbreviations: COR, class of recommendation; LOE, level of evidence; LV, left ventricular; LVEF, left ventricular ejection fraction; NYHA, New York Heart Association; RV, right ventricular.

Adapted from Khairy P, Van Hare GF, Balaji S, et al. PACES/HRS expert consensus statement on the recognition and management of arrhythmias in adult congenital heart disease: developed in partnership between the Pediatric and Congenital Electrophysiology Society (PACES) and the Heart Rhythm Society (HRS). Endorsed by the governing bodies of PACES, HRS, the American College of Cardiology (ACC), the American Heart Association (AHA), the European Heart Rhythm Association (EHRA), the Canadian Heart Rhythm Society (CHRS), and the International Society for Adult Congenital Heart Disease (ISACHD). Heart Rhythm 2014;11(10):e135; with permission.

and more than 2-fold higher in the setting of complex lesions compared with those without CHD.[24] Also, long-term complications, such as lead fracture or dislodgment, venous obstruction, endocarditis, and thromboembolic events in the presence of intracardiac shunts, are highly prevalent in these young patients, occurring in greater than 25% at 4 years of follow-up.[25,26] These are alarming figures considering that some complications are time-dependent and increase in prevalence with duration of follow-up, which may be lengthy in young patients. Another major concern is the high rate of inappropriate shocks (∼25%) mainly due to supraventricular arrhythmias.[26] Optimization of programming parameters, including long detection times and high detection

rates, may significantly reduce inappropriate therapies.[27,28]

The subcutaneous ICD may overcome several limitations and could be an attractive option, particularly for patients in whom transvenous access is not feasible or desired, provided that pacing is not required (**Fig. 3**).[29] To date, no lead failures have been reported. The largest series of adults with CHD and subcutaneous ICDs included 21 subjects from 7 North American centers.[30] The most common reasons for selecting a subcutaneous device were limited transvenous access and right-to-left shunts. Over a median follow-up of 14 months, 21% received inappropriate shocks and 1 subject (5%) had multiple appropriate shocks. The only arrhythmic death was attributable to severe

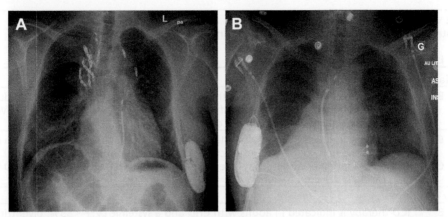

Fig. 3. Subcutaneous ICD in patients with complex CHD following resuscitated cardiac arrests: cyanotic non-Eisenmenger heart disease palliated with a bidirectional Glenn (*A*); and tricuspid atresia, dextrocardia, and extracardiac total cavopulmonary connection (*B*). Note the presence of a concomitant epicardial pacemaker in panel B.

bradycardia manifesting as asystole in the absence of bradycardia pacing. Moreover, the subject with multiple appropriate shocks could potentially have benefited from antitachycardia pacing. Such issues should be carefully considered before recommending this therapy.

Modified surgical approaches, which reflect the recognition of long-term sequelae, may also contribute substantially to reducing the incidence of SCD. For example, identification of anatomic isthmuses responsible for VT, in part created by surgical ventricular scars, have made surgeons adapt their approach by avoiding ventriculotomy incisions whenever possible. Other examples include offering corrective surgery at an earlier age, avoidance of palliative shunts, and prophylactic surgical ablation lesions. The value of electrophysiologically guided surgical approaches to preventing lethal arrhythmias is a topic of active investigation.[31,32]

Tetralogy of Fallot

Since initial descriptions in the 1970s of SCD and its relationship to ventricular arrhythmias in patients with repaired tetralogy of Fallot, a wealth of literature has emerged on the topic.[14] Today, SCD due to ventricular arrhythmias remains the leading cause of mortality in tetralogy of Fallot, with an incidence of approximately 2% per decade in adults.[33] Accordingly, tetralogy of Fallot is the most common CHD diagnosis in ICD recipients.[26]

It was soon appreciated that ventricular scars created during surgical repair had potential proarrhythmic effects. Anatomic isthmuses between electrical conduction barriers produced by ventriculotomy incisions, ventricular septal defect

patches, and pulmonary and tricuspid annuli represent critical channels capable of supporting macroreentrant circuits. These anatomic corridors are the most common pathophysiological substrate for VT in this population and can be targeted by ablation (see **Fig. 1**).[34]

Combining observations from multiple studies, a relatively consistent image of risk features related to ventricular arrhythmias and SCD in tetralogy of Fallot has emerged. These include clinical and surgical factors, parameters of left and right ventricular function, and electrocardiographic and electrophysiological metrics, as summarized in **Box 1**. However, no single factor, with the exception of severe left ventricular systolic dysfunction, seems to have strong enough predictive power to alone justify ICD implantation. The clinical history should also be carefully assessed for symptoms of syncope or rapid palpitations and to identify nonsustained VT.[35,36] In a North American multicenter study, a combination of factors was retained in a risk score to predict appropriate ICD shocks in patients with primary prevention ICDs. These factors had a cumulative effect on risk prediction and proved useful in stratifying patients into low-risk, moderate risk, and high-risk categories.[37] However, this risk score has not been prospectively validated and does not consider newer parameters derived from cardiac magnetic resonance imaging, such as extent of fibrosis and right ventricular mass.[38,39] For patients at intermediate risk, electrophysiological evaluation can further improve risk stratification. Inducibility of VT by programmed ventricular stimulation, when applied in combination with other factors, carries independent prognostic value and can be helpful in reclassifying patients into

---

Box 1
Factors associated with sudden cardiac death in tetralogy of Fallot

Surgical factors

Older age at repair

Prior palliative shunt

Ventriculotomy incision

Transannular patch

Clinical parameters

Syncope or rapid palpitations

History of atrial arrhythmias

Advanced NYHA functional class symptoms

Electrocardiographic and electrophysiological metrics

QRS duration ≥180 ms

Nonsustained VT (particularly if symptomatic)

Inducible sustained monomorphic or polymorphic VT

Prolonged QT or JT dispersion

Decreased heart rate variability

Frequent ventricular ectopic beats

Morphofunctional parameters

RV systolic dysfunction

RV mass to volume ratio ≥0.3 g/mL

LV diastolic dysfunction or LVEDP ≥12 mm Hg

LV systolic dysfunction

RV or LV fibrosis

Severe pulmonary regurgitation

Increased cardiothoracic ratio

Abbreviations: LV, left ventricle; LVEDP, left ventricle end-diastolic pressure; NYHA, New York Heart Association; RV, right ventricle; VT, ventricular tachycardia.

---

low-risk or high-risk groups. Importantly, it is not indicated in low-risk patients[40] and its predictive value beyond 5 to 7 years remains unknown.

Although severe pulmonary regurgitation and right ventricular dilatation and dysfunction have been correlated with higher risk in some studies, pulmonary valve replacement does not reliably protect against ventricular arrhythmias and SCD.[41] Reverse remodeling benefits associated with pulmonary valve replacement do not eradicate long-standing arrhythmogenic structural and electrical changes and do not directly address known substrates for ventricular macroreentry.[39,42]

Considering the totality of evidence, current recommendations state that primary prevention ICDs are reasonable in selected adults with tetralogy of Fallot and multiple risk factors for SCD, such as left ventricular systolic or diastolic dysfunction, nonsustained VT, QRS duration 180 ms or longer, extensive right ventricular scarring, or inducible sustained VT at electrophysiologic study (class IIa, level of evidence B) (see **Table 2**).[13]

Systemic Left Ventricle with Biventricular Physiology

Akin to other cardiomyopathies and based on clinical trials, such as the Sudden Cardiac Death in Heart Failure Trial (SCD-HeFT), patients with systemic left ventricular dysfunction and biventricular physiology should be considered for primary prevention ICDs if they meet standard criteria, that is, a left ventricular ejection fraction equal to or lower than 35% and New York Heart Association (NYHA) functional class II or III symptoms, regardless of the underlying defect.[43] This includes patients with simple forms of CHD, such as atrial or ventricular septal defects, who develop left ventricular dysfunction.[26] This recommendation was also included in the consensus document (see **Table 2**).[13]

Several studies have reported that SCD is an important cause of mortality in patients with aortic stenosis and coarctation, even if the defect was repaired.[5,7–9,12,44] Although the underlying mechanism is not well established, left ventricular enlargement, hypertrophy, and fibrosis can produce maladaptive remodeling changes in ion channel function, with shortened ventricular refractory periods, increased dispersion of refractoriness, and enhanced electrical excitability.[45] It also seems likely that a portion of sudden deaths are not related to arrhythmias, with causes such as myocardial infarction, aortic dissection, and cerebrovascular hemorrhage. In the largest study of SCD to date, no risk factor was identified in patients with left-side obstructive lesions.[10] Nevertheless, it is generally thought that left ventricular systolic dysfunction, severe outflow tract obstruction, aortic regurgitation, and ventricular hypertrophy incurs increased risk. Diastolic dysfunction and pulmonary hypertension have also been associated with higher mortality in this population.[46]

Systemic Right Ventricle

The 2 main lesions included in this category are TGA with atrial switch surgery and congenitally corrected TGA. In both groups of patients, the morphologic right ventricle is subaortic and, hence, prone to failure over time. Although the incidence of SCD in patients with congenitally corrected TGA is less certain, TGA with atrial switch surgery is among the highest risk lesions, with an incidence of SCD in the order of 5 to 10 per 1000 patient-years.[5,9]

Unfortunately, identification of high-risk patients has been less successful than with tetralogy of Fallot, as reflected by a low rate of appropriate shocks in subjects selected for primary prevention ICDs in multicenter studies.[47] For subjects with TGA and atrial switch surgery, the most consistent risk factors identified include severe systemic ventricular dysfunction, atrial arrhythmias, prolonged QRS duration, and at least moderate systemic AV valve (ie, tricuspid) regurgitation.[9,10,15] Similar high-risk features have been proposed in patients with congenitally corrected TGA. Even though severe systemic right ventricular dysfunction is associated with SCD, it should not be assumed that an ejection fraction threshold of 35%, as for a left ventricle, is the ideal cut-off value. The normal range of values for a morphologic right ventricle is approximately 20% lower than for a left ventricle.[23] Some degree of systemic right ventricular dysfunction is inevitable decades after atrial switch surgery.[48] In contrast to tetralogy of Fallot, inducibility of ventricular arrhythmias by means of programmed stimulation does not seem to identify high-risk patients.[47] In patients with atrial switch surgery, it has been hypothesized that an abnormal hemodynamic response to increased heart rates (eg, from atrial or sinus tachycardia) can result in a myocardial supply-and-demand mismatch, which triggers ischemia-related ventricular tachyarrhythmias.[17]

Although recommendations are less definitive, a primary prevention ICD may be reasonable in adults with a systemic right ventricular ejection fraction less than 35%, particularly in the presence of additional risk factors such as complex ventricular arrhythmias, unexplained syncope, NYHA functional class II or III symptoms, QRS duration 140 ms or longer, or severe systemic AV valve regurgitation (class IIb, level of evidence C) (see **Table 2**).

Univentricular Hearts

Most deaths in patients with Fontan palliation are related to heart failure, thromboemboli, or cardiac surgery, with SCD accounting for 9% to 13% of all deaths.[4,49] Although these patients account for a small proportion of ICD recipients with CHD (<2%),[26] they are disproportionately represented in case-series with subcutaneous devices.[30]

No clear risk factors have been associated with SCD in this subgroup of patients, although unexplained syncope and severe systolic ventricular dysfunction should always raise concerns.[15,49] It has been well-described that atrial arrhythmias can be poorly tolerated in patients with Fontan physiology and can be responsible for cardiac arrest.[49] However, unlike patients with TGA and atrial switch surgery in which atrial arrhythmias seem to trigger a substantial proportion of SCDs, this is thought to be a rare event. In contrast, ventricular arrhythmias have not been well-studied in this population. Although a recent single center study reported clinically significant ventricular arrhythmias in 10% of subjects an average of 15 years after Fontan surgery, no independent predictor of VT was identified.[50] A high frequency of premature ventricular contractions is commonly encountered on 24-hour Holter monitors in patients with Fontan surgery. Nevertheless, nonsustained VT has not been convincingly linked to SCD.[51]

According to recent recommendations, ICD therapy may be considered in patients with a single ventricle when the ejection fraction is less than 35%, particularly in the presence of other risk factors (class IIb, level of evidence C) or unexplained syncope, especially if thorough invasive and noninvasive tests have failed to define a cause (see **Table 2**).[13] It is worth emphasizing that if an ICD is considered, transvenous access to the ventricle is not feasible in patients with Fontan surgery, such that an epicardial or subcutaneous approach is required.

SUMMARY

Prevention of SCD is a major preoccupation for clinicians involved in the care of adults with CHD. Lessons learned from the first cohorts of adult survivors with moderate and complex forms of CHD have informed efforts to identify patients at high risk for SCD and have contributed to refining surgical approaches to improve outcomes. Unlike relatively homogeneous forms of heart disease (eg, hypertrophic and arrhythmogenic right ventricular cardiomyopathy), risk stratification for SCD in CHD is hampered by a vast assortment of congenital defects, surgical approaches, and residual hemodynamic lesions. Whereas some risk factors, such as severely impaired systemic ventricular function, are relatively ubiquitous, others, such as inducible ventricular arrhythmias, are more lesion-specific. Over the past decades, a clearer image of the high-risk patient with tetralogy of Fallot has emerged. In contrast, the high-risk profile is obscure in those with systemic right ventricles or univentricular hearts. Continued research is likely to shed light on knowledge gaps and contribute to further lowering the incidence of SCD for subsequent generations.

REFERENCES

1. Khairy P, Ionescu-Ittu R, Mackie AS, et al. Changing mortality in congenital heart disease. J Am Coll Cardiol 2010;56(14):1149–57.

2. Marelli AJ, Ionescu-Ittu R, Mackie AS, et al. Lifetime prevalence of congenital heart disease in the general population from 2000 to 2010. Circulation 2014;130(9):749–56.

3. Webb G, Mulder BJ, Aboulhosn J, et al. The care of adults with congenital heart disease across the globe: current assessment and future perspective: a position statement from the International Society for Adult Congenital Heart Disease (ISACHD). Int J Cardiol 2015;195:326–33.

4. Diller GP, Kempny A, Alonso-Gonzalez R, et al. Survival prospects and circumstances of death in contemporary adult congenital heart disease patients under follow-up at a large tertiary centre. Circulation 2015;132(22):2118–25.

5. Silka MJ, Hardy BG, Menashe VD, et al. A population-based prospective evaluation of risk of sudden cardiac death after operation for common congenital heart defects. J Am Coll Cardiol 1998; 32(1):245–51.

6. Oechslin EN, Harrison DA, Connelly MS, et al. Mode of death in adults with congenital heart disease. Am J Cardiol 2000;86(10):1111–6.

7. Verheugt CL, Uiterwaal CS, van der Velde ET, et al. Mortality in adult congenital heart disease. Eur Heart J 2010;31(10):1220–9.

8. Zomer AC, Vaartjes I, Uiterwaal CS, et al. Circumstances of death in adult congenital heart disease. Int J Cardiol 2012;154(2):168–72.

9. Gallego P, Gonzalez AE, Sanchez-Recalde A, et al. Incidence and predictors of sudden cardiac arrest in adults with congenital heart defects repaired before adult life. Am J Cardiol 2012;110(1):109–17.

10. Koyak Z, Harris L, de Groot JR, et al. Sudden cardiac death in adult congenital heart disease. Circulation 2012;126(16):1944–54.

11. Engelings CC, Helm PC, Abdul-Khaliq H, et al. Cause of death in adults with congenital heart disease - an analysis of the German National Register for congenital heart defects. Int J Cardiol 2016;211:31–6.

12. Raissadati A, Nieminen H, Haukka J, et al. Late causes of death after pediatric cardiac surgery: a 60-year population-based study. J Am Coll Cardiol 2016;68(5):487–98.

13. Khairy P, Van Hare GF, Balaji S, et al. PACES/HRS expert consensus statement on the recognition and management of arrhythmias in adult congenital heart disease: developed in partnership between the Pediatric and Congenital Electrophysiology Society (PACES) and the Heart Rhythm Society (HRS). Endorsed by the governing bodies of PACES, HRS, the American College of Cardiology (ACC), the American Heart Association (AHA), the European Heart Rhythm Association (EHRA), the Canadian Heart Rhythm Society (CHRS), and the International Society for Adult Congenital Heart Disease (ISACHD). Heart Rhythm 2014;11(10):e102–65.

14. Garson A Jr, Nihill MR, McNamara DG, et al. Status of the adult and adolescent after repair of tetralogy of Fallot. Circulation 1979;59(6):1232–40.

15. Walsh EP. Sudden death in adult congenital heart disease: risk stratification in 2014. Heart Rhythm 2014;11(10):1735–42.

16. Chaix MA, Marcotte F, Dore A, et al. Risks and benefits of exercise training in adults with congenital heart disease. Can J Cardiol 2016;32(4):459–66.

17. Khairy P. Sudden cardiac death in transposition of the great arteries with a Mustard or Senning baffle: the myocardial ischemia hypothesis. Curr Opin Cardiol 2016;32(1):101–7.

18. Opic P, Utens EM, Cuypers JA, et al. Sports participation in adults with congenital heart disease. Int J Cardiol 2015;187:175–82.

19. Budts W, Borjesson M, Chessa M, et al. Physical activity in adolescents and adults with congenital heart defects: individualized exercise prescription. Eur Heart J 2013;34(47):3669–74.

20. Mondesert B, Khairy P. Implantable cardioverter-defibrillators in congenital heart disease. Curr Opin Cardiol 2014;29(1):45–52.

21. Kapel GF, Reichlin T, Wijnmaalen AP, et al. Re-entry using anatomically determined isthmuses: a curable ventricular tachycardia in repaired congenital heart disease. Circ Arrhythm Electrophysiol 2015;8(1): 102–9.

22. van Zyl M, Kapa S, Padmanabhan D, et al. Mechanism and outcomes of catheter ablation for ventricular tachycardia in adults with repaired congenital heart disease. Heart Rhythm 2016;13(7):1449–54.

23. Khairy P. Ventricular arrhythmias and sudden cardiac death in adults with congenital heart disease. Heart 2016;102(21):1703–9.

24. Hayward RM, Dewland TA, Moyers B, et al. Device complications in adult congenital heart disease. Heart Rhythm 2015;12(2):338–44.

25. Khairy P, Landzberg MJ, Gatzoulis MA, et al. Transvenous pacing leads and systemic thromboemboli in patients with intracardiac shunts: a multicenter study. Circulation 2006;113(20):2391–7.

26. Vehmeijer JT, Brouwer TF, Limpens J, et al. Implantable cardioverter-defibrillators in adults with congenital heart disease: a systematic review and meta-analysis. Eur Heart J 2016;37(18):1439–48.

27. Khairy P, Mansour F. Implantable cardioverter-defibrillators in congenital heart disease: 10 programming tips. Heart Rhythm 2011;8(3):480–3.

28. Garnreiter JM, Pilcher TA, Etheridge SP, et al. Inappropriate ICD shocks in pediatrics and congenital heart disease patients: risk factors and programming strategies. Heart Rhythm 2015;12(5):937–42.

29. Bordachar P, Marquie C, Pospiech T, et al. Subcutaneous implantable cardioverter defibrillators in children, young adults and patients with congenital heart disease. Int J Cardiol 2016;203:251–8.

30. Moore JP, Mondesert B, Lloyd MS, et al. Clinical experience with the subcutaneous implantable cardioverter-defibrillator in adults with congenital heart disease. Circ Arrhythm Electrophysiol 2016;9:e004338.

31. Sabate Rotes A, Connolly HM, Warnes CA, et al. Ventricular arrhythmia risk stratification in patients with tetralogy of Fallot at the time of pulmonary valve replacement. Circ Arrhythm Electrophysiol 2015; 8(1):110–6.

32. Shivapour JK, Sherwin ED, Alexander ME, et al. Utility of preoperative electrophysiologic studies in patients with Ebstein's anomaly undergoing the Cone procedure. Heart Rhythm 2014;11(2):182–6.

33. Gatzoulis MA, Balaji S, Webber SA, et al. Risk factors for arrhythmia and sudden cardiac death late after repair of tetralogy of Fallot: a multicentre study. Lancet 2000;356(9234):975–81.

34. Zeppenfeld K, Schalij MJ, Bartelings MM, et al. Catheter ablation of ventricular tachycardia after repair of congenital heart disease: electroanatomic identification of the critical right ventricular isthmus. Circulation 2007;116(20):2241–52.

35. Koyak Z, de Groot JR, Bouma BJ, et al. Symptomatic but not asymptomatic non-sustained ventricular tachycardia is associated with appropriate implantable cardioverter therapy in tetralogy of Fallot. Int J Cardiol 2013;167(4):1532–5.

36. Walsh EP, Gonzales C, Atallah J. Multicenter case-control study of ventricular arrhythmia in tetralogy of Fallot [Abstract]. Heart Rhythm 2013;10(5):S46.

37. Khairy P, Harris L, Landzberg MJ, et al. Implantable cardioverter-defibrillators in tetralogy of Fallot. Circulation 2008;117(3):363–70.

38. Babu-Narayan SV, Kilner PJ, Li W, et al. Ventricular fibrosis suggested by cardiovascular magnetic resonance in adults with repaired tetralogy of Fallot and its relationship to adverse markers of clinical outcome. Circulation 2006;113(3):405–13.

39. Valente AM, Gauvreau K, Assenza GE, et al. Contemporary predictors of death and sustained ventricular tachycardia in patients with repaired tetralogy of Fallot enrolled in the INDICATOR cohort. Heart 2014;100(3):247–53.

40. Khairy P, Landzberg MJ, Gatzoulis MA, et al. Value of programmed ventricular stimulation after tetralogy of fallot repair: a multicenter study. Circulation 2004; 109(16):1994–2000.

41. Harrild DM, Berul CI, Cecchin F, et al. Pulmonary valve replacement in tetralogy of Fallot: impact on survival and ventricular tachycardia. Circulation 2009;119(3):445–51.

42. Khairy P. Melody and rhythm in congenital heart disease. Heart Rhythm 2016;13(11):2142–3.

43. Bardy GH, Lee KL, Mark DB, et al. Amiodarone or an implantable cardioverter–defibrillator for congestive heart failure. N Engl J Med 2005;352(3):225–37.

44. Khairy P, Harris L, Landzberg MJ, et al. Sudden death and defibrillators in transposition of the great arteries with intra-atrial baffles: a multicenter study. Circ Arrhythm Electrophysiol 2008;1(4):250–7.

45. Cuypers JA, Eindhoven JA, Slager MA, et al. The natural and unnatural history of the Mustard procedure: long-term outcome up to 40 years. Eur Heart J 2014;35(25):1666–74.

46. Khairy P, Fernandes SM, Mayer JE Jr, et al. Long-term survival, modes of death, and predictors of mortality in patients with Fontan surgery. Circulation 2008;117(1):85–92.

47. Pundi KN, Johnson JN, Dearani JA, et al. 40-Year Follow-Up After the Fontan Operation: Long-Term Outcomes of 1,052 Patients. J Am Coll Cardiol 2015;66(15):1700–10.

48. Czosek RJ, Anderson J, Khoury PR, et al. Utility of ambulatory monitoring in patients with congenital heart disease. Am J Cardiol 2013;111(5):723–30.

49. Keane JF, Driscoll DJ, Gersony WM, et al. Second natural history study of congenital heart defects. Results of treatment of patients with aortic valvar stenosis. Circulation 1993;87(2 Suppl):I16–27.

50. Nattel S, Maguy A, Le Bouter S, et al. Arrhythmogenic ion-channel remodeling in the heart: heart failure, myocardial infarction, and atrial fibrillation. Physiol Rev 2007;87(2):425–56.

51. Oliver JM, Gallego P, Gonzalez AE, et al. Pulmonary hypertension in young adults with repaired coarctation of the aorta: an unrecognised factor associated with premature mortality and heart failure. Int J Cardiol 2014;174(2):324–9.

Specific Congenital Heart Defects: Clinical Aspects and Ablation

Arrhythmias in Patients with Atrial Defects

Tahmeed Contractor, MD*, Ravi Mandapati, MD, FHRS, FACC

KEYWORDS

- Atrial septal defect • Atrial arrhythmia • Patent foramen ovale • Atrial fibrillation

KEY POINTS

- Atrial arrhythmias are common in patients with atrial septal defects.
- A myriad of factors are responsible for these that include remodeling related to the defect and scar created by the repair or closure.
- An understanding of potential arrhythmias, along with entrainment and high-density activation mapping can result in accurate diagnosis and successful ablation.
- Atrial fibrillation is being seen increasingly after patent foramen ovale closure and may be primary etiology of recurrent stroke in these patients.

INTRODUCTION

Atrial septal defects (ASDs) are one of the most common congenital heart defects[1]; these can lead to significant left-to-right shunting with resultant right-sided chamber enlargement and pulmonary hypertension. Surgical and percutaneous closure of ASDs is commonly performed. Atriotomy scar along with the underlying substrate due to remodeling predisposes these patients to atrial arrhythmias[2–4] that increase morbidity and mortality.[5] Patent foramen ovales (PFOs) also are common in the general population. Closure of these defects is done to prevent strokes,[6] and atrial arrhythmias can be seen after closure.

In this article, we outline the mechanisms of atrial arrhythmias in patients with ASDs and PFOs. We then describe the management of these arrhythmias with an emphasis on interventional cardiac electrophysiology techniques.

ATRIAL SEPTAL DEFECTS AND PATENT FORAMEN OVALES: PATHOLOGY AND GENERAL MANAGEMENT

The atrial septum is a complex structure that is formed by the embryologic septum primum (that

grows from caudal to cranial direction) and septum secundum (that grows from cranial to caudal direction). Abnormalities in formation of this atrium septum can lead to the presence of ASD (primum [15%–20% of ASDs] or secundum [75% of ASDs])[7] or a PFO (seen in 25% of general population).[6] Other types of ASDs are rare and have a more complicated embryologic development (sinus venosus ASD and the unroofed coronary sinus).

An ASD leads to shunting of blood from the left to right side. This can lead to right atrial as well as ventricular dilation as well as increased pulmonary blood flow resulting in right-sided heart failure and pulmonary vasoconstriction. As such, closure is usually recommended when there is evidence of right-sided chamber dilation.[8] Closure of PFO is generally performed when it is thought to be a cause of recurrent stroke or thromboembolism.[9]

ELECTROCARDIOGRAPHIC CHANGES SEEN WITH ATRIAL SEPTAL DEFECTS

A host of atrial tachyarrhythmias can be seen in patients with ASDs, as outlined later in this article. However, even in the absence of tachyarrhythmias,

Arrhythmia Center, Loma Linda University International Heart Institute, Department of Cardiology, 11234 Anderson Street, Loma Linda, CA 92354, USA
* Corresponding author.
E-mail address: TContractor@llu.edu

Card Electrophysiol Clin 9 (2017) 235–244
http://dx.doi.org/10.1016/j.ccep.2017.02.006
1877-9182/17/© 2017 Elsevier Inc. All rights reserved.

cardiacEP.theclinics.com

several electrocardiographic (ECG) abnormalities can be seen (**Fig. 1**)[10]:

1. A superior P-wave axis due to an abnormality in the sinus node, that can be seen in a sinus venosus defect.[11]
2. Evidence of right atrial abnormality may be seen due to right atrium enlargement.
3. A prolonged PR interval can be seen usually in primum ASD, but also in older patients with a secundum ASD.
4. The QRS axis is deviated to the right in secundum ASD, and leftward or extremely to the right in ostium primum ASDs.

Right ventricular hypertrophy and incomplete right bundle branch block can be seen, especially in the presence of pulmonary hypertension.

ATRIAL ARRHYTHMIAS WITH ATRIAL SEPTAL DEFECTS/PATENT FORAMEN OVALES

In general, the mere presence of a PFO is not associated with an increased risk of atrial arrhythmias. However, there is a significantly increased incidence of atrial arrhythmias post-PFO closure. Most patients undergoing PFO closure have recurrent "cryptogenic" stroke; it is possible that these patients have atrial arrhythmias that were underdiagnosed before PFO closure and were likely the cause of stroke[12] (**Fig. 2**).

On the other hand, ASDs, whether repaired or unrepaired, are associated with an increased risk of atrial arrhythmias.[4] In general, the incidence of atrial flutter/fibrillation increases with age, and although atrial flutter is the most common arrhythmia in younger patients, atrial fibrillation is more common in older patients.[10] Untreated ASDs have an incidence of atrial arrhythmias of greater than 10% after the age of 40 years. If patients undergo closure of the ASD at a younger age (<25 years), the incidence of atrial arrhythmias (new onset and persistence of prior atrial arrhythmias) is much less than in patients who undergo closure at an older age (>40 years). This is likely because of shunt-related remodeling of the atria leading to arrhythmias (described in the next section).

PATHOPHYSIOLOGY OF ARRHYTHMIAS WITH ATRIAL SEPTAL DEFECTS
Before Closure/Repair of an Atrial Septal Defect

1. Geometric remodeling: Due to the left-to-right shunt, the right atrium undergoes stretching

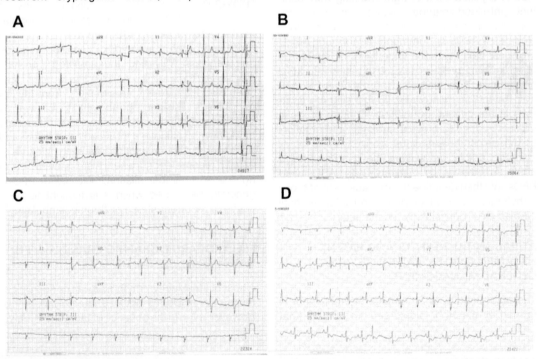

Fig. 1. ECG features of ASDs. (*A*) Ostium secundum ASD. Mild right-axis deviation, voltage evidence of right ventricular hypertrophy. (*B*) Sinus venosus ASD. Inverted inferior P-waves, right-axis deviation. (*C*) Ostium primum ASD. First-degree AV block, left-axis deviation, voltage evidence of right ventricular hypertrophy. (*D*) Eisenmenger ASD. Marked right-axis deviation, right atrial overload, right ventricular hypertrophy with extensive repolarization abnormalities ("strain pattern"). (*Reproduced with permission from* Webb G, Gatzoulis MA. Atrial septal defects in the adult: recent progress and overview. Circulation 2006;114(15):1645–53.)

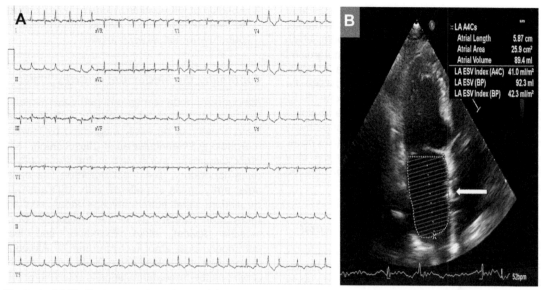

Fig. 2. Atrial fibrillation post-PFO closure. (*A*) Development of atrial fibrillation after PFO closure requiring pharmacologic cardioversion. (*B*) Echocardiogram showing severe LA dilation likely related to diastolic dysfunction predisposing patient to atrial fibrillation. Arrow is pointing to PFO closure device.

and remodeling; this results in interstitial fibrosis, increased size of the cardiac myocytes, and ultrastructural changes predisposing patients to atrial arrhythmias.[13] In addition to the right atrium, the left atrium also undergoes morphologic changes[14] leading to arrhythmias.

2. Electrical remodeling: Alongside the geometric remodeling, there is also electrical remodeling[15] that includes an increased sinus node recovery time, intra-atrial conduction delay, and increased atrial effective refractory period. These predispose to not only bradyarrhythmias, but also reentrant atrial arrhythmias. The ASD serves as a barrier to conduction; slowing around the defect has resulted in peri-ASD flutters even without prior surgery or device closure.[16]

After/Post Device/Surgical Closure

Based on the amount of remodeling and the age of closure (closure at older age may not lead to significant reverse remodeling), the aforementioned factors can still play a role in arrhythmogenesis. However, after closure, new factors are introduced that may predispose to arrhythmias. These factors are described in the following sections.

Local irritation

Due to postprocedure inflammation around the surgery or device site, focal tachycardias may occur. Usually these arrhythmias are short lived. Rarely, postprocedure pericarditis may predispose

patients to atrial arrhythmias including atrial fibrillation.

Atriotomy scar after surgical closure

The presence of an atriotomy scar as well as the ASD closure patch results in areas of anisotropic conduction close to areas with complete conduction block. This can lead to atriotomy-related flutters, cavotricuspid isthmus (CTI)-dependent flutter, and peri-patch reentrant flutters.[17] Dual-loop and multiple-loop reentrant arrhythmias also have been reported. Focal arrhythmias from abnormal automaticity, triggered activity and micro-reentry also can occur due to the presence of atrial scar and inhomogeneous conduction.[18] Cannulation of the superior vena cava instead of the right atrial appendage has been proposed as a method to reduce the risk of arrhythmias[19]; however, there are no prospective studies comparing these 2 approaches.

If possible, it will be very helpful to the electrophysiologist to obtain the surgical report before invasive electrophysiology study. The type of atriotomy can predict the circuit of atrial flutter and can help plan the mapping as well as ablation strategy. An elegant study from the Bordeaux group found that atriotomies that are vertical, long, anteriorly placed, and not extending to the inferior vena cava are more likely to result in peri-atriotomy atrial flutters.[20]

Presence of occlusion device

Although the central barrier of nonconduction remains unchanged after device deployment, peri-device inflammation and scarring can lead to anisotropic conduction and macro-reentry around the device.[21] The Bachmann bundle, which lies in the roof of the atrium, may be compromised by defect closure resulting in intra-atrial conduction block and delay providing a substrate for reentry and tachycardia.[18,22] Indeed, in one study, patients with P-wave prolongation were at higher risk of atrial tachyarrhythmias.[23] The fast pathway inputs to the compact atrioventricular (AV) node, which courses along the anterior margins of a PFO or secundum ASD,[24] and also can be affected and worsen heart block.[23]

A Mechanism Independent of Atrial Septal Defect?

Patients with ASDs may have atrial arrhythmias that are not related to the ASD itself. Atrial fibrillation is an important example of this. This is indirectly proven by the lack of efficacy of right-sided MAZE procedures to prevent postoperative atrial fibrillation[25]; triggers from the pulmonary veins and left atrium substrate likely play a role in these patients independent of ASD and right-sided overload.

A similar phenomenon is seen in patients with PFO. Atrial arrhythmias, commonly atrial fibrillation, can be seen after closure, which is usually done in patients with "cryptogenic" strokes.[12] Many of these patients have enlarged left atria due to diastolic dysfunction that predisposes them to atrial fibrillation (which may be the cause of stroke). Thus, the atrial fibrillation seen post-PFO closure may be a preexistent arrhythmia that could have been diagnosed before closure with long-term monitoring.

MANAGEMENT OF ARRHYTHMIAS

Although early postprocedure arrhythmias can be managed with electrical or pharmacologic cardioversion, the more chronic arrhythmias are typically managed by catheter ablation. The success rate of catheter ablation of atrial arrhythmias in patients with surgical ASD closure approaches 87% after multiple procedures over long-term follow-up.[26] Antiarrhythmic drugs can be used, but in general, have a low success rate.[27]

The electrophysiological approach to atrial arrhythmias in patients with ASD/PFO and postclosure include the following:

1. Confirming the mechanism of arrhythmia
2. Mapping: entrainment and activation mapping
3. Ablation

4. Ablation of left atrial arrhythmias in patients after ASD repair/closure: issues with transseptal puncture for left-sided access

Confirming the Mechanism of Arrhythmia

Although AV node reentry and pathway-mediated tachycardias can occur in patients with atrial defects, these can be easily diagnosed by P-wave morphology, ventricular-atrial dissociation, and other diagnostic maneuvers in the electrophysiology laboratory. The most common late-onset atrial arrhythmias in patients with ASD are CTI-dependent atrial flutter, atypical atrial reentrant tachycardia (which may involve incision, ASD, or closure device), atrial fibrillation, and less commonly focal atrial tachycardia.[28,29] Although uncommon, it is essential to rule out a focal mechanism, as the target for ablation is different for this (a presystolic early potential) as opposed to a macro-reentrant circuit (mid-diastolic potential).

Clinical clues indicating a focally emanating mechanism (abnormal automaticity or triggered activity) include warm-up initiation and cool-down termination as well as an isoelectric segment between the P-waves. It should be noted that scar-related slow conduction can result in an isoelectric segment even in macro-reentrant flutter. In the electrophysiology laboratory, demonstration of progressive fusion and fusion with reset are diagnostic of macro-reentry. Lack of fusion and postpacing suppression are markers of a focally emanating mechanism. **Table 1** outlines the major differences between the various mechanisms of atrial arrhythmias.

Mapping the Arrhythmia

In the era of high-density activation mapping, many have questioned the value of entrainment mapping. We continue to routinely perform entrainment mapping to define the circuit in macro-reentrant atrial flutter after completion of a high-density activation map (postpacing interval [PPI] minus tachycardia cycle length [TCL] typically <30 ms) and rarely in focally emanating tachycardias to define the exit site ("PPI" usually equals TCL). Entrainment mapping helps corroborate activation maps, confirm dual-loop reentry circuits, identify critical isthmuses, and perform ablation more confidently.[30–32]

Electroanatomic mapping has greatly helped electrophysiologists define tachycardia circuits, identify areas of scar, and "design" ablation lesions while reducing fluoroscopic exposure. The newer mapping technologies result in high-density maps with automatic acquisition. These include the CONFIDENSE Mapping Module in CARTO 3 (Biosense

Table 1
Clinical and electrophysiological differences between atrial arrhythmias based on mechanism

| Type of Arrhythmia | Focally Emanating | | | Macro-Reentry |
	Automaticity	Triggered Activity	Micro-Reentry	
Electrocardiogram		Discrete P-waves Prolonged isoelectric time		Continuous P-waves Minimal isoelectric time
Clinical arrhythmia	Nonsustained bursts	Nonsustained bursts	Sustained	Sustained
Adenosine	Termination	Termination	No effect	No effect
Overdrive pacing	Suppression	Acceleration	Concealed entrainment	Entrainment
Cycle length mapped	Partial	Partial	Complete	Complete
Electroanatomic map	Centrifugal	Centrifugal	Centrifugal	Circuit
Ablation/lesion	Presystolic/focal ablation	Presystolic/focal ablation	Diastolic/focal ablation	Mid-diastolic/linear ablation

Webster, Diamond Bar, CA) and RHYTHMIA mapping system (Boston Scientific, Marlborough, MA).[33] Using closely spaced multi-electrode catheters (PentaRay NAV for CARTO; Orion High-Resolution Mapping Catheter for RHYTHMIA), mapping with these automatic systems helps obtain very high-density maps in a relatively short period. **Figs. 3** and **4** are examples of atriotomy-related macro-reentrant atrial flutter and post-ASD repair focal atrial tachycardia, respectively.

Ablation

Planning radiofrequency ablation lesions/lines depends on the mechanism of the arrhythmia. Although focal ablation is usually required for

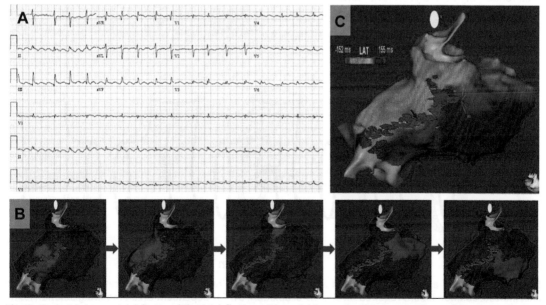

Fig. 3. Peri-atriotomy atrial flutter. (*A*) Atrial flutter with variable conduction in a patient with prior atriotomy. (*B*) High-density propagation map showing atrial flutter circuit around the atriotomy scar. (*C*) High-density activation mapping confirming macro-reentrant flutter involving atriotomy scar (PPI-TCL <30 ms at site of *arrow*; termination during ablation in that area). The reentry appeared to occur between the scars; the "gap" is either an incisional gap or an area between the atriotomy scar and scar below the atriotomy from remodeling. The flutter was noninducible after creating a line of block between the atriotomy and the inferior vena cava (IVC).

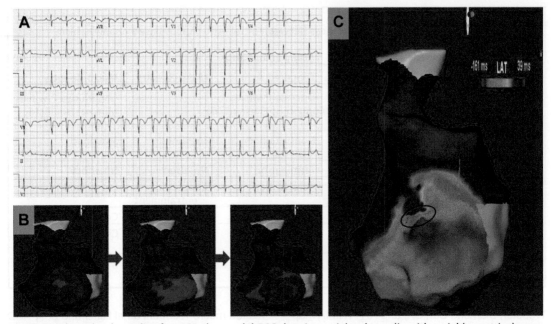

Fig. 4. Focal atrial tachycardia after ASD closure. (*A*) ECG showing atrial tachycardia with variable ventricular conduction (Wenckebach). (*B*) Propagation map showing focal emanation of tachycardia. (*C*) Activation map showing focal atrial tachycardia. Note anisotropic conduction from area of focal emanation. Black oval indicates area of slowest conduction superior to area of focal emanation.

the non–macro-reentrant flutters/tachycardias, linear lesions connecting 2 electrically silent areas are required to terminate and prevent recurrence of macro-reentrant atrial flutters. **Fig. 5** delineates potential circuits and ablation lesions required.

After ablation is performed, it is essential to confirm the presence of bidirectional block across the linear lesion. Using differential pacing, block is usually easily confirmed across the CTI. Similar principles can be used to confirm block across other linear lesions (**Fig. 6**). High-density activation

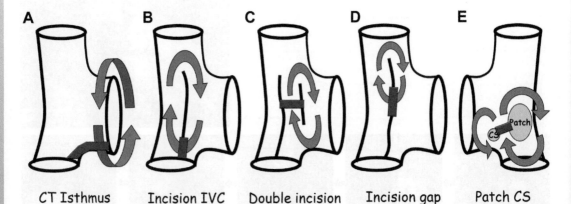

CT Isthmus   Incision IVC   Double incision   Incision gap   Patch CS

Fig. 5. Atrial flutters after ASD closure and ablation lesions required. Gray arrows indicate flutter circuits; red lines indicate ablation lesions required for successful ablation. (*A*) CTI-dependent circuit requiring ablation lesion from the tricuspid valve annulus to the IVC; (*B*) Atriotomy incision to IVC isthmus circuit requiring ablation lesion from the atriotomy to the IVC. (*C*) Flutter between 2 incisions requiring ablation lesions from one incision to another. (*D*) Incisional gap flutter requiring ablation lesion in the gap; line of block should be demonstrated across atriotomy. (*E*) Peri-ASD patch flutter (double loop with one circuit around patch and the other circuit around coronary sinus os) requiring ablation lesion from the patch of the coronary sinus os. (*Reproduced with permission from Dr E Aliot, MD and Dr C de Chillou, MD, CHU de Nancy, France.*)

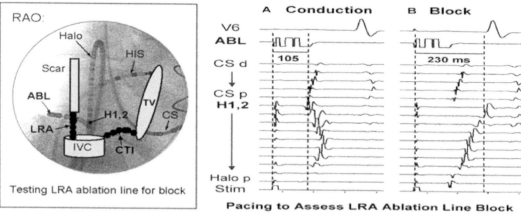

Fig. 6. The right panel shows the catheter configuration used to test the low lateral ablation line (LRA) for block. The ablation catheter (ABL) is located in the low lateral RA posterior to the LRA line, while the duodeca catheter (Halo) has been positioned between the free wall scar and the tricuspid valve (TV) annulus, so that the distal electrodes lay in the low lateral RA anterior to the LRA. The left panel shows pacing from the ablation catheter and the sequence and timing of activation anterior to the line on a duodeca catheter with LRA line block. (*Reproduced with permission from* Snowdon RL, Balasubramaniam R, Teh AW, et al. Linear ablation of right atrial free wall flutter: demonstration of bidirectional conduction block as an endpoint associated with long-term success. J Cardiovasc Electrophysiol 2010;21(5):526–31.)

mapping also can be used to confirm block: when pacing is performed close to one side of the line, the atrial tissue on the other side of the line should be activated last.

Ablation of Left Atrial Arrhythmias in Patients After Atrial Septal Defect Repair/Closure: Issues with Transseptal Puncture

Transseptal puncture can pose significant problems in patients who have had prior ASD repair. In the era of intracardiac echocardiography, the loss of the second "jump" of the needle into the fossa ovalis is not a major issue. However, in patients who have undergone surgical closure, the patch or native septum is thickened and fibrotic, making conventional puncture with a BRK needle difficult.

If operators are unable to cross with a standard BRK needle, conventional Bovie can be used keeping a short segment of the needle out of the sheath. There are also specialized needles using radiofrequency energy (Baylis needle) that can be used.[34] Alternatively, a Safe Sept transseptal guide wire (Pressure Products, Inc., San Pedro, CA, USA) can be used, which is a 0.014-inch nitinol wire with a sharp distal tip and preformed "J" shape.[35] It can be introduced through the inner lumen of a standard Brockenbrough transseptal needle to penetrate the interatrial septum into the left atrium. On crossing the septum, the wire immediately returns to its preformed "J" shape, which renders it atraumatic.

After obtaining left atrial access with the needle and dilator, it is sometimes difficult to advance the sheath that buckles at the septal entry site. In these situations, a wire can be placed into the left superior pulmonary vein or the right superior pulmonary vein to allow advancement of the sheath. A coiled wire also can be placed into the left atrium (Toray Valvuloplasty wire or Baylis Pigtail wire) to help with advancement. Balloon dilation of the puncture site has also been described.[36]

Presence of a closure device can make transseptal puncture even more challenging.[37,38] If the entire septum is not covered, the key is to find a portion not covered by the device by using intracardiac echocardiography, transesophageal echocardiography, or computed tomography scan. Usually intracardiac echo–guided puncture of the "spared" septum (commonly the inferior-posterior aspect) can be performed; radiofrequency energy can be delivered to cross, but device damage can occur with this.[39] A steerable sheath (such as Agilis steerable sheath [St. Jude Medical Inc., St. Paul, MN, USA]) can be used if the precurved sheaths do not allow engagement of the desired location; the dilator/needle can be pulled back, the sheath can be "steered" to the right location, and the dilator/needle can be re-advanced to engage this location. If the septum is completely covered, transseptal access using a Brockenbrough needle through the device with or without balloon angioplasty[40] can be done (**Fig. 7**). Rarely, a retrograde

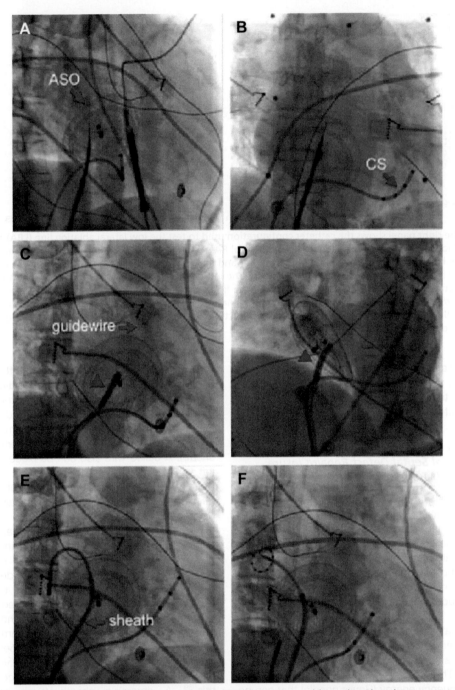

Fig. 7. Transseptal access through an ASD occluder. (*A, B*) Right anterior oblique (RAO) and anteroposterior projection showing transseptal puncture through the Amplatzer septal occluder. (*C, D*) dilatation of the left atrial access site with the angioplasty balloon (*arrowhead*) in RAO and left anterior oblique projections. (*E, F*) RAO projections showing radiofrequency ablation of the right pulmonary vein antrum and confirmation of pulmonary vein isolation with a circular mapping catheter. ASO, Amplatzer septal occluder; CS, coronary sinus. (*Reproduced with permission from* Chen K, Sang C, Dong J, et al. Transseptal puncture through Amplatzer septal occluder device for catheter ablation of atrial fibrillation: use of balloon dilatation technique. J Cardiovasc Electrophysiol 2012;23(10):1139–41.)

aortic approach is required using a magnetic navigation system.[41]

SUMMARY

Atrial arrhythmias are common in patients with ASDs. A myriad of factors are responsible for these that include remodeling related to the defect and scar created by the repair or closure. An understanding of potential arrhythmias, along with entrainment and high-density activation mapping can result in accurate diagnosis and successful ablation. Atrial fibrillation is being seen increasingly post-PFO closure and may be the primary etiology of recurrent stroke in these patients.

REFERENCES

1. Warnes CA, Williams RG, Bashore TM, et al. ACC/AHA 2008 guidelines for the management of adults with congenital heart disease: executive summary: a report of the American College of Cardiology/American Heart Association Task Force on Practice Guidelines (Writing Committee to Develop Guidelines for the Management of Adults With Congenital Heart Disease) Developed in Collaboration With the American Society of Echocardiography, Heart Rhythm Society, International Society for Adult Congenital Heart Disease, Society for Cardiovascular Angiography and Interventions, and Society of Thoracic Surgeons. J Am Coll Cardiol 2008;52(23): 1890–947.

2. Popper RW, Knott JM, Selzer A, et al. Arrhythmias after cardiac surgery. I. Uncomplicated atrial septal defect. Am Heart J 1962;64(4):455–61.

3. Reid J, Stevenson J. Cardiac arrhythmias following successful surgical closure of atrial septal defect. Br Heart J 1967;29(5):742.

4. Gatzoulis MA, Freeman MA, Siu SC, et al. Atrial arrhythmia after surgical closure of atrial septal defects in adults. N Engl J Med 1999;340(11): 839–46.

5. Murphy JG, Gersh BJ, McGoon MD, et al. Long-term outcome after surgical repair of isolated atrial septal defect: follow-up at 27 to 32 years. N Engl J Med 1990;323(24):1645–50.

6. Calvert PA, Rana BS, Kydd AC, et al. Patent foramen ovale: anatomy, outcomes, and closure. Nat Rev Cardiol 2011;8(3):148–60.

7. McCarthy K, Ho S, Anderson R. Defining the morphologic phenotypes of atrial septal defects and interatrial communications. Images Paediatric Cardiol 2003;5(2):1.

8. Warnes CA, Williams RG, Bashore TM, et al. ACC/AHA 2008 guidelines for the management of adults with congenital heart disease: a report of the American College of Cardiology/American Heart Association Task Force on Practice Guidelines (Writing Committee to Develop Guidelines on the Management of Adults With Congenital Heart Disease) developed in collaboration with the American Society of Echocardiography, Heart Rhythm Society, International Society for Adult Congenital Heart Disease, Society for Cardiovascular Angiography and Interventions, and Society of Thoracic Surgeons. J Am Coll Cardiol 2008; 52(23):e143–263.

9. Messé SR, Gronseth G, Kent DM, et al. Practice advisory: recurrent stroke with patent foramen ovale (update of practice parameter) report of the guideline development, dissemination, and implementation subcommittee of the American Academy of Neurology. Neurology 2016;87(8):815–21.

10. Egeblad H, Berning J, Efsen F, et al. Non-invasive diagnosis in clinically suspected atrial septal defect of secundum or sinus venosus type. Value of combining chest x-ray, phonocardiography, and M-mode echocardiography. Br Heart J 1980;44(3): 317–21.

11. Davia JE, Cheitlin MD, Bedynek JL. Sinus venosus atrial septal defect: analysis of fifty cases. Am Heart J 1973;85(2):177–85.

12. Bronzetti G, D'Angelo C, Donti A, et al. Role of atrial fibrillation after transcatheter closure of patent foramen ovale in patients with or without cryptogenic stroke. Int J Cardiol 2011;146(1):17–21.

13. Ueda A, Adachi I, McCarthy KP, et al. Substrates of atrial arrhythmias: histological insights from patients with congenital heart disease. Int J Cardiol 2013; 168(3):2481–6.

14. Roberts-Thomson KC, John B, Worthley SG, et al. Left atrial remodeling in patients with atrial septal defects. Heart Rhythm 2009;6(7):1000–6.

15. Morton JB, Sanders P, Vohra JK, et al. Effect of chronic right atrial stretch on atrial electrical remodeling in patients with an atrial septal defect. Circulation 2003;107(13):1775–82.

16. Mikhaylov E, Gureev S, Szili-Torok T, et al. Atypical atrial flutter in a patient with atrial septal defect without previous surgery: the role of septal defect as a part of the arrhythmia substrate. Europace 2009;11(12):1705–8.

17. Teh AW, Medi C, Lee G, et al. Long-term outcome following ablation of atrial flutter occurring late after atrial septal defect repair. Pacing Clin Electrophysiol 2011;34(4):431–5.

18. Chubb H, Whitaker J, Williams SE, et al. Pathophysiology and management of arrhythmias associated with atrial septal defect and patent foramen ovale. Arrhythm Electrophysiol Rev 2014;3(3):168.

19. Bink-Boelkens MTE, Meuzelaar KJ, Eygelaar A. Arrhythmias after repair of secundum atrial septal defect: the influence of surgical modification. Am Heart J 1988;115(3):629–33.

20. Shah D, Jaïs P, Haïssaguerre M. Electrophysiological evaluation and ablation of atypical right atrial flutter. Card Electrophysiol Rev 2002;6(4):365–70.

21. Marai I, Suleiman M, Lorber A, et al. Iatrogenic intra-atrial macro-reenterant tachycardia following trans-catheter closure of atrial septal defect treated by radiofrequency ablation. Ann Pediatr Cardiol 2011; 4(2):192.

22. Lemery R, Guiraudon G, Veinot JP. Anatomic description of Bachmann's bundle and its relation to the atrial septum. Am J Cardiol 2003;91(12): 1482–5.

23. Johnson JN, Marquardt ML, Ackerman MJ, et al. Electrocardiographic changes and arrhythmias following percutaneous atrial septal defect and patent foramen ovale device closure. Catheter Cardiovasc Interv 2011;78(2):254–61.

24. Anderson RH, Ho SY, Becker AE. Anatomy of the human atrioventricular junctions revisited. Anat Rec 2000;260(1):81–91.

25. Kobayashi J, Yamamoto F, Nakano K, et al. Maze procedure for atrial fibrillation associated with atrial septal defect. Circulation 1998;98(19 Suppl): II399–402.

26. Scaglione M, Caponi D, Ebrille E, et al. Very long-term results of electroanatomic-guided radiofrequency ablation of atrial arrhythmias in patients with surgically corrected atrial septal defect. Europace 2014;16(12):1800–7.

27. Walsh EP, Saul JP, Triedman JK. Cardiac arrhythmias in children and young adults with congenital heart disease. Philadelphia: Lippincott Williams & Wilkins; 2001.

28. Berger F, Vogel M, Kramer A, et al. Incidence of atrial flutter/fibrillation in adults with atrial septal defect before and after surgery. Ann Thorac Surg 1999;68(1):75–8.

29. Wasmer K, Köbe J, Dechering DG, et al. Isthmus-dependent right atrial flutter as the leading cause of atrial tachycardias after surgical atrial septal defect repair. Int J Cardiol 2013;168(3):2447–52.

30. Kalman JM, VanHare GF, Olgin JE, et al. Ablation of 'incisional' reentrant atrial tachycardia complicating surgery for congenital heart disease Use of entrainment to define a critical isthmus of conduction. Circulation 1996;93(3):502–12.

31. Nakagawa H, Shah N, Matsudaira K, et al. Characterization of reentrant circuit in macroreentrant right atrial tachycardia after surgical repair of congenital heart disease isolated channels between scars allow "focal" ablation. Circulation 2001;103(5):699–709.

32. Delacretaz E. Exploring atrial macroreentrant circuits. J Cardiovasc Electrophysiol 2005;16(7): 688–9.

33. Winner MW III. Mapping and ablation of an atypical left atrial flutter in a patient with a mechanical mitral valve repair. Bloomfield Hills: EP Lab Digest; 2016. p. 17.

34. Esch JJ, Triedman JK, Cecchin F, et al. Radiofrequency-assisted transseptal perforation for electrophysiology procedures in children and adults with repaired congenital heart disease. Pacing Clin Electrophysiol 2013;36(5):607–11.

35. Wadehra V, Buxton AE, Antoniadis AP, et al. The use of a novel nitinol guidewire to facilitate transseptal puncture and left atrial catheterization for catheter ablation procedures. Europace 2011; 13(10):1401–5.

36. Lakkireddy D, Rangisetty U, Prasad S, et al. Intracardiac echo-guided radiofrequency catheter ablation of atrial fibrillation in patients with atrial septal defect or patent foramen ovale repair: a feasibility, safety, and efficacy study. J Cardiovasc Electrophysiol 2008;19(11):1137–42.

37. Li X, Wissner E, Kamioka M, et al. Safety and feasibility of transseptal puncture for atrial fibrillation ablation in patients with atrial septal defect closure devices. Heart Rhythm 2014;11(2):330–5.

38. Santangeli P, Di Biase L, Burkhardt JD, et al. Transseptal access and atrial fibrillation ablation guided by intracardiac echocardiography in patients with atrial septal closure devices. Heart Rhythm 2011; 8(11):1669–75.

39. Pedersen ME, Gill JS, Qureshi SA, et al. Successful transseptal puncture for radiofrequency ablation of left atrial tachycardia after closure of secundum atrial septal defect with Amplatzer septal occluder. Cardiol Young 2010;20(02):226–8.

40. Chen K, Sang C, Dong J, et al. Transseptal puncture through Amplatzer septal occluder device for catheter ablation of atrial fibrillation: use of balloon dilatation technique. J Cardiovasc Electrophysiol 2012; 23(10):1139–41.

41. Miyazaki S, Nault I, Haïssaguerre M, et al. Atrial fibrillation ablation by aortic retrograde approach using a magnetic navigation system. J Cardiovasc Electrophysiol 2010;21(4):455–7.

Ebstein Anomaly

Elizabeth D. Sherwin, MD[a], Dominic J. Abrams, MD, MRCP[b],*

KEYWORDS

- Ebstein anomaly • Congenital heart disease • Arrhythmia • Radiofrequency catheter ablation

KEY POINTS

- Ebstein anomaly is a rare form of congenital heart disease with a uniquely high prevalence of arrhythmias.
- The most prevalent arrhythmia mechanisms are intrinsic to the underlying embryologic defects and may manifest at any stage.
- Current electrophysiological and surgical strategies are well equipped to address these arrhythmia mechanisms, yet despite available technology and a robust understanding of the mechanisms, these cases remain challenging.
- Surgical techniques that render arrhythmia substrates unreachable mandate comprehensive pre-surgical electrophysiological assessment and potential ablation.
- As in all forms of adult congenital heart disease, as the population ages the need to address atrial fibrillation management and risk stratification for sudden cardiac death becomes ever more pertinent.

INTRODUCTION

Ebstein anomaly is a rare variant of congenital heart disease, with a prevalence of 5.2 per 100,000 live births, representing only 1% of all congenital cardiac lesions.[1] Symptoms may occur at any stage from fetal life to old age: early presentation is often driven by more severe tricuspid valve insufficiency and associated structural anomalies, such as functional or anatomic right ventricular outflow tract obstruction,[2] whereas presentation in adult life is often arrhythmic. In a proportion of patients, it may be found incidentally. Historical population analyses found an infant mortality rate of 23.4%,[1] although improved peri-operative care and surgical techniques have increased survival significantly.

Ebstein anomaly was eponymously described in 1866 in a 19-year-old patient admitted to Allerheiligen Hospital in Breslau, Germany (now Wroclaw, Poland), where Wilhelm Ebstein was in his early career as an assistant physician having recently qualified from medical school. The patient reported increasing dyspnea and palpitations since childhood, and on examination had "marked jugular venous pulsations synchronous with the heart beat," dullness to percussion across a large area of the chest, and systolic and diastolic murmurs. The patient died a few days later; at autopsy, Ebstein found the right atrium and right ventricle to be extremely dilated and the tricuspid valve profoundly abnormal.[3]

Ebstein anomaly arises from embryologic failure of the posterior and septal tricuspid valve leaflets to delaminate from the underlying myocardium in the inlet portion of the right ventricle (RV), to which they remain fused. This displaces the leaflet attachment (functional annulus) toward the RV apex to varying degrees, creating a thin-walled "atrialized" area within the RV. The posterior and anterior leaflets are typically fused such that they

a Division of Cardiology, Children's National Health System, 111 Michigan Avenue NW, Washington, DC 20010, USA; b Division of Cardiac Electrophysiology, Boston Children's Hospital, Harvard Medical School, 300 Longwood Avenue, Boston, MA 02115, USA
* Corresponding author.
E-mail address: dominic.abrams@cardio.chboston.org

Card Electrophysiol Clin 9 (2017) 245–254
http://dx.doi.org/10.1016/j.ccep.2017.02.007
1877-9182/17/© 2017 Elsevier Inc. All rights reserved.

cardiacEP.theclinics.com

cannot be distinguished visually, whereas the septal leaflet is frequently underdeveloped, described by Ebstein as "discoid" or representing a "3 penny piece."[4] The anterior leaflet is enlarged and often fenestrated,[5] with thickened valve leaflets and abnormal chordae and papillary muscles. In severe cases, the posterior and septal leaflets are completely fused to the ventricular myocardium, and associated chordae and papillary muscles may be completely absent,[4] and redundant anterior leaflets prolapse into the RV outflow tract causing functional obstruction. Associated structural lesions may be present, most commonly pulmonary valve stenosis or atresia and atrial septal defects.[2]

The anatomic malformation of the tricuspid valve and the myocardial structural changes result in multiple important electrophysiologic alterations in Ebstein anomaly. The compact atrioventricular (AV) node is frequently displaced inferiorly toward the coronary sinus os, although the penetrating His bundle is normally located within the central fibrous body at the apex of the triangle of Koch.[4] The PR interval may be prolonged due to right atrial dilation and delayed interatrial conduction. Intrinsic AV nodal conduction may be prolonged in a minority.[6] Electrocardiographically, RV conduction delay is common, caused by delayed activation of the atrialized RV and by abnormalities of the His-Purkinje system. Histologically, the right bundle branch may be abnormal and underdeveloped or completely absent, potentially related to malformation of the septal leaflet and medial papillary muscle.[4] The QRS duration has been shown to reflect the degree of RV dilatation and dysfunction. The presence of fractionation, defined as a distinct low-amplitude wave in the terminal QRS or early ST segment, is a marker of a greater right atrialized portion of the ventricle.

PRACTICAL CONSIDERATIONS IN ELECTROPHYSIOLOGICAL PROCEDURES IN EBSTEIN ANOMALY

- Review prior operative reports detailing valve surgery and atrial incisions.
- Vascular occlusion from recurrent access in childhood is common in adult congenital heart disease; ultrasound confirmation of femoral venous patency can be helpful before the case.
- Determine ventricular function and anticipate potential hemodynamic complications to establish periprocedural management strategies.
- Right-to-left shunting across patent foramen ovale or atrial septal defect (ASD) is common and should be assessed before the procedure to determine optimal anticoagulation strategies. Fatal thromboembolic complications have been reported.[7]
- Angiography of the right atrium can provide fluoroscopic delineation of the true annulus, atrialized RV, and displaced valve leaflets (**Fig. 1**). The right coronary artery and the tricuspid valve fat pad also identify the position of the tricuspid annulus.

ARRHYTHMIA MECHANISMS
Accessory Pathway–Mediated Tachycardia

Structural and histologic abnormalities around the right atrioventricular junction precipitate a high prevalence of right-sided accessory pathways (APs). The vast majority of APs are located on the inferior tricuspid valve: posteroseptal approximating the coronary sinus os and posterolateral concordant with the posterior and septal leaflets. A minority of right-sided pathways is located in a

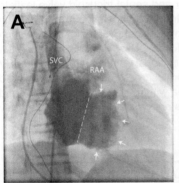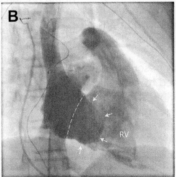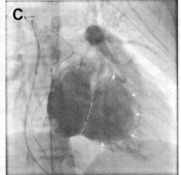

Fig. 1. Angiographic visualization of the tricuspid annulus and valve leaflets. Three fluoroscopic images of the right atrium (RA) and RV from the right anterior oblique view during angiographic injection in the RA. The images captured during ventricular diastole (*A, C*) and systole (*B*) demonstrate the position of the true tricuspid annulus (*dashed line*) and displaced valve leaflets (*white arrows*) separated by the atrialized right ventricle (ARV). RAA, right atrial appendage.

more superior septal or lateral position; rarely APs can be located on the mitral annulus.[8,9] Up to 50% of patients will have multiple pathways.[8–10] The 12-lead electrocardiogram (ECG) will typically show ventricular preexcitation indicative of manifest anterograde AP conduction, although concealed pathways also occur. In 3 series incorporating 43 patients all with symptomatic arrhythmia undergoing electrophysiology study, 40 (93%) had electrocardiographically manifest pathways,[8,9] whereas in an unselected population, preexcitation was found in only 43 (20%) of 220.[2] An apparently normal QRS morphology and duration may be seen in patients with clear anatomic evidence of Ebstein anomaly on cardiac imaging as the result of pseudo normalization: anterograde activation of the atrialized RV via a right lateral pathway may offset the typical right bundle branch block pattern due to delayed conduction via the His-Purkinje, thereby shortening the PR interval and QRS duration and thus "normalizing" the ECG (**Fig. 2**).[11]

Atrioventricular reentrant tachycardia (AVRT) may be poorly tolerated in Ebstein anomaly relating to the severity of the underlying hemodynamics, and syncope has been reported in approximately 30% of patients with symptomatic arrhythmia.[8,9] In 12 of 17 patients with induced preexcited atrial fibrillation or flutter, the shortest R-R interval was ≤250 ms, reflecting rapid conduction; sustained AVRT degenerating to fatal ventricular fibrillation has been reported.[9]

Intracardiac electrograms (EGM) recorded at the true annulus and within the atrialized RV often show significant fractionation, reflecting the abnormal underlying myocardium, making differentiation of the atrial, accessory pathway, and ventricular components challenging. This appearance lessens laterally on the annulus, anatomically distant from the posterior and septal leaflets.[8] Most pathways display typical AP characteristics; however, a proportion are "Mahaim" or atriofascicular fibers (AFF). The anatomic appearance of an AFF was reported by Becker and colleagues[12] in 1978 in a 31-year old woman with atrial fibrillation and AVRT who died during surgery. At autopsy, she was found to have Ebstein anomaly and an AP on anterolateral aspect of the tricuspid valve. A nodelike structure was identified at the atrial aspect of the true valve annulus and extending 10 mm into the atrialized RV, consistent histologically with specialized conduction system reminiscent of the normal atrioventricular node.[12] Debate continues as to whether the distal insertion point of these Mahaim fibers is the distal right bundle (ie, a true atriofascicular connection) or distal RV cavity (long atrioventricular connection). In a combined 81 patients with AFF diagnosed at electrophysiology study, 14 (17%) had Ebstein anomaly.[13,14]

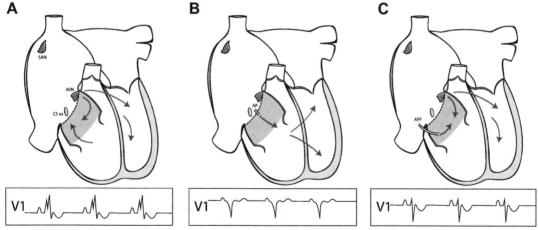

Fig. 2. Patterns of atrioventricular cardiac activation in Ebstein anomaly. A 4-chamber view of the heart in Ebstein anomaly. The posterior and septal leaflets are adherent to the underlying myocardium, displacing the functional tricuspid valve annulus toward the apex. The true annular position is depicted by a dotted line and the ARV shown in gray. (*A*) Activation of the ventricles via the atrioventricular node (AVN) (*red arrows*) leads to a typical right bundle branch QRS morphology due to a combination of slowed conduction within the ARV and structural anomalies of the right bundle branch. (*B*) Anterograde activation via a posteroseptal AP produces a preexcited QRS with a negative delta wave and QRS polarity in V1. The degree of preexcitation varies depending on the relative conduction velocities of the AP and AVN. (*C*) In the presence of an AFF on the lateral wall, activation of the RV occurs simultaneously via the AFF and AVN; preexcitation of the lateral ARV via the AFF offsets the typical right bundle branch block and "pseudo normalizes" the QRS morphology. CS, coronary sinus; SAN, sinoatrial node.

Historically, success of AP ablation is typically lower in Ebstein than in the structurally normal heart, a factor that has been related to pathway location within the atrialized RV and signal complexity.[8] Acute initial procedural success is between 75% and 80%, with recurrence reported in 25% to 50%.[8,10] Whether these figures are improved by the use of 3-dimensional mapping technology or intracardiac echocardiography to better define anatomic sites is uncertain.

The following are practical considerations in ablation of APs:

- Selective right coronary angiography identifies the true tricuspid valve annulus, the ideal site for ablation. Ablation on the ventricular aspect within the thinned wall of the atrialized RV runs the risk of coronary artery stenosis.[15]
- A decapolar reference catheter within the coronary sinus provides local ventricular excitation times in the posteroseptal region. Access to the coronary sinus can be challenging due to right atrial size and a prominent Eustachian ridge. A long SL3 sheath can provide anterior and septal reach from the inferior vena cava to the coronary sinus os.[16]
- Long deflectable sheaths provide mapping catheter stability on the lateral tricuspid annulus, especially in the face of severe right atrial dilatation and tricuspid regurgitation.
- A multipolar (eg, duodecapolar) in the right atrium approximating the tricuspid annulus may guide detailed mapping and ablation. Alternatively, a micro catheter within the right coronary artery can be helpful in localizing lateral tricuspid annulus pathways.[8,17]
- During AVRT via typical APs, the ventriculoatrial timing is often prolonged due to slowed conduction within the atrialized RV.[9,18]
- Consider a right lateral AFF causing pseudonormalization in a patient with a normal QRS duration. To confirm, pacing from the right atrial free wall or coronary sinus will produce left and right bundle patterns, respectively, due to preferential engagement of the atriofascicular pathway or AV node.[11]
- Atrioventricular reentry with anterograde conduction via an AFF produces a left bundle branch QRS morphology and negative HV interval. Dependence of the circuit on the AFF can be proven by introduction of a late-coupled atrial extrastimulus coincident with low right atrium activation that advances subsequent ventricular and atrial activation with an identical QRS morphology and intracardiac activation sequence (Fig. 3).[19]

- AFFs demonstrate automaticity both spontaneously, which may initiate atrioventricular reentry, and also during ablation, a factor suggesting embryologic origins similar to the atrioventricular node and His-Purkinje system.[14]

Atrial Flutter and Other Atrial Arrhythmias

In numerous series of adult patients who have undergone prior biventricular repair, the dominant macroreentrant atrial tachycardia is cavotricuspid isthmus (CTI)-dependent atrial flutter (Figs. 4 and 5). Long-term hemodynamic stress coupled with surgical intervention and natural obstacles create an ideal electroanatomic substrate fulfilling criteria for reentry: central barriers to wave front propagation with narrow corridors of slowly conducting myocardium; circuit length that exceeds effective refractoriness of atrial myocardium; and the potential for unidirectional block of initiating impulses.[20]

Right atrial enlargement is almost ubiquitous in Ebstein anomaly, permitting the development of reentrant atrial tachycardias, including CTI-dependent and nondependent circuits, the latter more common in patients who have undergone prior cardiac surgery.[10] In experimental models with the septal tricuspid valve leaflet removed and resulting atrial enlargement, sustained arrhythmia with surface and intracardiac electrogram morphology and activation sequence consistent with atrial flutter could be induced. Myocardial fibrosis was evident on histologic analysis, although arrhythmia inducibility appeared independent of changes in underlying atrial electrophysiology.[21] The relationship between right atrial dilatation and CTI-dependent atrial flutter has been studied in patients with unrepaired ASDs but no prior arrhythmic history. Widely spaced double potentials indicative of conduction delay were recorded along the crista terminalis, which persisted despite ASD closure and elimination of the left-to-right shunt. Functional conduction block at the crista with or without persistent right atrial dilation are fundamental prerequisites for the development of atrial flutter late after ASD closure.[22]

Other atrial arrhythmias have been reported, including atrial fibrillation and focal atrial tachycardia.[10] As adult patients with congenital heart disease age, the prevalence of atrial fibrillation (AF) will escalate rapidly and become a significant clinical burden. A comprehensive analysis of patients with a variety of congenital lesions, including Ebstein anomaly, found age of AF onset to be considerably less than other forms

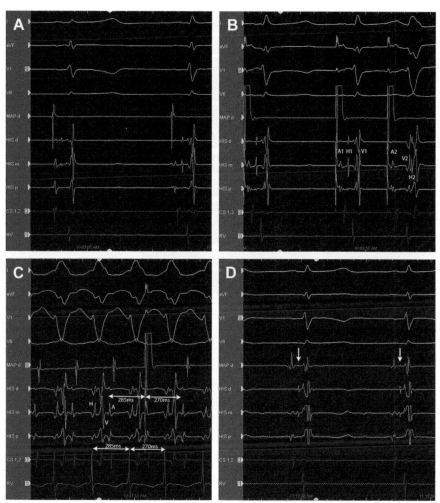

Fig. 3. Electrophysiology study in a patient with Ebstein anomaly and AFF. In a patient with Ebstein anomaly who presented with an irregular broad complex tachycardia, 4 surface ECG leads (I, aVF, V1, and V6) are shown along with EGMs recorded from a quadripolar mapping catheter (MAP), hexapolar His catheter, decapolar coronary sinus catheter, and quadripolar right ventricular catheter. (*A*) During sinus rhythm with MAP positioned in the high RA, the QRS in V1 shows normal duration and morphology, with normal intracardiac intervals. (*B*) Extrastimulus pacing (S1-S1 700 ms; S1-S2 400 ms) from the lateral wall of the RA shows a left bundle morphology, which is exacerbated by shorter S2 coupling intervals, associated with prolongation of the AH interval (A2-H2), a negative HV interval (V2-H2). (*C*) Continued pacing induced a wide complex tachycardia (cycle length 285 ms) with identical left bundle QRS morphology. Earliest intracardiac activation was seen on the RV catheter, followed by the His bundle, His ventricular electrogram, and a concentric pattern of retrograde atrial activation. Introduction of a premature atrial stimulus timed with low atrial activation (His atrial EGM) advances subsequent ventricular and atrial activation, confirming anterograde activation via an AFF integral to the tachycardia circuit with retrograde nodal conduction. (*D*) Mapping on the lateral tricuspid annulus identified balanced atrial and ventricular EGMs separated by a discrete AFF potential (*whitearrows*), coincidental with the His potential. Ablation here led to AFF automaticity before success, determined by change to a right bundle QRS morphology. This confirms the narrow QRS in sinus to have been pseudo normalized by simultaneous activation of the ARV via the AFF and AVN.

of structural heart disease and related to lesion complexity. Importantly, there was a high incidence of thromboembolic disease, which may precede arrhythmia onset, and a rapid progression to long-standing persistent AF.[23] The temporal relationship between organized reentry and AF has been studied for many years and clearly exists in adult congenital heart disease, although to what degree pulmonary vein activity has in initiating and sustaining AF in patients with severe right-sided disease remains to be seen. In one historical series of Ebstein anomaly, all 4 patients who developed AF died within 5 years.[24]

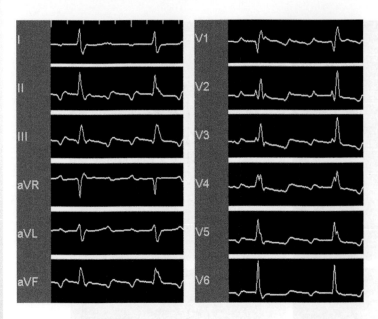

Fig. 4. A 12-lead ECG in Ebstein anomaly. A 12-lead ECG recorded in a 42-year-old patient with Ebstein anomaly with prior tricuspid valve replacement. With a 2-week history of lethargy and exertional dyspnea, atrial flutter with variable atrioventricular conduction was seen on ECG. Flutter wave morphology is negative in II, III, and aVF, and positive in V1, consistent with a peri-annular cavotricuspid isthmus dependent circuit.

The following are practical considerations in ablation of atrial flutter:

- Three-dimensional imaging and cardiac reconstruction by MRI or computed tomography can help case planning, including choice of sheaths and catheters (**Fig. 6**), and can be merged with nonfluoroscopic electroanatomical maps during ablation procedures.
- Long sheaths improve ablation catheter stability and reach in the face of right atrial and CTI dilatation and tricuspid regurgitation.
- A reference catheter positioned within the coronary sinus is helpful, as detailed previously.
- A J-curve ablation catheter is frequently needed to ensure adequate ablation lesions at the tricuspid valve aspect of the CTI.
- Reduced power should be considered in areas of potentially thinned atrial or atrialized ventricular myocardium to reduce the risk of cardiac perforation.

Ventricular Tachycardia

Despite the significant right ventricular dilatation and underlying abnormal myocardium, clinical ventricular tachycardia is rare in Ebstein anomaly, although it may be more commonly inducible at electrophysiology study.[25] The abnormal atrialized RV myocardium may lead to automatic tachycardias or produce sites of conduction block adjacent to the tricuspid annulus creating a narrow channel of slow conduct and allowing a peri-annular reentrant circuit.[26,27]

Sudden Cardiac Death

Sudden cardiac death is well recognized in all variants of congenital heart disease, including Ebstein anomaly. Although the refractory periods of a significant proportion of APs are sufficient to support rapidly conducted AF or flutter, no patient with known preexcitation has been reported to die suddenly. In 220 cases of Ebstein anomaly, sudden death occurred in 8 (3.6%), compared with 26 deaths related to heart failure and 17 perioperative deaths. Four patients who died suddenly had prior documented arrhythmias: atrial in 3 after prior tricuspid valve surgery and ventricular in 1. One patient died after hemodynamic deterioration, and in 3 no precedent event could be identified. None of the 18 patients with ventricular preexcitation died suddenly.[2]

A multicenter, international analysis reported 1189 cases of sudden death in adult congenital heart disease of proven or presumed arrhythmia, including 42 cases (3.5%) of Ebstein anomaly. All cases were compared with 2 controls matched by diagnosis, age, gender, and surgical intervention. Although specific details of the Ebstein cases were not available, sudden death was associated with a prior history of supraventricular tachycardia, moderate-to-severe systemic or subpulmonary ventricular dysfunction, increased QRS duration, and QT dispersion.[28]

Implantable cardioverter-defibrillators (ICD) have been used in a small number of patients with Ebstein anomaly. A meta-analysis of ICD use in adult congenital heart disease identified ICD implantation in 4 (1%) of 412 patients

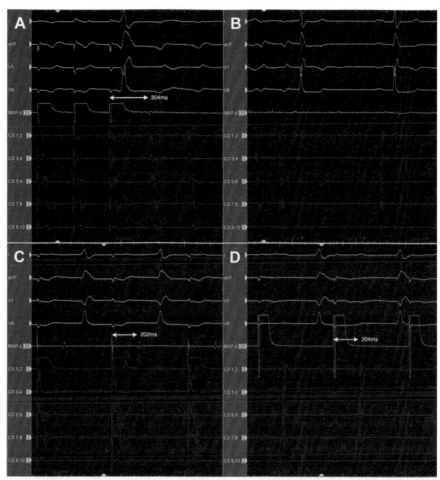

Fig. 5. Electrophysiology study and radiofrequency ablation in Ebstein anomaly. Surface ECG and intracardiac EGMs from an electrophysiology study in the same patient depicted in **Fig. 4**. Four surface ECG leads (I, aVF, V1, and V6) are shown along with EGMs recorded from a J-curve irrigated mapping catheter and a reference decapolar catheter positioned on the medial aspect of the tricuspid valve with distal poles approximating the coronary sinus os. (*A*) During clinical tachycardia (cycle length 300 ms), pacing lateral to the CTI adjacent to the tricuspid valve prosthesis demonstrated concealed entrainment with a postpacing interval almost identical to tachycardia cycle length. (*B*) A linear ablation lesion (45 W/50°C) was successful in terminating tachycardia; subsequent pacing from the (*C*) medial and (*D*) lateral aspects of the CTI demonstrated bidirectional conduction block.

with Ebstein anomaly in 15 studies; none received appropriate ICD therapy.[29] Technical issues with ICD implantation relate to lead stability in the face of severe right atrial and ventricular dilatation and placing (and extracting) leads following tricuspid valve repair or replacement. The presence of a right-to-left shunt places the patient at risk of paradoxic embolus despite formal anticoagulation.[30] Extravascular subcutaneous ICD may overcome these problems and was reported in a single patient with Ebstein anomaly,[31] although suitability for this device may be impeded by the typical low R-wave to T-wave amplitude limiting appropriate

sensing vectors. An alternative is placement of a high-voltage lead within the pericardial space with atrial and ventricular pace/sense epicardial leads at the time of tricuspid valve surgery.

Preoperative Assessment and Arrhythmia Surgery

Interest in surgical intervention in Ebstein anomaly has been reinvigorated by the cone reconstruction of the tricuspid valve, although, like tricuspid valve replacement, this limits postoperative access to the right atrioventricular junction for transcatheter

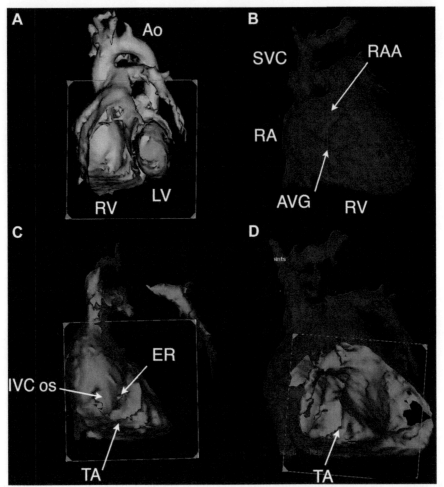

Fig. 6. Three-dimensional reconstructions in a patient with Ebstein anomaly using cardiac MRIs. Three-dimensional reconstructions from cardiac MRI in a 24-year-old with Ebstein anomaly, created with the Carto-Merge system (Biosense Webster, Diamond Bar, CA) before electrophysiology study and ablation. The patient with no prior cardiac interventions presented with palpitations, and on 12-lead electrocardiogram was found to have atrial flutter. (A) A view from the cardiac apex with a clipping plane applied at a mid-ventricular level shows marked dilatation of the RV compared with the left ventricle (LV). (B) A right lateral view shows marked dilatation of the RA and RV, separated by the atrioventricular groove (AVG) marking the position of the true tricuspid annulus. (C) Application of the clipping plane angled from the superior RA to inferior RV shows internal structures: ostium of the inferior caval vein (IVC os), Eustachian ridge (ER), and inferior section of the true tricuspid annulus (TA). (D) A clipping plane applied to the lateral RA and RV demonstrates the inferoseptal aspect of the dilated TA.

ablation.[32] Shivapour and colleagues[25] reported the use of invasive electrophysiology studies and ablation before the cone procedure to define and eliminate arrhythmia mechanisms that may hinder the postoperative course and be impossible to ablate after the cone reconstruction. The same approach is equally applicable to tricuspid valve replacement. Forty-two patients (median age 13.8 years) underwent preoperative electrophysiological studies that identified 56 different arrhythmia mechanisms in 29 patients (69%). Arrhythmias were inducible in 8 (42%) of

19 patients with no prior arrhythmic history or electrocardiographic features suggestive of an underlying substrate, suggesting symptoms and electrocardiography do not identify all patients at risk of postprocedural arrhythmia. An AP was present in 21 patients, of whom 14 (66%) had a second identifiable mechanism, including additional AP or AFF, atrial tachycardia, atrioventricular nodal reentry tachycardia, AF, and ventricular tachycardia.[25]

Arrhythmia substrates can be successfully eliminated via transcatheter ablation, with a reported

94% acute success rate in a contemporary cohort.[25] Patient age, complex and fractionated electrograms, and thin myocardium may result in obstacles to or inordinate risk with transcatheter ablation. Surgical arrhythmia therapies may be indicated, including right or biatrial maze procedure, ventricular tachycardia ablation lines, or ICD placement. In 604 surgeries on 539 patients with Ebstein anomaly, 144 arrhythmia surgical interventions were performed, including accessory pathway ablation, right atrial maze, and ablation of atrioventricular nodal reentry tachycardia.[33] APs visualized as muscular strands crossing the annulus can be divided.[34] Right atrial reduction may decrease the likelihood of future atrial arrhythmias stemming from atrial dilation. To prevent or eliminate reentrant atrial tachycardia circuits, a right atrial cryoablation lesion set may be sufficient with lines across the CTI and previously identified critical corridors, such as atriotomy to superior vena cava (SVC), and atrial septal patch to tricuspid annulus or SVC.[10] For AF, right or biatrial maze procedures can be successful; Stulak and colleagues[35] reported 79% freedom from atrial flutter and AF without antiarrhythmic medications following surgical maze during Ebstein repair. To avoid placing a transvenous lead across a reconstructed tricuspid valve, epicardial defibrillator coil and pacing leads can be placed at the time of surgery for immediate or future use. Multidisciplinary discussions for planning of intraoperative arrhythmia intervention and anticipation of postoperative rhythm management are critical.

SUMMARY

Ebstein anomaly is a rare form of congenital heart disease with a uniquely high prevalence of arrhythmias. The most prevalent arrhythmia mechanisms are intrinsic to the underlying embryologic defects and may manifest at any stage: from fetal life as part of an overall deleterious hemodynamic picture, to adult life unmasking the diagnosis. Current electrophysiological and surgical strategies are well equipped to address these arrhythmia mechanisms, yet despite available technology and a robust understanding of the mechanisms, these cases remain challenging. Surgical techniques that render arrhythmia substrates unreachable mandate comprehensive presurgical electrophysiological assessment and potential ablation. As in all forms of adult congenital heart disease, as the population ages the need to address AF management and risk stratification for sudden cardiac death becomes ever more pertinent.

REFERENCES

1. Correa-Villasenor C, Ferencz C, Neill CA, et al, for the Baltimore-Washington Infant Study Group. Ebstein's malformation of the tricuspid valve: genetic and environmental factors. Teratology 1994;50: 137–47.
2. Celermajer DS, Bull C, Till JA, et al. Ebstein's anomaly: presentation and outcome from fetus to adult. J Am Coll Cardiol 1994;23:170–6.
3. van Son JA, Konstantinov IE, Zimmermann V. Wilhelm Ebstein and Ebstein's malformation. Eur J Cardiothorac Surg 2001;20:1082–5.
4. Ho S, Goltz D, McCarthy K, et al. The atrioventricular junction in Ebstein malformation. Heart 2000;83: 444–9.
5. Barbara DW, Edwards WD, Connolly HM, et al. Surgical pathology of 104 tricuspid vales (2000-2005) with classic right-sided Ebstein's malformation. Cardiovasc Pathol 2008;17:166–71.
6. Egidy Assenza G, Valente AM, Geva T, et al. QRS duration and QRS fractionation on surface electrocardiogram are markers of right ventricular dysfunction and atrialization in patients with Ebstein anomaly. Eur Heart J 2013;34(3):191–200.
7. Chetaille P, Walsh EP, Triedman JK. Outcomes of radiofrequency catheter ablation of atrioventricular reciprocating tachycardia in patients with congenital heart disease. Heart Rhythm 2004;1:168–73.
8. Cappato R, Schlüter M, Weiss C, et al. Radiofrequency current catheter ablation of accessory atrioventricular pathways in Ebstein's anomaly. Circulation 1996;94:376–83.
9. Smith WM, Gallagher JJ, Kerr CR, et al. The electrophysiologic basis and management of symptomatic recurrent tachycardia in patients with Ebstein's anomaly of the tricuspid valve. Am J Cardiol 1982; 49(5):1223–34.
10. Roten L, Lukac P, DE Groot N, et al. Catheter ablation of arrhythmias in Ebstein's anomaly: a multicenter study. J Cardiovasc Electrophysiol 2011; 22(12):1391–6.
11. Sherwin ED, Walsh EP, Abrams DJ. Variable QRS morphologies in Ebstein's anomaly: what is the mechanism? Heart Rhythm 2013;10:933–7.
12. Becker AE, Anderson RH, Durrer D, et al. The anatomical substrates of Wolff-Parkinson-White syndrome. A clinicopathologic correlation in seven patients. Circulation 1978;57(5):870–9.
13. Buber Y, Triedman JK, Alexander ME, et al. Atriofascicular fibers in young patients: a 25 year, single center experience. Heart Rhythm 2014;11(5):S49.
14. Sternick EB, Sosa E, Timmermans C, et al. Automaticity in Mahaim fibers. J Cardiovasc Electrophysiol 2004;15:738–44.
15. Bertram H, Boeknkamp R, Pester M, et al. Coronary artery stenosis after radiofrequency ablation of

accessory atrioventricular pathways in children with Ebstein's malformation. Circulation 2001;103: 538–43.

16. Shah M, Jones TK, Cecchin F. Improved localization of right-sided accessory pathways with microcatheter-assisted right coronary artery mapping in children. J Cardiovasc Electrophysiol 2004;15:1238–43.

17. Pepper CB, Davidson NC, Ross DL. Use of a long preshaped sheath to facilitate cannulation of the coronary sinus at electrophysiologic study. J Cardiovasc Electrophysiol 2001;12:1335–7.

18. Josephson ME, Wellens HJ. Young woman with a stroke and palpitations. Heart Rhythm 2015;12: 1398–9.

19. McClelland JH, Wang X, Beckman KJ, et al. Radiofrequency catheter ablation of right atriofascicular (Mahaim) accessory pathways guided by accessory pathway potentials. Circulation 1994;89:2655–66.

20. The Sicilian gambit. A new approach to the classification of antiarrhythmic drugs based on their actions on arrhythmogenic mechanisms. Task Force of the Working Group on Arrhythmias of the European Society of Cardiology. Circulation 1991;84(4): 1831–51.

21. Bowden PA, Hoffman BF. The effects on atrial electrophysiology and structure of surgically induced right atrial enlargement in dogs. Circ Res 1981; 49(6):1319–31.

22. Morton JB, Sanders P, Vohra JK, et al. Effect of chronic right atrial stretch on atrial electrical remodeling in patients with an atrial septal defect. Circulation 2003;107:1775–82.

23. Teuwen CP, Ramdjan TT, Götte M, et al. Time course of atrial fibrillation in patients with congenital heart defects. Circ Arrhythm Electrophysiol 2015;8: 1065–72.

24. Gentles T, Calder AL, Clarkson PM, et al. Predictors of long-term survival with Ebstein's anomaly of the tricuspid valve. Am J Cardiol 1992;69:377–81.

25. Shivapour JK, Sherwin ED, Alexander ME, et al. Utility of preoperative electrophysiologic studies in patients with Ebstein's anomaly undergoing the Cone procedure. Heart Rhythm 2014;11:182–6.

26. Obioha-Ngwu O, Milliez P, Richardson A, et al. Ventricular tachycardia in Ebstein's anomaly. Circulation 2001;104:E92–4.

27. Kumar S, Subramanian A, Selvaraj RJ. Peritricuspid reentrant ventricular tachycardia in Ebstein's anomaly. Europace 2014;16:1633.

28. Koyak Z, Harris L, de Groot JR, et al. Sudden cardiac death in adult congenital heart disease. Circulation 2012;126:1944–54.

29. Vehmeijer JT, Brouwer TF, Limpens J, et al. Implantable cardioverter-defibrillators in adults with congenital heart disease: a systematic review and meta-analysis. Eur Heart J 2016;37:1439–48.

30. Khairy P, Landzberg MJ, Gatzoulis MA, et al, Epicardial Versus ENdocardial Pacing and Thromboembolic Events Investigators. Transvenous pacing leads and systemic thromboemboli in patients with intracardiac shunts: a multicenter study. Circulation 2006;113:2391–7.

31. Moore JP, Mondésert B, Lloyd MS, et al, Alliance for Adult Research in Congenital Cardiology (AARCC). Clinical experience with the subcutaneous implantable cardioverter-defibrillator in adults with congenital heart disease. Circ Arrhythm Electrophysiol 2016;9(9) [pii:e004338].

32. da Silva JP, Baumgratz JF, da Fonseca L, et al. The cone reconstruction of the tricuspid valve in Ebstein's anomaly. The operation: early and midterm results. J Thorac Cardiovasc Surg 2007;133:215–23.

33. Brown ML, Dearani JA, Danielson GK, et al, Mayo Clinic Congenital Heart Center. The outcomes of operations for 539 patients with Ebstein anomaly. J Thorac Cardiovasc Surg 2008;135:1120–36.

34. Chavaud S, Brancaccio G, Carpentier A. Cardiac arrhythmia in patients undergoing surgical repair of Ebstein's anomaly. Ann Thorac Surg 2001;71: 547–52.

35. Stulak JM, Sharma V, Cannon BC, et al. Optimal surgical ablation of atrial tachyarrhythmias during correction of Ebstein anomaly. Ann Thorac Surg 2015;99:1700–5.

Arrhythmias Following the Mustard and Senning Operations for Dextro-Transposition of the Great Arteries
Clinical Aspects and Catheter Ablation

Sherrie Joy Baysa, MD, Melissa Olen, ARNP,
Ronald J. Kanter, MD*

KEYWORDS

- Mustard operation • Senning operation • Dextro-transposition of the great arteries
- Sinoatrial node dysfunction • Intraatrial reentry tachycardia

KEY POINTS

- The atrial switch procedures, Mustard and Senning Operations, for dextro-transposition of the great arteries, have been supplanted by the arterial switch operation, meaning that a finite number of adult patients are currently alive with this anatomical arrangement.
- Sinoatrial node dysfunction is common long-term after this operation and, when clinically severe, is successfully treated with pacemaker implantation.
- Atrial tachycardias, especially intraatrial reentry tachycardia, is also prevalent long-term after this operation, and may be successfully ablated in the great majority of cases.
- Although there is known to be an increased risk of systemic ventricular dysfunction and sudden death in this patient group, risk assessment and treatment are only beginning to be understood.

INTRODUCTION

Transposition of the great arteries (TGA) accounts for 5% of all congenital heart defects and is the most common cardiac cause of cyanosis in the newborn period (**Fig. 1**).[1]

Although the introduction of balloon atrial septostomy by Rashkind and Miller[2] in 1966 led to a dramatic change in the early survival of patients, TGA is ultimately a surgical disease. Early attempts at anatomic correction with arterial switch procedures showed dismal results, particularly because of the need for coronary artery transfer.[3] Thus, reversing the venous inflows, or so-called atrial switch procedures, became the mainstay of surgical treatment in dextro-TGA (d-TGA) for many years and remained so for more than a decade after Jatene and colleagues[4] reported the first successful arterial switch operation in 1976.[3]

Because the arterial switch and coronary artery translocation procedure supplanted the Mustard and Senning operations in most Western countries starting in the late 1980s, most surviving patients of the atrial switch are now at least 25 to 30 years old. However, there are rare anatomic conditions for which these operations are still used. These conditions primarily include congenitally corrected transposition in which a double switch (atrial and

Division of Cardiology, Nicklaus Children's Hospital, Miami, FL 33155, USA
* Corresponding author. 3100 Southwest 62 Avenue, 2nd Floor, Ambulatory Care Building, Miami, FL 33155.
E-mail address: Ronald.kanter@mch.com

Card Electrophysiol Clin 9 (2017) 255–271
http://dx.doi.org/10.1016/j.ccep.2017.02.008
1877-9182/17/© 2017 Elsevier Inc. All rights reserved.

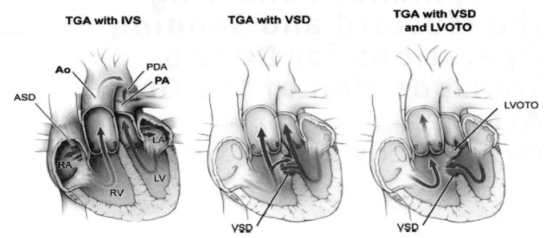

TGA with IVS

TGA with VSD

TGA with VSD and LVOTO

Fig. 1. Examples of anatomic variants of dextro-TGA. Arrows indicate direction of blood flow. Locations where arrows cross one another represents opportunities for mixing of systemic and pulmonary venous returns. It is only at those locations that effective blood flow may occur. Effective blood flow is defined as that portion of systemic venous return that is fully saturated by the lungs. Ao, aorta; ASD, atrial septal defect; IVS, intact ventricular septum; LA, left atrium; LV, left ventricle; LVOTO, left ventricular outflow tract obstruction; PA, pulmonary artery; PDA, patent ductus arteriosus; RA, right atrium; RV, right ventricle; TGA, transposition of the great arteries; VSD, ventricular septal defect. (*From* Qureshi Athar M, Justino H, Heinle Jeffrey S. Transposition of the great arteries. [Chapter 47]. In: Allen HD, Shaddy RE, Penny DJ, editors. Moss and Adams' heart disease in infants, children, and adolescents, including the fetus and young adult. 9th edition. Philadelphia: Lippincottt Williams and Wilkins; 2016. p. 1163; with permission.)

arterial switches) or atrial switch plus right ventricular (RV) outflow tract-to-pulmonary artery conduit are indicated. Even rarer are patients with isolated atrioventricular (AV) discordance, in whom there is AV discordance but ventriculoarterial concordance. In all of these conditions, the atrial switch will establish the anatomic left ventricle as the subaortic pumping chamber and the anatomic RV as the subpulmonic pumping chamber.

SURGICAL ANATOMY
Senning Operation

Senning[5] performed the first atrial switch procedure in 1958. In this procedure, an atrial baffle is created with autologous tissue to direct systemic venous return to the mitral valve and subpulmonic left ventricle. First, a vertical right atriotomy is made anterior to the crista terminalis (**Fig. 2**A, upper dotted line). Then, the anterior, inferior, and superior margins of the atrial septum are incised, creating an atrial septal flap (**Fig. 2**B, dotted line). The atrial septal flap is placed down into the left atrium and sutured around the pulmonary veins, separating the pulmonary venous return from the left atrium and forming the floor of the eventual systemic venous pathway (**Fig. 2**C). The posterior/lateral right atrial wall is then sutured around the superior and inferior vena cavae orifices and onto the anterior edge of the atrial septal remnant

between the AV valves (approximation of the 2 dotted lines in **Fig. 2**C). In this way, an intercaval tube representing the systemic venous pathway to the mitral valve is completed (**Fig. 2**D). A vertical left atriotomy is then made between the right pulmonary veins and the atrial septum (see **Fig. 2**A, lower dotted line). Finally, the anterior right atrial wall is used to complete the pulmonary venous pathway from the left atriotomy to the tricuspid valve and systemic RV (see **Fig. 2**D, dotted line of upper free wall flap is brought down to lower dotted line). Pericardium or artificial material may be required to bridge the gap between those incisions.

Mustard Operation

In 1963, Mustard[6] performed an atrial switch operation, using pericardium to create the intra-atrial baffle; this soon emerged as an alternative to the Senning procedure. In this operation, the atrial septum and most of the limbus are excised to create a large atrial septal defect, extending from the inferior to superior vena cava. An intra-atrial baffle, generally made of pericardium, is then placed, directing the systemic venous flow to the left-sided mitral valve and ultimately to the pulmonary artery (**Fig. 3**). Surgical details are described later in the section on the electrophysiologic anatomy.

The Mustard and Senning atrial switch procedures provided excellent early and midterm results;

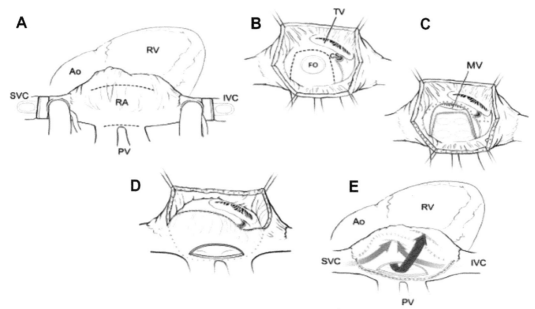

Fig. 2. The atrial switch operation as described by Senning. Images are from the surgeon's perspective from the right side of the table, with the head to the left and the feet to the right. See text for complete description. Ao, aorta; FO, foramen ovale; IVC, inferior vena cava; MV, mitral valve; PV, pulmonary veins; RA, right atrium; SVC, superior vena cava; TV, tricuspid valve. (*From* Qureshi Athar M, Justino H, Heinle Jeffrey S. Transposition of the great arteries. [Chapter 47]. In: Allen HD, Shaddy RE, Penny DJ, editors. Moss and Adams' heart disease in infants, children, and adolescents, including the fetus and young adult. 9th edition. Philadelphia: Lippincottt Williams and Wilkins; 2016. p. 1172; with permission.)

but with time, it became evident that both led to important long-term sequelae. As is further discussed later, common late findings include sinus node dysfunction and atrial tachyarrhythmias.[7–11] Sudden cardiac death (SCD) may also be seen in a subset of patients, which is presumed to be due to arrhythmia or myocardial failure.[7,10–12] Because the RV remains the systemic ventricle, RV dysfunction may develop with time, often coexisting with tricuspid regurgitation, which is usually progressive.[10,13,14] Other complications of the atrial switch operations include atrial baffle obstruction, particularly at the superior vena cava-baffle junction, as well as baffle leaks.[8,10,15]

ARRHYTHMIA BURDEN

Before the late 1980s most patients born with d-TGA underwent surgical palliation using the Mustard or Senning operation with encouraging early outcomes in terms of mortality and quality of life. However, the aging adult congenital heart population has revealed the consequences of intra-atrial baffling, which exposes the atria (especially the native right atrium) to extensive suture lines and fibrosis. The right atrial remodeling places the sinus node and atrial muscle at risk for cardiac rhythm abnormalities. Loss of sinus

rhythm, atrial tachyarrhythmias, and the risk of sudden death have been recognized as important sequelae following these operations.[11,16,17] Possibly or probably contributing to this burden are the added risk factors of RV dysfunction, AV regurgitation, systemic or pulmonary venous baffle obstruction, and pulmonary hypertension. A summary of the relative incidences of each arrhythmia type following the Mustard or Senning operation appears in **Table 1**.

Sinoatrial Node Dysfunction

The pathogenesis for the development of sinoatrial node dysfunction (SAND) following atrial redirection surgery is interruption of sinus node blood flow or damage to the sinus node itself. Determining the precise incidence of SAND is challenging and highly variable given the variations in operative techniques and surgical epochs. However, it has been reported that 20 years after Mustard or Senning repair, sinus node dysfunction can be present in as high as 47% of patients.[11] Similarly, Gelatt and colleagues[7] reported that 40% of patients over a 20-year period had SAND. Significant SAND requiring pacemaker implantation has been reported in 5% to 11% of patients.[7,8,18] The loss of sinus rhythm carries risk

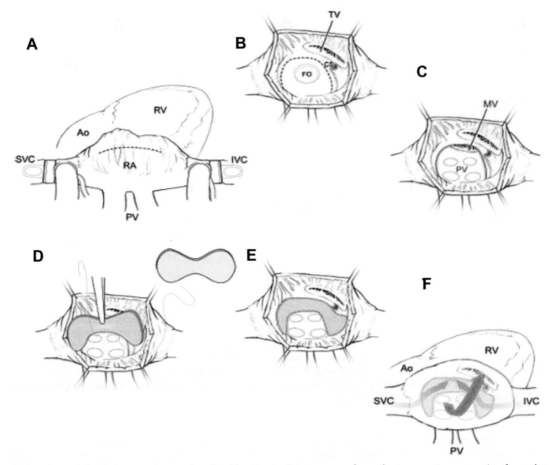

Fig. 3. The atrial switch operation as described by Mustard. Images are from the surgeon's perspective from the right side of the table, with the head to the left and the feet to the right. See text for complete description. Ao, aorta; FO, foramen ovale; IVC, inferior vena cava; MV, mitral valve; PV, pulmonary veins; RA, right atrium; SVC, superior vena cava; TV, tricuspid valve. (*From* Qureshi Athar M, Justino H, Heinle Jeffrey S. Transposition of the great arteries. [Chapter 47]. In: Allen HD, Shaddy RE, Penny DJ, editors. Moss and Adams' heart disease in infants, children, and adolescents, including the fetus and young adult. 9th edition. Philadelphia: Lippincottt Williams and Wilkins; 2016. p. 1174; with permission.)

beyond the obvious symptoms due to bradycardia. Gewilling and colleagues[19] reported a 2.4% per year loss of sinus rhythm following the Mustard operation, and the occurrence of junctional rhythm was associated with a 2.1-fold increased risk of developing supraventricular tachycardia ($P<.05$).

Intra-Atrial Reentry Tachycardia and Other Forms of Supraventricular Tachycardia

Following these operations, intra-atrial reentry tachycardia (IART) develops not only because of natural conduction barriers (crista terminalis, valve annuli, the superior/inferior caval orifices, pulmonary vein orifices) but also because of fibrosis related to suture lines and patches primarily within the native right atrium.[20] Compared with typical atrial flutter in the normal heart, IART is typically slower, with an atypical P-wave morphology. Because the AV relationship is most commonly 2:1, these patients may be asymptomatic at rest. This rhythm should be suspected when there is a monotonous ventricular rate of 100 to 140 beats per minute (bpm) with a nearly flat baseline.[20]

The incidence of supraventricular tachycardia is about 13% in both the Senning and Mustard cohorts at 5 to 10 years after repair.[11] Longer-term data 20 years after Mustard repair report incidences as high as 34%; in an exclusively adult group (>18 years old) reported by Puley and colleauges,[21] at least 48% had had at least one episode of supraventricular tachycardia. Independent risk factors include pulmonary hypertension,

Table 1
Relative incidences of arrhythmias long-term following Mustard and Senning operations for dextro-transposition of the great arteries

Type of Arrhythmia	Relative Prevalence	Comments
Bradyarrhythmias		
Sinus node dysfunction	*****	Mustard > Senning
AV block	**	Mostly with VSD or tricuspid valve surgery
Tachyarrhythmias		
IART	****	Most common atrial tachycardia
Peri-tricuspid valve	****	Usually involves pulmonary venous atrium
Other	**	Superior baffle line, peri-IVC, peri-pulmonary vein
Focal atrial tachycardia	***	Often coincident with IART; associated with suture lines
Automatic junctional tachycardia	**	—
AV nodal reentrant tachycardia	**	Slow AV nodal inputs on pulmonary venous side
Atrial fibrillation	*	—
Accessory-pathway mediated	*	Much less common than in l (levo)-TGA
Ventricular tachycardia/fibrillation	**	May be primary or secondary to atrial tachycardias

The number of asterisks represents the relative prevalence of the arrhythmia, from uncommon (*) to highly prevalent (*****).

Abbreviations: AV, atrioventricular; IART, intra-atrial reentry tachycardia; IVC, inferior vena cava; VSD, ventricular septal defect.

Adapted from Khairy P, Van Hare GF. Catheter ablation in transposition of the great arteries with Mustard or Senning baffles. Heart Rhythm 2009;6:284; with permission.

RV dysfunction, and junctional rhythm before the 18 years of age.[21]

As discussed later, IART is by far the most common form of supraventricular tachycardia in this patient group. The term *IART* is sometimes used interchangeably with atrial flutter, as both are macro-reentry rhythms. Its presence has been shown by Gewillig and colleagues[19] to increase the risk of sudden death as much as 4.7-fold (*P*<.01). The pathophysiology of sudden death is thought to be related to a rapid ventricular response to IART followed by ischemia-related ventricular tachycardia and fibrillation. Certain Mustard/Senning patients seem to have a particularly short AV nodal refractory period, hence, placing them at particular risk. This has been anecdotally, and tragically, observed during ambulatory rhythm monitoring. In summary, the diagnosis of IART after an atrial switch operation carries a worse prognosis than it would in most other conditions and certainly worse than it would in patients having a normal heart.

Sudden Cardiac Death

SCD is more common after atrial switch operation for d-TGA than following almost any other form of congenital heart surgery. The reported incidence is about 5.6 per 1000 patient-years (5.6% per decade).[7,11,12,16,18,19,22] In Kammeraad and colleagues'[16] case-control study of 34 SCD and near-miss SCD patients, significant associations included the presence of any symptoms (odds ratio [OR] = 6.45, 2.42–17.24; *P*<.0005), the presence of arrhythmic symptoms (OR = 21.6, 2.8–166.9; *P* = .003), prior heart failure symptoms (OR = 4.44, 1.85–10.62; *P* = .001), documented atrial tachycardias (OR = 4.87, 1.90–12.46; *P* = .001), and use of cardiac medications (OR = 5.16, 1.86–14.28; *P* = .002). In this group, 81% of events occurred during exercise.[16] It seems that the combination of diminished RV function and tachyarrhythmias represents the highest-risk patient group.[7,19,21] Bradyarrhythmias, such as SAND, are less important risk factors for SCD.[7,16,22,23] In all documented SCD or near-miss SCD, polymorphic VT/VF (ventricular tachycardia/ventricular fibrillation) was found to be the terminal rhythm.

Further insight into the mechanisms and associations with SCD in this patient group comes from Khairy and colleagues'[24] multicenter, retrospective cohort study of 37 patients who had already undergone implantation of implantable cardioverter-defibrillator (ICD) (23 for primary prevention). They found no association between the results of programmed ventricular stimulation and eventual appropriate ICD discharges but good association with secondary prevention as the reason for implantation (hazard ratio [HR] = 18; 1.2261; P = .034) and with *lack of treatment* with beta-blocker (HR = 16.7; 1.3, 185.2; P = .03).[24] They also concluded that a history of supraventricular tachycardia may be implicated in SCD.[24]

NONABLATIVE THERAPIES
Antiarrhythmic Drug Therapies

Before the emergence of ablation for postoperative supraventricular tachyarrhythmias, arrhythmias could only be managed pharmacologically. However, antiarrhythmic drugs were often incompletely effective and often had proarrhythmic and other untoward side effects.[25–28] It was also unclear whether or not antiarrhythmic medications conferred any protection against sudden death. In Kammeraad and colleagues'[16] report of 47 Mustard and Senning patients with sudden death or aborted sudden death, drug therapy did not reduce the risk of sudden death, despite 20 patients being on antiarrhythmic medications. However, as previously noted, Khairy and colleagues[24] demonstrated a possible protective effect of beta-blockers in atrial switch patients. They found that in patients with in situ ICDs, beta-blockers decreased the number of appropriate ICD shocks. The investigators posit that perhaps this is due to a combination of factors, including suppression of primary ventricular or supraventricular arrhythmias, slowing of ventricular response to atrial tachycardias, increase in diastolic filling time, and reduction of myocardial ischemia.

Antitachycardia Pacing for Atrial Tachyarrhythmias

Antitachycardia pacing (ATP) has been shown by some to successfully terminate reentrant atrial tachycardia in patients with a history of complex congenital heart disease. Stephenson and colleagues[29] showed that a second-generation permanent pacemaker with antitachycardia and DDDR pacing capabilities was able to appropriately detect and, in 50% of episodes, successfully pace terminate atrial arrhythmias in patients with congenital heart disease, some of whom were status-post Mustard or Senning operation. Earlier studies even suggested that ATP could facilitate reduction or cessation of medical therapy, but there has been concern for possible acceleration of tachycardia into new and even fatal rhythms.[28,30] Despite this caveat, ATP still remains a possible adjunctive therapy but only in a select subgroup of patients with transposition.

Other Nonablative Therapies: Bradycardia Pacing, Implantable Cardioverter-Defibrillators, Cardiac Resynchronization Therapy

Previously, it was thought that bradyarrhythmias were the main trigger for sudden death in atrial switch patients, but subsequent studies failed to show protection from implanted pacemakers.[16] Nevertheless, bradycardia accounts for significant morbidity. In this patient group, class I indications for permanent pacemaker implantation include symptomatic sinoatrial node dysfunction, either intrinsic or secondary to required drug therapy; symptomatic bradycardia related to second- or third-degree AV block; and third-degree AV block with a wide complex escape mechanism. Class IIa indications include sinus bradycardia or AV dissociation with impaired hemodynamics assessed by invasive or noninvasive means; sinus or junctional bradycardia to prevent recurrences of IART; and an awake heart rate less than 40 bpm or pauses greater than 3 seconds.[31]

Experience with implantable cardiac defibrillators after the Mustard or Senning operation is relatively limited.[24,32,33] In Khairy and colleagues'[24] previously noted report, there were 37 total patients with ICDs: 23 for primary prevention and 14 for secondary prevention. Interestingly, the rate of appropriate shocks in primary prevention patients was quite low, whereas a relatively high rate of appropriate shocks was noted in secondary prevention patients. This study highlights the difficulty in predicting which patients are at highest risk of sudden death and the need for better risk stratification in this patient population. It is also notable that in this study supraventricular tachyarrhythmias preceded or coexisted with 50% of the appropriate shocks for confirmed ventricular tachyarrhythmias. Class I indications for ICD implantation include survivors of cardiac arrest due to ventricular fibrillation or hemodynamically unstable ventricular tachycardia after evaluation has ruled out other completely reversible causes;

patients having had spontaneous sustained ventricular tachycardia; adults with an ejection fraction of 35% or less and New York Heart Association (NYHA) class II or III symptoms.[31]

Cardiac resynchronization therapy (CRT) for RV failure is of salient importance in patients with transposition after atrial switch operation, as their RV remains the systemic ventricle. In an early small study by Dubin and colleagues,[34] CRT resulted in improvement (as judged by ejection fraction) in patients with congenital heart disease with moderate to severe RV dysfunction. In another study, which included some Senning and Mustard patients, CRT led to acute improvement in systolic and diastolic RV function as well as improved NYHA class during midterm follow-up.[35] There was also confirmed synchrony of contraction by tissue Doppler imaging. This study did not, however, show significant improvement in tricuspid valve regurgitation. There are no class I indications for CRT in this patient group; but class IIa indications include systemic RV ejection fraction less than 35%, RV dilatation, NYHA class II to IV symptoms, complete right bundle branch block (RBBB) with intrinsic or paced QRS duration greater than 150 milliseconds, RV ejection fraction less than 35%, intrinsically narrow QRS complex, and patients with NYHA class I to IV who are getting a new or replacement device and expected ventricular pacing burden greater than 40%.[31]

CATHETER ABLATION STRATEGIES

Catheter ablation of any supraventricular tachyarrhythmias following atrial redirection surgery is worthwhile in patients having recurrent clinical episodes and is probably the therapy of choice in those having IART and a rapid ventricular response. The overall short-term success rate is well in excess of 80%,[36–40] and late recurrence rates are probably intermediate between those described in patients who had simple atrial septal defect surgery (<10%) and those who had Fontan-style operations (>40%).[36] The operator should have a thorough understanding of the surgical anatomy and how it applies to catheter course, the normal conduction system, and natural conduction obstacles. Electroanatomic mapping techniques are useful, especially when creating multi-chamber reconstructions. This section discusses the necessary preparation for this procedure followed by a more detailed description of mapping and catheter ablation of the usual tachycardia substrates.

Electrophysiological Anatomy

The Mustard operation is performed through a right atriotomy, which may be aligned vertically or horizontally. When vertical, it is usually anterior to the crista terminalis. Following this operation, the AV node and penetrating bundle are always segregated to the pulmonary venous/systemic ventricular side of the circulation. During the Mustard operation, the anterior portion of the atrial baffle (constructed of pericardium; Dacron, INVISTA North America S.A.R.L., Wichita, KS; or Gore-Tex, W.L. Gore & Associates, Inc, Newark, DE) is sutured to the anterior remnant of the atrial septum, just behind (posterior to) the AV node. (In the past, intraoperative heart block occurred in <5% of patients, related to this portion of the procedure.) The suture line then continues inferiorly where it anteriorly encircles the inferior vena cava orifice. This section necessarily bisects the medial cavotricuspid isthmus (CTI), but there is technical variability in how this is accomplished depending largely on how the coronary sinus ostium is handled: (1) When the suture line is placed anteriorly to the ostium, the coronary sinus drains into the system venous atrium, leaving a relatively large portion of the medial isthmus on that side. (2) Conversely, if the suture line is posterior to the ostium, more of the isthmus is on the same side as the tricuspid valve. (3) Most commonly, surgeons incised the proximal coronary sinus and sutured the baffle to the cut edge, leaving an intermediate portion of posteroseptal remnant/medial isthmus on each side (**Fig. 4**). In all cases, accessing the coronary sinus ostium is difficult if not impossible. The surgical technique chosen also determines what portion of the slow inputs to the AV node is accessible to a systemic venous catheter (see **Fig. 4**). Conduction delay in this area has been demonstrated by intraoperative activation mapping.[41]

As the baffle suture line is then extended posteriorly, it crosses the plane of the old atrial septum and passes inferior to the lower pulmonary veins, before laterally encircling the left pulmonary veins. This procedure results in bisection of the left lower pulmonary vein-mitral annulus isthmus. The suture line then passes superior to the upper pulmonary veins, recrossing the plane of the original atrial septum, and is then anteriorly directed to encircle the superior vena cava orifice. This portion of the suture line is responsible for damage to the sinoatrial node and/or its blood supply. The baffle suture line is completed as it passes through the pectinate muscles at the base of the right atrial appendage before reengaging the anterior septal remnant. When there are baffle leaks, which can theoretically pose a risk of paradoxic embolus, they usually occur in this area. A variable portion of right atrial appendage and all of the left atrial appendage remain on the

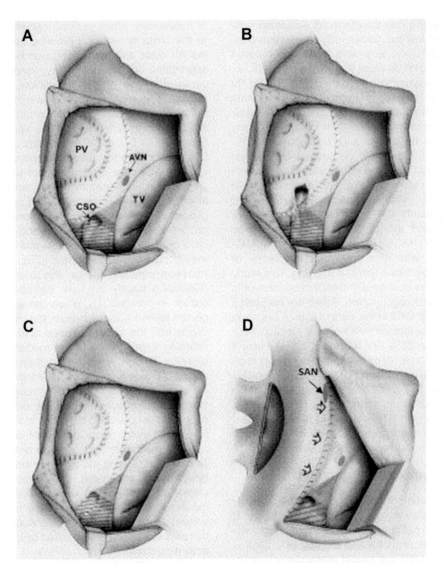

Fig. 4. Internal view of the pulmonary venous atrium from a right lateral perspective following the Mustard (*A–C*) and Senning (*D*) operations, showing the pertinent components of the conduction system, especially as relates to the variations in the inferior baffle suture line and the coronary sinus ostium (CSO). (*A*) The suture line is posterior to the CSO, leaving it to drain in the pulmonary venous atrium. (*B*) The CSO is incised, and the suture line includes the cut edge of the proximal coronary sinus. (*C*) The suture line is anterior to the CSO, leaving it to drain in the systemic venous atrium. The shaded area is the approximate region of the slow inputs to the AV node. The crosshatched area is the medial cavotricuspid isthmus. Arrowheads in (*D*) represent the suture line connecting the right atrial free wall with the anterior edge of the atrial septal remnant. AVN, atrioventricular node; PV, pulmonary veins; SAN, sinoatrial node; TV, tricuspid valve. (*Adapted from* Kanter RJ, Papagiannis J, Carboni MP, et al. Radiofrequency catheter ablation of supraventricular tachycardia substrates after Mustard and Senning operations for d-transposition of the great arteries. J Am Coll Cardiol 2000;35:431; with permission.)

systemic venous side, where they, plus the roof of the native left atrium, are favored places to insert permanent atrial leads. Left phrenic nerve stimulation is a well-known risk of lead placement in the left atrial appendage.

As previously discussed, the Senning operation involves 3 major incisions: (1) a vertical one in the posterior left atrium between the right pulmonary veins and the posterior attachment of the atrial septum; (2) a second vertical one in the anterolateral right atrium between the caval orifices; and (3) a horseshoe-shaped incision in the atrial septum, creating an anterior flap (still attached posteriorly). Following completion of this procedure, the coronary sinus ostium and AV node are on the pulmonary venous side, as is almost all of the CTI (see

Fig. 4D). Surgical scar in that region related to the incisions and infolding of the right atrial free wall can create the substrate for typical (CTI) atrial flutter. Conduction barriers related to the interposition material in the pulmonary venous atrium may contribute to other IARTs. Finally, the sinoatrial node may be displaced inferiorly and posteriorly, as the cavoatrial junction is brought toward the atrial septum.

Preparation

Planning for a possible catheter ablation in an adult who has undergone a Mustard or Senning operation requires 4 categories of consideration: anatomic variations, hemodynamic fragility, vascular access, and electrophysiologic substrates/data acquisition. These categories are considered separately.

Anatomic variations

Depending on the thoroughness of the surgeon, access to the original surgical report may provide valuable information, such as the direction of the right atriotomy and the handling of the coronary sinus in Mustard patients and the method of pulmonary venous atrial conduit completion in Senning patients. The authors have found that even nuances of native anatomy may influence the procedure. For example, when the aortic valve is in an oblique plane and tilted leftward, the catheter pass from the aorta retrograde across the tricuspid valve may be more difficult and may be prone to dangerously splinting both valves open. Meticulous preprocedure imaging is crucial to allow preparation for anatomic variations, baffle obstruction, and baffle leaks. Although undesirable for other reasons, a baffle leak may permit access to pulmonary venous atrial tachycardia substrates from the systemic venous side.

Hemodynamic fragility

The subaortic RV is thought to be especially vulnerable to myocardial ischemia, and the abbreviated diastole imposed by supraventricular tachycardias with a rapid ventricular response may be especially problematic. Even prolonged periods of rapid atrial pacing that may be required to induce the clinical arrhythmia may take its toll during the course of a study. If patients are known to only have IART, intravenous diltiazem may be used to reduce the ventricular response rate, thus, protecting RV function. This agent may suppress inducibility of other supraventricular tachycardias, however. When the procedure is performed under general anesthesia, a conversation with the anesthesiologist should include the anesthetic agents; those that reduce ventricular performance should

be used sparingly or not at all. The clinical conduct of these procedures should include continuous blood pressure surveillance with an indwelling arterial line; intermittent measurements of systemic perfusion (blood lactate levels and urine output); and, if under general anesthesia, monitoring of end-tidal carbon dioxide and scalp near-infrared spectroscopy. In patients known to be at especially high risk because of poor RV function, Fishberger and colleagues[42] reported the use of the transarterial ventricular assist device, Impella (Abiomed, Danvers, MA). For postprocedure care, a bed in an intensive care unit skilled in the management of adults with congenital heart disease should be arranged in advance.

Vascular access

Ideally, the authors prefer to have at least 3 catheters placed from the venous side (at least one of which is from a lower body approach): one for ventricular pacing, at least one multipole catheter for multiple atrial reference sites and atrial pacing, and a point-to-point mapping/ablation catheter. A single femoral artery sheath is required if pulmonary venous atrial mapping/ablation is to be performed using the retrograde transaortic approach. However, the operator should be prepared for limited vascular access because the high incidence of iliofemoral vein occlusion incurred during catheter-based procedures way back in infancy. Internal jugular, subclavian, and hepatic veins are alternatives. The last two veins will also be unavailable if there is complete superior vena caval baffle obstruction, another well-known sequelae of the Mustard operation. Determination of baffle patency is another role of preprocedure imaging. Intraprocedural transesophageal echocardiography and angiography are alternative strategies.

Electrophysiologic substrates/data acquisition

Electroanatomic mapping is useful during these procedures to help create anatomic shells of the systemic and pulmonary venous atria. Modern technologies allow simultaneous display of both chambers. Preprocedural imaging by computerized tomography or magnetic resonance may be used to enable image merging, but this is not critical. The anatomic shell ideally will include the AV valve annuli, vena caval orifices, and pulmonary vein orifices. Once tachycardia is induced, point-to-point mapping, perhaps using newer systems that record multiple points simultaneously, is acceptable; these tachycardia circuits tend to be stable over time. A local activation (LAT) map facilitates understanding of the tachycardia mechanism (head-meets-tail activation for macro-reentry and centrifugal activation for focal atrial tachycardia). Voltage mapping will identify scar as areas with bipolar voltage less than 0.05 V. Newer force-contact catheters verify the validity of low-voltage areas when at least 10 g of force is observed. Classic electrophysiologic techniques may then be applied as necessary, such as manifest and concealed entrainment, postpacing intervals, and V-A-V versus V-A-A-V responses to ventricular pacing. The authors prefer to have in place a duodecapolar electrode catheter spanning the intercaval tube, generally from the proximal superior caval baffle down to the right atrial–inferior vena caval orifice. Although this will display activity, especially in the medial isthmus portion of the systemic venous side, it must be recognized that the middle bipoles will be recording signals from the posterior native left atrium in the case of the Mustard operation and the atrial septal flap in the case of the Senning operation (**Fig. 5**). Some operators prefer, in addition, to have a stable multiple catheter with its tip in the left atrial appendage. This catheter will provide a more reliable opportunity for atrial capture than might be achieved from the intercaval multipole catheter, and it will generate additional reference recording sites (mostly from the posterior native left atrium).

The operator should be prepared to access the pulmonary venous atrium. Unless there is a known baffle leak, this may only be accomplished using the retrograde, transaortic valve, transtricuspid valve approach or by performing a baffle perforation, analogous to a transseptal puncture. The retrograde approach enables mapping and ablation of the native lateral right atrium, areas around the right pulmonary veins, and the inferior half of the peri-tricuspid valve region. The catheter should be flexed and prolapsed across the aortic valve to avoid valve damage. It usually crosses the valve with the tip pointed anteriorly. Clockwise torque brings the catheter rightward and posterior. Opening up the flexion will then direct the tip across the tricuspid valve and to the low lateral native right atrium. A combination of catheter withdrawal and tip extension will engage the pulmonary venous component of the lateral CTI right up to the tricuspid valve annulus. Clockwise torque, catheter pullback, and tip extension will engage the septal tricuspid valve where slow pathway mapping is possible (see **Fig. 7**). Flexion will then direct the tip superiorly toward the His bundle region. This technique is not robust for mapping other portions of the pulmonary venous atrium because of the energy lost in catheter flexion around the aortic arch and the RV-to-tricuspid valve bend.

Transbaffle perforation may safely be performed in these patients and is the only method of pulmonary venous atrial access in patients who have undergone artificial tricuspid valve replacement.[37] When baffle perforation is performed from the inferior vena caval approach, the transseptal needle is directed anteriorly and sometimes slightly rightward[37,43,44] (**Fig. 6**). If a standard BRK XS needle (30° angle) (St. Jude Medical, St Paul, MN) is used, and sliding is encountered, it has been suggested that the angulation should be manually adjusted to 80° to 140°.[37] The authors prefer the NRG RF Transseptal Needle (Baylis Medical, Saint Laurent, QC, Canada)[45]; but even after successful perforation, advancement of a long sheath may be difficult and require dilation techniques. The authors have found the 7F or 8F Mullins transseptal sheath (Medtronic Inc, Minneapolis, MN) to most easily follow the needle across the puncture site, although use of stiffer deflectable sheaths has been described. This procedure should be guided by intracardiac or esophageal echocardiography, whenever possible.[37] This approach permits mapping of the pulmonary venous side of the entire native right atrium and the right pulmonary veins. It most naturally engages the mid-CTI from the tricuspid valve to the baffle suture line. With hard clockwise torque, the septal tricuspid valve can be accessed; with counterclockwise torque, the left pulmonary veins all the way to the peri-vein suture line can be reached. Systemic heparinization is necessary after entry to the pulmonary venous atrium, and the activated clotting time should be maintained at greater than 250 seconds.

Remote magnetic navigation technology uses a very flexible mapping/ablation catheter that is guided through the cardiovascular system by external manipulation of magnetic fields. Because these systems are extremely expensive, they are not widely used. However, when available, they have been used for retrograde access to the pulmonary venous atrium and successful ablation of supraventricular tachyarrhythmia substrates.[36,38,46] In 2 small series, 13 of 15 tachycardias were successfully treated by this method.[38,46]

Ablation of Intra-Atrial Reentry Tachycardia

In published series, catheter ablation of IART was acutely successful in 71 of 83 (86%) patients. Long-term recurrences have been reported to occur in up to 33% of patients.[36,37] In the larger published experiences, the critical zone of slow conduction that was successfully targeted for catheter ablation was the CTI in 77% to 88% of circuits.[40,47,48] When using standard techniques of concealed entrainment mapping with a

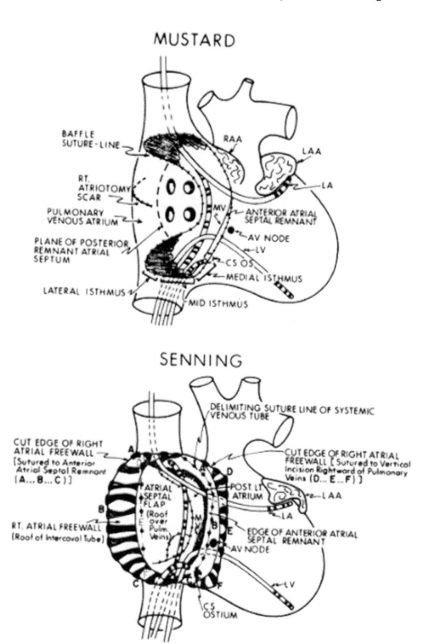

Fig. 5. A right anterior oblique view showing the internal anatomy of both the systemic and pulmonary atria following the Mustard operation (*top*) and of the system venous atrium following the Senning operation (*bottom*), with special attention to the physical relationship between the usual location of electrode catheters and the surgically revised structures. In particular, note the relationship between the multipole catheter and the medial cavotricuspid isthmus (lower electrodes) and with the posterior native left atrium after the Mustard operation and the atrial septal flap after the Senning operation (middle electrodes). CS OS, coronary sinus ostium; LA, left atrium; LAA, left atrial appendage; LV, left ventricle; RAA, right atrial appendage; RT, right. (*From* Kanter RJ, Papagiannis J, Carboni MP, et al. Radiofrequency catheter ablation of supraventricular tachycardia substrates after Mustard and Senning operations for d-transposition of the great arteries. J Am Coll Cardiol 2000;35:432; with permission.)

postpacing interval similar to the tachycardia cycle length, both sides of the baffle suture line are usually shown to be included in the circuit.[49] In case series, successful ablation from only the systemic venous atrium was much less common (10%)[36,40] than from only the pulmonary venous atrium (47%–73%)[36,40] or from both sides (18%–100%).[36,40,49] The authors are reluctant to

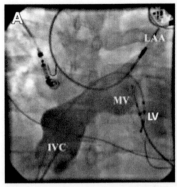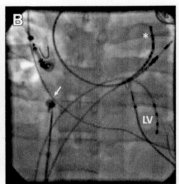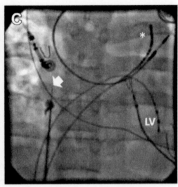

Fig. 6. Posteroanterior fluoroscopic images demonstrating transbaffle puncture. (*A*) Contrast injection in the inferior systemic venous baffle with contrast in the proximal inferior vena cava (IVC) up to the region of the mitral valve (MV). (*B*) Transseptal needle-pointed superior and anterior and with staining of the wall (*arrow*). (*C*) Following successful perforation of the wall and entry of the needle tip (*arrowhead*) into the pulmonary venous atrium. If only fluoroscopy is used, lateral projection is also required to assure anterior angulation of the needle. There is a quadripolar electrode catheter in the left ventricle (LV in *A–C*), a multipole catheter in the left atrial appendage (LAA) (*asterisk, B, C*), and a permanent pacing lead also in the LAA. (*Adapted from* Khairy P, Van Hare GF. Catheter ablation in transposition of the great arteries with Mustard or Senning baffles. Heart Rhythm 2009;6:287; with permission.)

ablate the systemic venous side (only medial isthmus tends to be available) in those occasional patients having first-degree AV block and no VA conduction at baseline. The authors suspect that during the original surgery they incurred damage to their fast AV nodal inputs and depend on the slow inputs for AV conduction. The authors have created second-degree AV block during ablation in the medial CTI in one such patient.[40]

The authors' approach to mapping IART circuits in these patients is to first identify atrial diastole. Because the cycle length of IART in these patients is usually between 220 and 300 milliseconds, typically, there is a 2:1 AV relationship. The surface P wave (flutter wave) may be low amplitude and is frequently buried in the T and QRS waves when there is a 2:1 AV relationship. Placement of premature ventricular beats or brief rapid ventricular pacing will allow identification of the P waves and the isoelectric periods between them. The relationship of intracardiac electrograms from the multipole electrode catheter to these surface electrocardiogram events allows them to be surrogates for atrial systole/diastole. A point-to-point electroanatomic map is then constructed and concentrated in regions of putative atrial diastole. Areas of scar are carefully identified. An LAT map showing a head-meets-tail pattern with dense isochrones between conduction obstacles will generally be associated with diastole-spanning fractionated potentials or discrete double potentials (**Fig. 7**). Once the mechanism of macro-reentry is confirmed, these regions are fertile for concealed entrainment mapping and catheter ablation.

IART circuits other than the CTI have been reported to exist around a pulmonary vein, the inferior vena caval orifice, and (presumably) between the native right atriotomy and crista terminalis.[47] The authors have also identified the region between the superior vena caval orifice and the posterior edge of the atrial septectomy as a critical zone of slow conduction in 2 Senning patients.[40] The authors are also aware of IART involving the mitral isthmus in these patients.

There is no particular contraindication to use an irrigated tip catheter for IART, but the authors have not generally found it to be necessary in these patients. This circumstance is unlike Fontan patients, in whom the atrial wall is unusually thick and deep energy delivery is almost always required. If an open irrigated tip catheter is used and excessive ablation times are required, notation of the total fluid delivery should be considered, especially in smaller patients who have congestive heart failure. Because the tachycardia target may be in the lateral native RV, damage to the right phrenic nerve by endocardial energy delivery is a theoretic concern. This structure may be displaced by epicardial fibrosis and not in the usual location. High-output pacing from the ablation catheter at those sites before radiofrequency energy delivery is, therefore, advised. That said, the authors are unaware of phrenic nerve injury during catheter ablation in these patients.

Most published experiences have defined acute success as termination of IART during energy delivery followed by noninducibility with variably

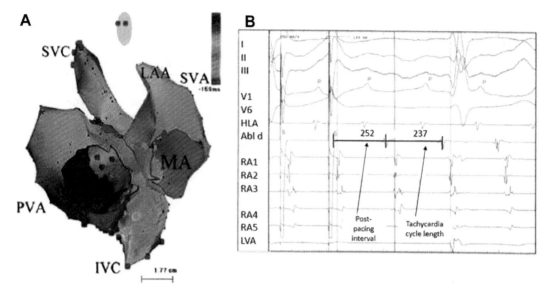

Fig. 7. Typical atrial flutter following Mustard operation. (*A*) Left anterior oblique view of an electroanatomic rendering of the systemic and pulmonary venous atria. Color coding of isochrones demonstrates slow conduction in the cavotricuspid isthmus of both atria. (*B*) Concealed entrainment with a postpacing interval that is within 30 milliseconds of the tachycardia cycle length. Pacing was from the systemic venous atrial side near the baffle suture line of the medial cavotricuspid isthmus. The right atrial bipolar (systemic venous) recording sites (RA1-5) channels are also recorded from the inferior baffle of the systemic venous atrium and, along with the pacing site, seem to be in midatrial diastole. Despite this, successful ablation was not achieved until lesions were also placed at the lateral cavotricuspid isthmus by the tricuspid valve annulus in the pulmonary venous atrium. ABl d, distal ablation bipole (and pacing); HLA, high left atrium; IVC, inferior vena cava; LAA, left atrial appendage; LVA, left ventricular apex; MA, mitral annulus; P, P or flutter wave; PVA, pulmonary venous atrium; SVA, systemic venous atrium; SVC, superior vena cava; TA, tricuspid annulus. (*Adapted from* Zrenner B, Dong J, Schreieck J, et al. Delineation of intra-atrial reentrant tachycardia circuits after Mustard operation for transposition of the great arteries using biatrial electroanatomic mapping and entrainment mapping. J Cardiovasc Electrophysiol 2003;14:1305; with permission.)

aggressive atrial extrastimulus and burst pacing with or without isoproterenol influence. Demonstration of bidirectional block is the gold standard for successful ablation of the CTI in patients with a normal heart; in those patients, this may be accomplished with a multipole catheter alone. This procedure may be difficult to achieve in Mustard/Senning patients because ideally it requires electroanatomic propagation mapping during pacing from each side of the ablation line, and this requires sampling from both the pulmonary and venous atrial sides. Balaji and colleagues[50] published a small experience of such patients in whom they thought that bidirectional block was shown by recording from both the systemic venous side of the superior baffle and from either the systemic or pulmonary venous side of the CTI while pacing from the opposite side of the CTI. Compared with preablation, postablation block was associated with a longer transbaffle interval in the CTI versus the interval from the CTI to the superior baffle.

Focal Atrial Tachycardia

Focal atrial tachycardia (FAT) is a paroxysmal rhythm that may be discriminated from IART by a combination of findings: (1) the P wave tends to be more discrete than that observed during IART, though this is not a reliable finding; (2) intracardiac electrograms from the chamber of interest tend to occupy at least 70% of the atrial cycle in IART, but less so in FAT; (3) a centrifugal atrial activation pattern during electroanatomic mapping characterizes FAT, compared with a head-meets-tail pattern in IART; and (4) manifest and concealed entrainment criteria are demonstrated with IART but not FAT. The presence of atrial diastole-spanning fractionated electrograms is a sensitive but not a specific finding in IART. That is, a damaged area remote from a clinically important FAT source may show this finding and mislead the operator; concealed entrainment will not be demonstrated at that site. The cycle length of FAT in these patients tends to be slower than that of IART.

The mechanism of FAT in Mustard/Senning patients is thought to be micro-reentry, although this is difficult to prove; a triggered mechanism is also possible. This arrhythmia has been described in 8 of 47 patients (17%) undergoing catheter ablation for supraventricular tachycardias in 3 relatively large studies.[40,47,48] The FAT foci seem to mostly be adjacent to suture lines on either the systemic or pulmonary venous sides. Discrete electrograms preceding the surface P wave by at least 30 milliseconds are targeted, and the acute success rate approaches 100%, with rare long-term recurrences.[40] The authors have observed new FAT foci in subsequent studies in 2 patients, suggesting that FAT may have a dynamic pathophysiology in certain patients.

Atrioventricular Nodal Reentrant Tachycardia

This tachycardia has been described in 12 of 53 patients (23%) in 2 relatively large series of Mustard/Senning patients undergoing catheter ablation for supraventricular tachycardia.[36,40] The cycle length is often quite long, sometimes greater than 400 milliseconds; only the typical variety (slow/fast) has been described. The diagnosis is based on the following: (1) the presence of concentric (as best can be determined) atrial

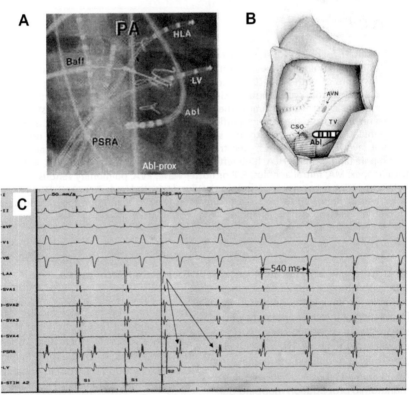

Fig. 8. Typical variety (slow/fast) of AV nodal reentrant tachycardia (tAVNRT). (*A*) Posteroanterior fluoroscopic view from a Senning patient showing the ablation catheter (Abl) retrogradely passed across the aortic and tricuspid valves and engaging the region of the slow inputs to the AV node. (*B*) Right lateral view of the pulmonary venous atrium after a Mustard operation showing the catheter in the approximate location as in (*A*). Shaded area represents region of slow inputs to the AV node. Crosshatched area represents medial cavotricuspid isthmus. (*C*) Intracardiac electrograms showing the initiation of tAVNRT in a Senning patient. Atrial extrastimulus testing results in double ventricular activation by S2(A2) using fast and slow inputs to the AV node, which is associated with a supraventricular tachycardia having 1:1 AV relationship and an ultrashort V-A interval. Note how slow the tachycardia is. Abl-prox, proximal ablation catheter in the descending aorta; AVN, AV node; Baff, multipole electrode catheter in the intercaval tube of a Senning patient; CSO, coronary sinus ostium; HLA, high left atrium; LAA, left atrial appendage bipolar recording; LV, left ventricular bipolar recording; PSRA, posteroseptal right atrial channel bipolar recordings from a second multipole catheter; SVA1–4, systemic venous atrial channel bipolar recordings; TV, tricuspid valve. (*Adapted from* Kanter RJ, Papagiannis J, Carboni MP, et al. Radiofrequency catheter ablation of supraventricular tachycardia substrates after Mustard and Senning operations for d-transposition of the great arteries. J Am Coll Cardiol 2000;35:433; with permission.)

activation during ventricular pacing; (2) mode of initiation during atrial extrastimulus testing: V1-V2 dependent, not A1-A2 dependent, and sometimes associated with double ventricular activation after A2; (3) mode of termination, following atrial electrogram; (4) very short VA interval during tachycardia (<70 milliseconds when septal atrial electrograms can be mapped); and (5) V-A-V response during tachycardia and ventricular pacing. The PR interval is usually normal during sinus rhythm, and dual AV nodal physiology is not often demonstrated.[39]

Anatomically, the location of the coronary sinus ostium can only be estimated in these patients. Although the slow inputs to the AV node may be apportioned to both sides of the inferior baffle suture line, the tricuspid valve annulus, compact AV node, and His bundle electrograms are always on the pulmonary venous side. Jongbloed and colleagues[51] recommend placing a catheter on the systemic venous side near the expected location of the coronary sinus ostium as an anatomic reference. The arterial, retroaortic approach of the ablation catheter is favored in most reports[40,51] (**Fig. 8**). After a His bundle electrogram cloud is created, the flexion on the catheter is relaxed, the aforementioned reference catheter is targeted, and characteristic electrograms are sought as one would in a normal heart. Radiofrequency energy has been reported to cause junctional acceleration on both sides of the baffle,[39] but elimination of tachycardia inducibility is reported to only be accomplished from the pulmonary venous side[39,40] along the tricuspid valve annulus. The authors are aware of one Senning patient in whom successful modification of the slow inputs could only be accomplished from the systemic venous side. The acute success rate is reported to be 100% in small series.[36,39,40]

SUMMARY

Within the next 30 years, the contents of this section will largely be of historical interest only, as the population of adults having undergone the Mustard or Senning operation will have passed on or undergone cardiac transplantation. Medium- and now long-term outcomes suggest that the arterial switch operation has successfully supplanted the atrial switch. That said, the tenets of procedural planning, customization of catheter courses, and use of electrophysiologic principles to nontraditional substrates, which are so critical in this patient group, may be applied throughout the spectrum of postoperative complex congenital heart disease.

REFERENCES

1. Perry LW, Neill CA, Ferencz C, et al. Infants with congenital heart disease: the cases. In: Ferencz C, Rubin JD, Loffredo CA, et al, editors. Epidemiology of congenital heart disease. The Baltimore-Washington infant study 1981-1989. Mount Kisco (NY): Futura Publishing; 1993. p. 33–62.
2. Rashkind WJ, Miller WW. Creation of an atrial septal defect without thoracotomy: a palliative approach to complete transposition of the great arteries. JAMA 1966;196:991–2.
3. Evans W. The arterial switch operation before Jatene. Pediatr Cardiol 2009;30:119–24.
4. Jatene AD, Fontes VF, Paulista PP, et al. Anatomic correction of transposition of the great vessels. J Thorac Cardiovasc Surg 1976;72:364–70.
5. Senning A. Surgical correction of transposition of the great arteries. Surgery 1959;45:966–80.
6. Mustard WT. Successful two-stage correction of transposition of the great arteries. Surgery 1964; 55:469–72.
7. Gelatt M, Hamilton RM, McCrindle BW, et al. Arrhythmia and mortality after the Mustard procedure: a 30-year single-center experience. J Am Coll Cardiol 1997;29:194–201.
8. Turley K, Hanley FL, Verrier ED, et al. The Mustard procedure in infants (less than 100 days of age). Ten-year follow-up. J Thorac Cardiovasc Surg 1988;96:849–53.
9. Kanter RJ, Garson A Jr. Atrial arrhythmias during chronic follow-up of surgery for complex congenital heart disease. Pacing Clin Electrophysiol 1997;20: 502–11.
10. Moons P, Gewillig M, Sluysmans T, et al. Long term outcome up to 30 years after the Mustard or Senning operation: a nationwide multicentre study in Belgium. Heart 2004;90:307–13.
11. Dos L, Teruel L, Ferreira IJ, et al. Late outcome of Senning and Mustard procedures for correction of transposition of the great arteries. Heart 2005;91: 652–6.
12. Wilson NJ, Clarkson PM, Barratt-Boyes BG, et al. Long-term outcome after the Mustard repair for simple transposition of the great arteries: 28-year follow-up. J Am Coll Cardiol 1998;32:758–65.
13. Warnes CA, Somerville J. Transposition of the great arteries: late results in adolescents and adults after the Mustard procedure. Br Heart J 1987;58:148–55.
14. Hagler DJ, Ritter DG, Mair DD, et al. Right and left ventricular function after the Mustard procedure in transposition of the great arteries. Am J Cardiol 1979;44:276–83.
15. Warnes CA. Transposition of the great arteries. Circulation 2006;114:2699–709.
16. Kammeraad JA, Van Deurzen CH, Sreeram N, et al. Predictors of sudden cardiac death after Mustard or

Senning repair for transposition of the great arteries. J Am Coll Cardiol 2004;44:1095–102.

17. Deanfield J, Camm J, Macauley F, et al. Arrhythmia and late mortality after Mustard and Senning operation for transposition of the great arteries. An eight-year prospective study. J Thorac Cardiovasc Surg 1988;96:569–76.

18. Turina M, Siebenmann R, Nussbaumer P, et al. Long-term outlook after atrial correction of transposition of great arteries. J Thorac Cardiovasc Surg 1988;95:828–35.

19. Gewillig M, Cullen S, Mertens B, et al. Risk factors for arrhythmia and death after Mustard operation for simple transposition of the great arteries. Circulation 1991;84:III187–92.

20. Walsh E, Cecchin F. Arrhythmias in adult patients with congenital heart disease. Circulation 2007;115:534–5.

21. Puley G, Siu S, Connelly M, et al. Arrhythmia and survival in patients >18 years of age after the Mustard procedure for complete transposition of the great arteries. Am J Cardiol 1999;83:1080–4.

22. Flinn CJ, Wolff GS, Dick M II, et al. Cardiac rhythm after the Mustard operation for complete transposition of the great arteries. N Engl J Med 1984;310:1635–8.

23. Helbing WA, Hansen B, Ottenkamp J, et al. Long-term results of atrial correction for transposition of the great arteries: comparison of Mustard and Senning operations. J Thorac Cardiovasc Surg 1994;108:363–72.

24. Khairy P, Harris L, Landzberg MJ, et al. Sudden death and defibrillators in transposition of the great arteries with intra-atrial baffles: a multicenter study. Circ Arrhythm Electrophysiol 2008;1:250–7.

25. Hammermeister KE, Boerth RC, Warbasse JR. The comparative inotropic effects of six clinically used antiarrhythmic agents. Am Heart J 1972;5:643–52.

26. The Cardiac Arrhythmia Suppression Trial Investigators. Preliminary report: effect of encainide and flecainide on mortality in a randomized trial of arrhythmia suppression after myocardial infarction. N Engl J Med 1989;321:406–12.

27. Kingma JH, Suttorp MJ. Acute pharmacologic conversion of atrial fibrillation and flutter: the role of flecainide, propafenone, and verapamil. Am J Cardiol 1992;70:A56–61.

28. Rhodes LA, Walsh EP, Gamble WJ, et al. Benefits and potential risks of atrial antitachycardia pacing after repair of congenital heart disease. Pacing Clin Electrophysiol 1995;18:1005–16.

29. Stephenson EA, Casavant D, Tuzi J, et al. Efficacy of atrial antitachycardia pacing using the Medtronic AT500 pacemaker in patients with congenital heart disease. Am J Cardiol 2003;92:871–6.

30. Gillette PC, Zeigler VL, Case CL, et al. Atrial antitachycardia pacing in children and young adults. Am Heart J 1991;122:844–9.

31. Khairy P, Van Hare GF, Balaji S, et al. PACES/HRS expert consensus statement on the recognition and management of arrhythmias in adult congenital heart disease: developed in partnership between the Pediatric and Congenital Electrophysiology Society (PACES) and the Heart Rhythm Society (HRS). Endorsed by the governing bodies of PACES, HRS, the American College of Cardiology (ACC), the American Heart Association (AHA), the European Heart Rhythm Association (EHRA), the Canadian Heart Rhythm Society (CHRS), and the International Society for Adult Congenital Heart Disease (ISACHD). Heart Rhythm 2014;11:e102–65.

32. Michael KA, Veldtman GR, Paisey JR, et al. Cardiac defibrillation therapy for at risk patients with systemic right ventricular dysfunction secondary to atrial redirection surgery for dextro-transposition of the great arteries. Europace 2007;9:281–4.

33. Bouzeman A, Marijon E, de Guillebon M, et al. Implantable cardiac defibrillator among adults with transposition of the great arteries and atrial switch operation: case series and review of literature. Int J Cardiol 2014;177:301–6.

34. Dubin AM, Feinstein JA, Reddy VM, et al. Electrical resynchronization: a novel therapy for the failing right ventricle. Circulation 2003;107:2287–9.

35. Janoušek J, Tomek V, Chaloupecký V, et al. Cardiac resynchronization therapy: a novel adjunct to the treatment and prevention of systemic right ventricular failure. J Am Coll Cardiol 2004;44:1927–31.

36. Wu J, Deisenhofer I, Ammar S, et al. Acute and long-term outcome after catheter ablation of supraventricular tachycardia in patients after the Mustard or Senning operation for D-transposition of the great arteries. Europace 2013;15:886–91.

37. Jones DG, Jarman JW, Lyne JC, et al. The safety and efficacy of trans-baffle puncture to enable catheter ablation of atrial tachycardias following the Mustard procedure: a single centre experience and literature review. Int J Cardiol 2013;168:1115–20.

38. Wu J, Pflaumer A, Deisenhofer I, et al. Mapping of atrial tachycardia by remote magnetic navigation in postoperative patients with congenital heart disease. J Cardiovasc Electrophysiol 2010;21:751–9.

39. Greene AE, Skinner JR, Dubin AM, et al. The electrophysiology of atrioventricular nodal reentry tachycardia following the Mustard or Senning procedure and its radiofrequency ablation. Cardiol Young 2005;15:611–6.

40. Kanter RJ, Papagiannis J, Carboni MP, et al. Radiofrequency catheter ablation of supraventricular tachycardia substrates after Mustard and Senning operations for d-transposition of the great arteries. J Am Coll Cardiol 2000;35:428–41.

41. Wittig JH, deLeval MR, Stark J, et al. Intraoperative mapping of atrial activation before, during, and after

the Mustard operation. J Thorac Cardiovasc Surg 1977;73:1–13.

42. Fishberger SB, Asnes JD, Rollinson NL, et al. Percutaneous right ventricular support during catheter ablation of intra-atrial reentrant tachycardia in an adult with a mustard baffle–a novel use of the Impella device. J Interv Card Electrophysiol 2010; 29:69–72.

43. Khairy P, Van Hare GF. Catheter ablation in transposition of the great arteries with Mustard or Senning baffles. Heart Rhythm 2009;6:283–9.

44. Perry JC, Boramanand NK, Ing FF. "Transseptal" technique through atrial baffles for 3-dimensional mapping and ablation of atrial tachycardia in patients with d-transposition of the great arteries. J Interv Card Electrophysiol 2003;9:365–9.

45. Esch JJ, Triedman JK, Cecchin F, et al. Radiofrequency-assisted transseptal perforation for electrophysiology procedures in children and adults with repaired congenital heart disease. Pacing Clin Electrophysiol 2013;36:607–11.

46. Ernst S, Babu-Narayan SV, Keegan J, et al. Remote-controlled magnetic navigation and ablation with 3D image integration as an alternative approach in patients with intra-atrial baffle anatomy. Circ Arrhythm Electrophysiol 2012;5:131–9.

47. Zrenner B, Dong J, Schreieck J, et al. Delineation of intra-atrial reentrant tachycardia circuits after mustard operation for transposition of the great arteries using biatrial electroanatomic mapping and entrainment mapping. J Cardiovasc Electrophysiol 2003;14:1302–10.

48. Lukac P, Pedersen AK, Mortensen PT, et al. Ablation of atrial tachycardia after surgery for congenital and acquired heart disease using an electroanatomic mapping system: which circuits to expect in which substrate? Heart Rhythm 2005; 2:64–72.

49. Dong J, Zrenner B, Schreieck J, et al. Necessity for biatrial ablation to achieve bidirectional cavotricuspid isthmus conduction block in a patient following Senning operation. J Cardiovasc Electrophysiol 2004;15:945–9.

50. Balaji S, Stajduhar KC, Zarraga IG, et al. Simplified demonstration of cavotricuspid isthmus block after catheter ablation in patients after Mustard's operation. Pacing Clin Electrophysiol 2009;32: 1294–8.

51. Jongbloed MR, Kelder TP, DEN Uijl DW, et al. Anatomical perspective on radiofrequency ablation of AV nodal reentry tachycardia after Mustard correction for transposition of the great arteries. Pacing Clin Electrophysiol 2012;35:e287–90.

Development of Tachyarrhythmias Late After the Fontan Procedure
The Role of Ablative Therapy

Natasja M.S. de Groot, MD, PhD*, Ad J.J.C. Bogers, MD, PhD

KEYWORDS

• Ablative therapy • Fontan procedure • Tachyarrhythmia • Atrial • Ventricular

KEY POINTS

- Patients with a Fontan circulation seem to be at high risk of developing a variety of atrial tachyarrhythmias (ATs) and ventricular tachycardias (VTs) at a relatively young age.
- The mechanisms underlying AT are variable, including both ectopic activity and reentry.
- Over time, successive AT may be caused by different mechanisms.
- The acute success rate of ablative therapy for AT is considerably high, yet, during long-term follow-up, recurrences frequently occur.
- It is most likely that these recurrences are caused by a progressive atrial cardiomyopathy rather than arrhythmogenicity of prior ablative lesions.

INTRODUCTION

In 1971, Francis Fontan and colleagues[1,2] from Bordeaux were the first to report on a new operation for patients with a single functional ventricle. The initial procedure was aimed at redirecting systemic venous blood directly into the pulmonary circulation without passing through the subpulmonary ventricle by constructing a connection between the right atrium and pulmonary artery.[1,2] Ever since, numerous modifications have been made to this procedure. Patients with a Fontan circulation are at high risk for developing a variety of cardiac dysrhythmias after cardiac surgery.[3] These dysrhythmias are most often supraventricular tachyarrhythmias (SVTs) but ventricular tachyarrhythmias may occur as well.[4] The quality of life of Fontan patients with tachyarrhythmias is often seriously affected by recurrent symptoms, such as fatigue, palpitations, and syncope. In addition, they may cause severe complications, such as hemodynamic deterioration, thromboembolic events, and even sudden cardiac death. In Fontan patients who died of heart failure, approximately 90% had SVTs.[5] The morbidity and mortality associated with tachyarrhythmias in this patient group justify close follow-up and aggressive arrhythmia therapy.

INDICATIONS FOR THE FONTAN PROCEDURE

In patients with single ventricle physiology, the most commonly applied therapy is surgical palliation by a Fontan procedure.[1,2] In this regard, the term *Fontan procedure* includes all variants of circulation in which the systemic venous return passes through the pulmonary vascular bed without the driving force of a subpulmonary ventricle. Over time, several determinants for successful outcome have been defined.[6] Essentially, the most important determinant is the pulmonary vascular bed. Preferably, the pulmonary vascular

Department of Cardiology, Erasmus Medical Center, s'Gravendijkwal 230, Rotterdam 3015CE, Netherlands
* Corresponding author.
E-mail address: n.m.s.degroot@erasmusmc.nl

Card Electrophysiol Clin 9 (2017) 273–284
http://dx.doi.org/10.1016/j.ccep.2017.02.009
1877-9182/17/© 2017 Elsevier Inc. All rights reserved.

bed should have normal anatomy and a low or normal vascular resistance and the systemic ventricle should have a good function with no regurgitation of the atrioventricular valves. In combination with sinus rhythm, this provides the best pull function of the systemic ventricle with limited increase of central venous (pulmonary arterial) pressure as the driving force of the pulmonary circulation.

DIFFERENT TYPES OF FONTAN PROCEDURES

Originally, Fontan and Baudet[1] described their operation for palliation of tricuspid atresia as a single-stage atriopulmonary or atrioventricular connection. Although a Fontan circulation with an atriopulmonary or atrioventricular connection may be initially successful, many patients developed complications during long-term follow-up. Most of all, this concerns progressive right atrial dilatation and consequently atrial tachyarrhythmias (ATs), resulting in a loss of atrial transport function and a further decrease of cardiac output in these patients.

The total cavo-pulmonary connection (TCPC) was introduced in an attempt to overcome this problem.[7] Designed as a single-stage operation, nowadays most surgical centers apply the staged approach, with a partial cavo-pulmonary connection (of which several variants exist) in the first year of life to divert the superior caval blood directly to the pulmonary circulation. The Fontan circulation is completed in a separate operation to a TCPC by directing the inferior caval blood to the pulmonary circulation as well.[8]

This procedure is accomplished by an intra-atrial lateral tunnel, which has the advantage of growth potential. However, it needs intracardiac surgery with extracorporal circulation. Fontan completion can also be done with an extracardiac conduit, which has the disadvantage of a fixed (sometimes gradually declining) diameter and may lead to suboptimal hemodynamics.

However, an extracardiac conduit does not require open-heart surgery or extracorporal circulation. Apart from the scars of previous surgical procedures and the closing line of the superior and inferior caval vein, no additional intra-atrial scars are introduced. Whether the extracardiac conduit approach truly reduces the incidence of late atrial arrhythmias is still a matter of debate.[9,10]

Atrial dilatation and supraventricular arrhythmias were increasingly observed during long-term follow-up of patients with an atriopulmonary and atrioventricular Fontan circulation.

One option for patients who develop significant hemodynamic or arrhythmic problems after a classic atriopulmonary or atrioventricular Fontan is to perform an operation to convert them to a TCPC, either with a lateral intra-atrial tunnel or with an extracardiac conduit.[11–15]

PATHOPHYSIOLOGY OF SUPRAVENTRICULAR TACHYARRHYTHMIAS

Tachyarrhythmias are generally caused by abnormalities in either impulse formation (ectopic activity caused by triggered activity or enhanced automaticity) or impulse conduction (reentry). In patients with a Fontan circulation, SVTs are most often ATs, including intra-atrial reentrant tachycardia (IART), type I typical atrial flutter (AFL) or atrial fibrillation (AF); focal atrial tachycardias (FATs) have been less frequently observed.[16,17] Atrioventricular (nodal) reentrant tachycardia has, to the authors' knowledge, only been described in case reports.[18,19] Risk factors for SVT in patients with a Fontan circulation include right atrial enlargement, elevated atrial pressure, dispersion of atrial refractoriness, sinus node dysfunction, older age at the time of cardiac surgery, elevation of pulmonary pressure, low oxygen saturation, preoperative arrhythmias, prior palliation with an atrial septectomy, atrioventricular valve replacement, and aging.[20–22] The type of surgical technique used may also be related with the incidence of SVT. In 1991, Balaji and colleagues[23] found a lower incidence of late postoperative AT in patients who underwent a total cavo-pulmonary connection compared with patients who had a direct atriopulmonary connection. This observation was attributed to the lower right atrial pressure and subsequent atrial wall distension in patients with a total cavo-pulmonary connection.

In patients with a Fontan circulation, precipitating factors for development of reentrant tachycardias are the presence of prosthetic materials, electropathologic alterations of the atrial myocardium and chronic bradycardia due to damage to the sinus node, the sinus node artery, or usage of β-blocking drugs.[4,24] The myocardium is further affected by an ongoing pressure/volume overload and progressive scarring along suture lines or atriotomies. These structural changes cause intra-atrial conduction delay and regional differences in dispersion of atrial refractoriness. Local conduction abnormalities combined with a higher incidence of premature atrial beats due to stretch of myocardial fibers make these patients more prone to development of SVT.

MACRO-REENTRANT TACHYCARDIAS

As demonstrated in the left panel of **Fig. 1**, endovascular mapping studies before ablation of AT in patients with a Fontan circulation described as peri-tricuspid, counterclockwise rotation of a

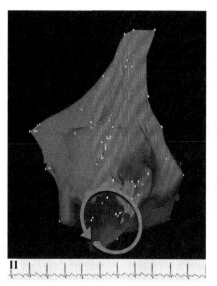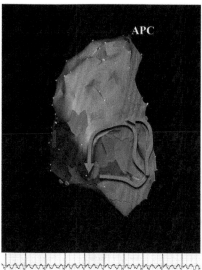

Fig. 1. Macro-reentrant tachycardias observed in patients with a Fontan circulation include typical, cavo-tricuspid isthmus-dependent AFL (*left panel*, *left-anterior-oblique view*), and IARTs involving areas of scar tissue (*right panel*, *anteroposterior view*) and corresponding surface electrocardiograms (lead II). The blue arrows indicate the main activation direction, and the gray areas indicate sites with peak-to-peak amplitudes of 0.1 mV or less. APC, atriopulmonary conduit.

reentrant wave front activating the septum and posterior wall in a caudo-cranial direction and the lateral and anterior wall in a craniocaudal direction.[17,25] The anterior and posterior boundaries of this circuit consisted of areas of conduction block between the venae cava. Thus, this typical counterclockwise AFL, which also occurs in humans without congenital heart disease, can develop in patients with a Fontan circulation as well, although in a minority of the cases.[17]

Most ATs in Fontan patients are due to macro-reentrant circuits bordered by prosthetic materials, scar tissue, suture lines, or anatomic structures (see right panel of **Fig. 1**).[16,17]

A so-called IART is shown in **Fig. 2**. The reentrant circuit of an IART often contains numerous corridors and dead-end pathways embedded within areas of scar tissue. Because of the extensiveness of multiple areas of scar tissue scattered throughout the dilated atria, multiple reentrant circuits are often possible. In 21 patients with a Fontan circulation who underwent ablative therapy for symptomatic drug-refractory SVT, crucial pathways of the reentrant circuits targeted for ablation were bordered by either areas of scar tissue (N = 18, 86%) or by areas of scar tissue and anatomic structures, such as the inferior caval vein (N = 3, 14%).

FOCAL ATRIAL TACHYCARDIAS

FATs have also been observed in patients with a Fontan circulation, though they occur less frequently

then macro-reentrant tachycardias. A FAT is defined as an AT originating from a circumscribed region from where it expands centrifugally to the remainder of the atrium, as demonstrated in **Fig. 3**.[26] Spread of the activation from the focal area does not necessarily have to be radially as conduction can be interrupted and directed by barriers such as areas of scar tissue or surgically prosthetic materials. When intra-atrial conduction is severely impaired, the surface electrocardiogram (ECG) may show

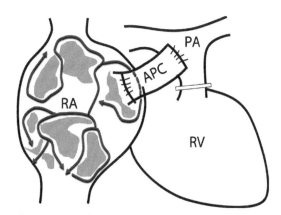

Fig. 2. The cardiac anatomy of a patient with a Fontan circulation. In the enlarged atria, there are multiple corridors bordered by areas of scar tissue. Hence, there are numerous circuits possible, as indicated by the red arrows. APC, atriopulmonary conduit; PA, pulmonary artery; RA, right atrium; RV, right ventricle.

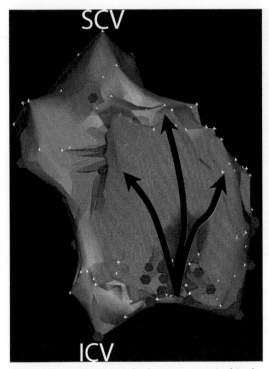

Fig. 3. Three-dimensional electro-anatomic bipolar activation map of the right atrium of a Fontan patient demonstrating a FAT originating in the lower part of the anterior wall. The electrical activation originates from a small, circumscribed region from where it spreads in all directions. ICV, inferior caval vein; SCV, superior caval vein.

more flutterlike patterns without isoelectric intervals between the consecutive ectopic P waves.

The mechanism underlying FAT in patients with congenital heart disease, whether it is due to ectopic activity or microreentry, is still a matter of debate. FAT in Fontan patients may be caused by triggered activity in response to atrial stretch due to the ongoing pressure/volume overload. Mapping studies have demonstrated that in patients with a Fontan circulation, FAT not only arise from the known predilection sites of FAT in normal hearts but also from sites nearby surgically created barriers.[26] It has been suggested that FAT originates from areas with nonuniform anisotropic properties where cell-to-cell uncoupling by, for example, deposition of fibrotic tissue diminishes electrotonic inhibition thereby allowing a rapidly discharging focus to become apparent. The role of microreentry as the underlying mechanism is supported by the observation that electrograms recorded from the earliest site of activation during FAT consist of fractionated, low amplitude potentials or even continuous electrical activity, as shown in **Figs. 4** and **5**.[27]

These fractionated potentials are caused by asynchronous activation of neighboring cardiomyocytes. In patients with congenital heart disease and FAT, including patients with a Fontan circulation, comparison of electrogram morphologies obtained from the area of earliest activation with sites located at a distance of at least 2 cm away showed that electrograms from the focal area were indeed characterized by higher incidences of fractionated potentials, prolonged fractionation durations, and lower peak-to-peak amplitudes.[27]

ATRIAL FIBRILLATION

Teuwen and colleagues[28] examined the time course of AF episodes in a large cohort of patients with a various congenital heart defects including 11 patients with uni-ventricular hearts who were palliated with a Fontan circulation. As shown in **Fig. 6**, AF in these patients was first documented at 28 ± 9 years of age and occurred 23 ± 9 years after the first surgical procedure. Thus, AF in patients with a Fontan circulation develops at a much younger age than in the normal population. So far, only one study has reported on the mechanism underlying AF in a patient with a Fontan circulation.[29] The patient presented with a surface ECG of AF and had an area of continuous electrical activity at the interatrial septum. By creating a circular lesion around the area of continuous electrical activity, AF was eliminated. This observation suggests the presence of a microreentrant circuit causing fibrillatory conduction.

COEXISTENT ATRIAL FIBRILLATION AND ATRIAL TACHYARRHYTHMIA

Teuwen and coinvestigators[28] also found that in 7 Fontan patients, episodes of AF and regular AT were alternatingly documented; an example is given in **Fig. 7**. The upper panel shows the surface ECG obtained from a 26-year-old Fontan patient who presented with collapse at the emergency department. She was born with tricuspid valve atresia, transposition of the great arteries, atrial septal defect, multiple ventricular septal defects, and pulmonary stenosis and had undergone a modified Fontan procedure (connection between the right atrium and pulmonary artery). The ECG clearly showed AF. After electrical cardioversion, she had sinus rhythm and was discharged from the hospital without any antiarrhythmic drugs. Four months later, she presented again at the emergency department with complaints of palpitations, dyspnea, and near collapse. Interestingly, her ECG then showed a regular AT, as demonstrated in the lower panel

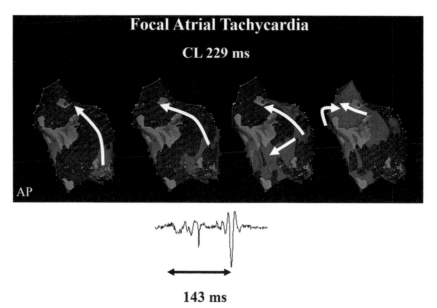

Focal Atrial Tachycardia

CL 229 ms

AP

143 ms

Fig. 4. Three-dimensional electro-anatomic propagation map of the right atrium obtained from a patient with a Fontan circulation shown in an anteroposterior (AP) view. Mapping revealed an FAT with a cycle length (CL) of 229 milliseconds. The red color indicates propagation of the activation wave front, and the white arrows indicate the main activation direction. The duration of the electrogram recorded at the site of earliest activation was considerably prolonged and had a duration of 143 milliseconds, thereby covering 62% of the tachycardia CL.

of **Fig. 7**. At ablation, mapping revealed an IART around an area of scar tissue. However, despite a successful ablation procedure, she still regularly presents at the emergency department with either episodes of AF or a regular AT, despite the use of antiarrhythmic drugs.

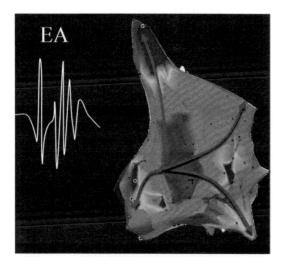

EA

Fig. 5. Three-dimensional electro-anatomic bipolar activation map of the right atrium obtained from a Fontan patient (*right lateral view*) demonstrating an FAT originating from the lateral free wall. The bipolar electrogram recorded from the earliest activated (EA) site is clearly fractionated. Red arrows indicate the main activation directions.

THERAPY FOR ATRIAL TACHYARRHYTHMIAS

ATs after the Fontan procedure are difficult to manage.[23] Treatment modalities for AT in Fontan patients include antiarrhythmic drug therapy, an atrial defibrillator, antitachycardia pacing, conversion surgery, and catheter ablation. Most ATs in Fontan patients are drug refractory; in addition to this, antiarrhythmic drugs may be proarrhythmic, negative inotropic, and may aggravate sinus and AV node dysfunction. Antitachycardia pacing is also frequently ineffective; it can accelerate the AT and increases the risk of conversion of AT to AF. Considering the low success rates of these treatment modalities combined with the ongoing evolution in mapping and ablation technologies, catheter ablation is a good alternative therapy for elimination of postoperative AT in Fontan patients.

ELECTRO-ANATOMIC ACTIVATION MAPPING

Catheter ablation of AT in patients with a Fontan circulation is challenging because of the enlarged atria and the distorted anatomy. The success rate of ablative therapy is determined by the capability to accurately identify the arrhythmogenic substrate and to depict target sites for ablation. This can, however, be time consuming and difficult in this specific patient group. In the past decades, numerous tools to facilitate both mapping and

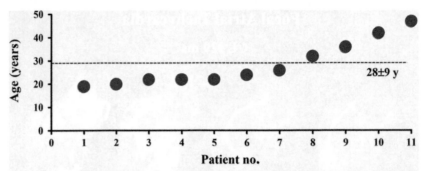

Fig. 6. Age at first documented AF episode in 11 Fontan patients; patients are ranked according to an increase in age. The average age of AF onset was 28 years.

ablative therapy have been introduced in order to improve procedural outcomes.[30,31] Three-dimensional electro-anatomic contact or noncontact mapping systems visualize the activation wave front in a 3-dimensional reconstruction of the atria, including the presence of areas of scar tissue, prior incision sites, or prosthetic materials, such as atriopulmonary conduits. In addition, fusion with computed tomography scan images further facilitates real-time navigation of the ablation catheter through the atria by demonstrating their true anatomy.

As most ATs in patients with a Fontan circulation are caused by intra-atrial reentry circuits embedded within scar tissue, accurate delineation of scar tissue is an essential step in the mapping procedure before selection of suitable target sites for ablation.

ELECTRO-ANATOMIC VOLTAGE MAPPING

In literature, different cutoff values of peak-to-peak amplitudes of bipolar electrograms have been used for identification of areas of scar tissue.[32,33]

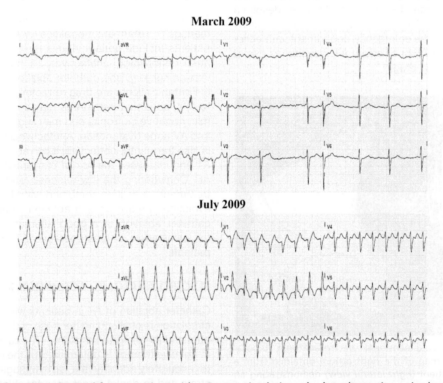

Fig. 7. Surface ECGs obtained from a patient with a Fontan circulation who has alternating episodes of AF and regular AT. Initially, she presented with AF, which was successfully cardioverted to sinus rhythm. As this was her first episode, she did not receive any antiarrhythmic drugs. A few months later, she presented again, with a regular AT. Mapping of this AT revealed an IART as the underlying mechanism.

By comparing atrial bipolar voltage distributions during various SVTs between patients with and without congenital heart disease, it seemed that bipolar voltages of 0.1 mV or less were never recorded in the latter group (**Fig. 8**).[32] This value was, therefore, used as the upper limit of the lowest voltage areas in patients with congenital heart disease in order to discriminate between healthy and diseased myocardium. Scar tissue delineation with the 0.1-mV cutoff value combined with activation mapping and entrainment techniques were used to accurately facilitate selection of target sites for ablation. Voltage-based scar tissue delineation was only possible with bipolar electrograms and was not possible with unipolar electrograms. **Fig. 9** shows an example of a right atrial bipolar voltage maps constructed during IART obtained from a patient with a tricuspid atresia palliated with an atriopulmonary conduit, shown in an anterior and posterior view. The gray colored areas (scar) represent sites from which bipolar electrograms with an amplitude of 0.1 mV or less were recorded. The lower panel shows that in a group of 5 patients with a Fontan circulation, the highest amount of scar tissue areas was found at

the posterior quadrants. A possible explanation could be that the elevated intra-atrial pressure stretches the thinner, posterior wall more than the thicker, trabeculated, anterolateral wall. Identification of scar tissue can be further improved by the use of contact force sensing catheters, which ensure stable contact between the atrial wall and the tip of the catheter.

OUTCOME OF ABLATIVE THERAPY

Though many studies have reported on the outcome of ablative therapy on SVT in large cohorts of patients with a variety of congenital heart defects including patients with Fontan circulation, only a few studies described success rates of ablative therapy and long-term outcome specifically in patients with a Fontan circulation.[16,23,34]

In a European multicenter study, 19 patients (aged 29 ± 9 years) with uni-ventricular hearts (tricuspid atresia: 13, mitral atresia and double outlet right ventricle: 3, double inlet ventricle: 3) and late, postoperative SVT were followed on average 53 ± 34 months after the first ablation procedure. SVTs developed 18 ± 9 years after the first surgical

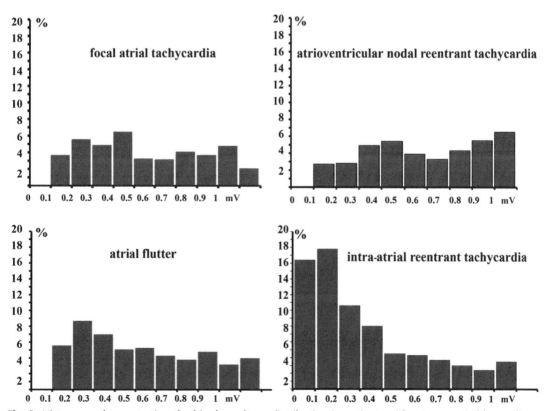

Fig. 8. Histograms demonstrating the bipolar voltage distribution in patients without congenital heart disease during AF, FAT, or atrioventricular nodal reentrant tachycardia and during IART in patients with a variety of congenital heart defects. Bipolar voltages of 0.1 mV or less were only recorded in patients with IARTs.

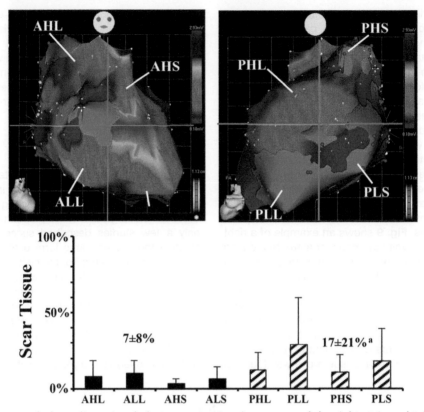

Fig. 9. Upper panel: three-dimensional electro-anatomic voltage maps of the right atrium obtained from a Fontan patient during an IART in an anteroposterior view (*left panel*) and the posterior-anterior view (*right panel*). Maps are subdivided into 8 quadrants, including anterior-high-lateral (AHL), anterior-high-septal (AHS), anterior-low-lateral (ALL), anterior-low-septal (ALS), posterior-high-lateral (PHL), posterior-high-septal (PHS), posterior-low-lateral (PLL), and posterior low-septal (PLS). Lower panel: The bars indicate the percentage of bipolar voltages less than 0.1 mV in each of the 8 quadrants in 5 Fontan patients; bipolar voltages recorded at the posterior quadrants were significantly lower than in the anterior quadrants. [a] $P<.001$.

procedure, and ablation was performed 6 ± 5 years after the initial SVT episode. In these 19 patients, a total of 41 SVTs were mapped and subsequently ablated during 38 different ablation procedures. Mechanisms underlying these SVTs were AFL (N = 4), IART (N = 30), FAT (N = 6), and AF (N = 1). Ten patients underwent multiple ablation procedures. Of interest is that mapping revealed that these SVTs were caused by different mechanisms in 6 patients. For example, a patient first presented with an IART that was successfully ablated during the next ablation procedure, mapping revealed an FAT originating from an area remote from the initial intraatrial reentry circuit. These observations suggest that the recurrent SVTs were caused by a progressive atrial cardiomyopathy instead of an unsuccessful ablation procedure or arrhythmogenicity of prior ablative lesions. However, despite many recurrences, 72% of the patients were still in sinus rhythm during long-term follow-up.

Yap and colleagues[16] also evaluated the long-term outcome of ablative therapy in 11 patients (aged 33 ± 9 years) with an atriopulmonary or atrioventricular connection during a follow-up period of 2.3 ± 1.6 years. All patients had an IART of which 6 were successfully ablated (defined as noninducibility), and the cumulative IART recurrence rate at 2 years was 50%.

A retrospective, 20 years' follow-up study of 162 Fontan patients with either an atriopulmonary or atrioventricular connection found that 18.5% (N = 30) of the Fontan survivors developed paroxysmal or incessant ATs. Mapping before ablation revealed that the critical isthmuses of these ATs were mainly located at the region between the inferior caval vein and either the tricuspid annulus or the inferior border of the lateral atriotomy scar. Ablative therapy was successful in 25 (83%) patients; at 3 years' follow-up, the Kaplan-Meier estimates for freedom of tachycardia in patients with an initially successful ablation was 81%.[34]

The long-term outcome of ablative therapy of AT in patients with a Fontan circulation is complicated by many recurrences during long-term follow-up. In one Fontan patient, even 7 procedures within 6 years have been described.[29] The development of different tachycardias in this Fontan patient during a follow-up period of 6 years is shown in **Fig. 10**. She was born in 1972 with a type IB tricuspid atresia and underwent a Fontan procedure at 6 years of age. The Fontan procedure consisted of placement of a conduit between the right atrium and right ventricular outflow tract. Ten years later she underwent a surgical procedure in order to modify a stenotic part of the conduit. She developed SVT at 23 years of age; 1 year later she underwent ablative therapy, as the arrhythmia could not be controlled with antiarrhythmic drugs. Between 1996 and 2005, she underwent ablative therapy for 9 different SVTs, including 5 IARTs, 3 FATs, and 1 AF. In this patient, focal activity not only resulted in an FAT but also in AF. Except for 2 IARTs, all ATs were successfully ablated. Two years after the last ablation procedure, she underwent cardiac surgery during which an extracardiac conduit was placed between the superior caval vein and pulmonary artery and she has been free of AT ever since.

The bars in **Fig. 10** demonstrate a steady increase in the amount of scar tissue from ATs No. 2 to 9. (The IART was ablated without the use of a 3-dimensional electro-anatomic mapping technique.) The locations of all successful target sites for ablation are depicted in the schematic presentation of the right atrium. As can be seen, the arrhythmogenic substrate of the 9 successive ATs are located at different sites, indicating that these recurrent ATs are caused by a progressive cardiomyopathy.

Moore and colleagues[35] recently investigated the arrhythmogenic substrate underlying AT in 36 patients who had an extracardiac TCPC. A total of 46 ablation procedures in these patients showed that most of the ATs were IARTs with a crucial pathway of conduction located between the atrioventricular valve annulus and the oversewn inferior caval vein. The reported success rate was 83%, with a 17% recurrence rate during a median follow-up duration of 0.4 years.

SURGICAL MAZE IN FONTAN PATIENTS

The TCPC, either with a lateral intra-atrial tunnel or with an extracardiac conduit, is used as a conversion option for the failing atriopulmonary connection or atrioventricular connection.[11–15,36]

At the moment of conversion, ATs are additionally being treated by excision of a greater part of

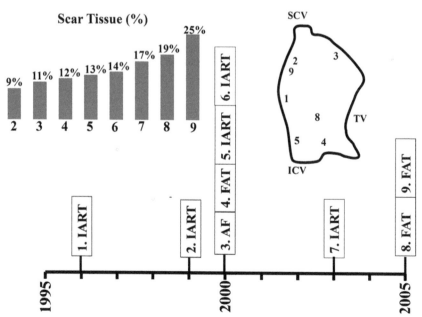

Fig. 10. Timeline demonstrating development of 9 different types of AT over time. The bars in the upper right corner demonstrate the percentage of electrograms with peak-to-peak voltages 0.1 mV or less recorded during the AT. The right atrium demonstrates all successful ablation sites. ICV, inferior caval vein; SCV, superior caval vein; TV, tricuspid valve.

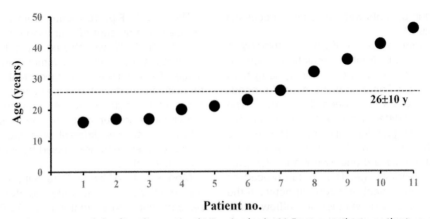

Fig. 11. Age at the moment of the first documented VT episodes in 11 Fontan patients; patients are ranked according to an increase in age. The average age of VT onset was 26 years.

the dilated right atrial free wall and by intraoperative ablation of potential circuits of ATs. Intraoperative ablation consists of a right-sided maze operation for AFL or the Cox-Maze-III procedure for AF.[37] In addition, some investigators recommend placement of an epicardial pacemaker system for further management of arrhythmias.[13,15] The rationale is that transvenous access to the heart after surgery is not possible anymore and that frequent conversion concerns a more than once repeated sternotomy. After conversion to a TCPC, most patients improve in New York Heart Association class.[12] This improvement may, however, take up to a year after surgery. Without antiarrhythmia surgery, the reported recurrence rate of AT is up to 76%. In addition, conversion surgery appears to be able to restore atrial transport function, which is essential in the Fontan circulation.[38]

Important issues that may limit the success rate of surgical ablation in this regard are the type of AF, the duration of AF, the size of the (remaining) left and right atria or single atrium, the anatomy and function of the systemic ventricle, the technique and procedure applied for curing AF, and the presence of clots in the left or single atrial appendage.

VENTRICULAR TACHYARRHYTHMIAS

Reports on development of ventricular tachyarrhythmias after Fontan repair are rare. It is generally assumed that most sudden cardiac arrests in patients with congenital heart defects are caused by ventricular tachycardias (VTs), ventricular fibrillation, or atrioventricular conduction block.

A recent study reported that 13% of the 180 patients with a Fontan circulation had a sudden cardiac arrest at an average of 28 years of age (23–36 years) during a long-term follow-up period of 22 years.[4]

In a cohort of 32 patients undergoing Fontan repair, 24-hour Holter monitoring 1 day before and after the surgical procedure showed VT in only one patient.[24]

Teuwen and colleagues[39] investigated the development of late postoperative VT after Fontan repair. The time course of VT was retrospectively studied in 145 patients with a variety of congenital heart defects, including 11 patients with univentricular hearts who had a Fontan repair. These 11 patients presented first with either nonsustained VTs (N = 8) or sustained VTs (N = 3). As demonstrated in **Fig. 11**, these VTs developed at 26 ± 10 years of age (16–46 years). An implantable cardiac defibrillator (ICD) was implanted in 3 patients with sustained VTs. During a follow-up period of 4 years on average after the initial presentation with VTs, none of the patients had sustained VTs. Only one patient received an ICD shock, which was inappropriate and caused by SVT.

SUMMARY

Patients with a Fontan circulation seem to be at high risk of developing a variety of ATs and VTs at a relatively young age. The mechanisms underlying AT are variable, including both ectopic activity and reentry. Over time, successive AT may be caused by different mechanisms. The acute success rate of ablative therapy of AT is considerably high, yet during long-term follow-up, recurrences frequently occur. It is most likely that these recurrences are caused by a progressive atrial cardiomyopathy rather than arrhythmogenicity of prior ablative lesions.

ACKNOWLEDGMENTS

The authors would like to thank Dr C. Teuwen for his help with this article.

REFERENCES

1. Fontan F, Baudet E. Surgical repair of tricuspid atresia. Thorax 1971;26(3):240–8.

2. Fontan F, Mounicot FB, Baudet E, et al. "Correction" de l'atresie tricuspidienne. Rapport de deux cas "corriges" par l'utilisation d'une technique chirurgicale nouvelle. Ann Chir Thorac Cardiovasc 1971; 10(1):39–47.

3. Driscoll DJ, Offord KP, Feldt RH, et al. Five- to fifteen-year follow-up after Fontan operation. Circulation 1992;85(2):469–96.

4. Pundi KN, Pundi KN, Johnson JN, et al. Sudden cardiac death and late arrhythmias after the Fontan operation. Congenit Heart Dis 2017;12(1):17–23.

5. Piran S, Veldtman G, Siu S, et al. Heart failure and ventricular dysfunction in patients with single or systemic right ventricles. Circulation 2002;105(10): 1189–94.

6. Fontan F, Kirklin JW, Fernandez G, et al. Outcome after a "perfect" Fontan operation. Circulation 1990; 81(5):1520–36.

7. de Leval MR, Kilner P, Gewillig M, et al. Total cavopulmonary connection: a logical alternative to atriopulmonary connection for complex Fontan operations. Experimental studies and early clinical experience. J Thorac Cardiovasc Surg 1988;96(5):682–95.

8. Talwar S, Nair VV, Choudhary SK, et al. The hemi-Fontan operation: a critical overview. Ann Pediatr Cardiol 2014;7(2):120–5.

9. Robbers-Visser D, Miedema M, Nijveld A, et al. Results of staged total cavopulmonary connection for functionally univentricular hearts; comparison of intra-atrial lateral tunnel and extracardiac conduit. Eur J Cardiothorac Surg 2010;37(4):934–41.

10. Bossers SS, Duppen N, Kapusta L, et al. Comprehensive rhythm evaluation in a large contemporary Fontan population. Eur J Cardiothorac Surg 2015; 48(6):833–40 [discussion: 40–1].

11. Park HK, Shin HJ, Park YH. Outcomes of Fontan conversion for failing Fontan circulation: mid-term results. Interact Cardiovasc Thorac Surg 2016;23(1):14–7.

12. Ono M, Cleuziou J, Kasnar-Samprec J, et al. Conversion to total cavopulmonary connection improves functional status even in older patients with failing Fontan circulation. Thorac Cardiovasc Surg 2015; 63(5):380–7.

13. Terada T, Sakurai H, Nonaka T, et al. Surgical outcome of Fontan conversion and arrhythmia surgery: need a pacemaker? Asian Cardiovasc Thorac Ann 2014;22(6):682–6.

14. Jang WS, Kim WH, Choi K, et al. The mid-term surgical results of Fontan conversion with antiarrhythmia surgery. Eur J Cardiothorac Surg 2014;45(5): 922–7.

15. Hiramatsu T, Iwata Y, Matsumura G, et al. Impact of Fontan conversion with arrhythmia surgery and pacemaker therapy. Eur J Cardiothorac Surg 2011; 40(4):1007–10.

16. Yap SC, Harris L, Downar E, et al. Evolving electroanatomic substrate and intra-atrial reentrant tachycardia late after Fontan surgery. J Cardiovasc Electrophysiol 2012;23(4):339–45.

17. de Groot NM, Lukac P, Blom NA, et al. Long-term outcome of ablative therapy of postoperative supraventricular tachycardias in patients with univentricular heart: a European multicenter study. Circ Arrhythm Electrophysiol 2009;2(3):242–8.

18. Arana-Rueda E, Pedrote A, Duran-Guerrero JM, et al. Simplified approach for ablation of nodal reentrant tachycardia in a patient with tricuspid atresia and extracardiac Fontan palliation. Rev Esp Cardiol (Engl Ed) 2013;66(4):314–6.

19. Arana-Rueda E, Pedrote A, Sanchez-Brotons JA, et al. Ablation of atrioventricular nodal reentrant tachycardia in a patient with tricuspid atresia guided by electroanatomic mapping. Pacing Clin Electrophysiol 2012;35(10):e293–5.

20. Cecchin F, Johnsrude CL, Perry JC, et al. Effect of age and surgical technique on symptomatic arrhythmias after the Fontan procedure. Am J Cardiol 1995; 76(5):386–91.

21. Gelatt M, Hamilton RM, McCrindle BW, et al. Risk factors for atrial tachyarrhythmias after the Fontan operation. J Am Coll Cardiol 1994;24(7):1735–41.

22. Agnoletti G, Borghi A, Vignati G, et al. Fontan conversion to total cavopulmonary connection and arrhythmia ablation: clinical and functional results. Heart 2003;89(2):193–8.

23. Balaji S, Gewillig M, Bull C, et al. Arrhythmias after the Fontan procedure. Comparison of total cavopulmonary connection and atriopulmonary connection. Circulation 1991;84(5 Suppl):III162–7.

24. Kurer CC, Tanner CS, Vetter VL. Electrophysiologic findings after Fontan repair of functional single ventricle. J Am Coll Cardiol 1991;17(1):174–81.

25. Akar JG, Kok LC, Haines DE, et al. Coexistence of type I atrial flutter and intra-atrial re-entrant tachycardia in patients with surgically corrected congenital heart disease. J Am Coll Cardiol 2001;38(2):377–84.

26. de Groot NM, Zeppenfeld K, Wijffels MC, et al. Ablation of focal atrial arrhythmia in patients with congenital heart defects after surgery: role of circumscribed areas with heterogeneous conduction. Heart Rhythm 2006;3(5):526–35.

27. De Groot NM, Schalij MJ. Fragmented, long-duration, low-amplitude electrograms characterize the origin of focal atrial tachycardia. J Cardiovasc Electrophysiol 2006;17(10):1086–92.

28. Teuwen CP, Ramdjan TT, Gotte M, et al. Time course of atrial fibrillation in patients with congenital heart defects. Circ Arrhythm Electrophysiol 2015;8(5):1065–72.

29. De Groot NM, Blom N, Vd Wall EE, et al. Different mechanisms underlying consecutive, postoperative

atrial tachyarrhythmias in a Fontan patient. Pacing Clin Electrophysiol 2009;32(11):e18–20.

30. Dorostkar PC, Cheng J, Scheinman MM. Electroanatomical mapping and ablation of the substrate supporting intraatrial reentrant tachycardia after palliation for complex congenital heart disease. Pacing Clin Electrophysiol 1998;21(9):1810–9.

31. Ellison KE, Friedman PL, Ganz LI, et al. Entrainment mapping and radiofrequency catheter ablation of ventricular tachycardia in right ventricular dysplasia. J Am Coll Cardiol 1998;32(3):724–8.

32. De Groot NM, Kuijper AF, Blom NA, et al. Three-dimensional distribution of bipolar atrial electrogram voltages in patients with congenital heart disease. Pacing Clin Electrophysiol 2001;24(9 Pt 1):1334–42.

33. de Groot NM, Schalij MJ, Zeppenfeld K, et al. Voltage and activation mapping: how the recording technique affects the outcome of catheter ablation procedures in patients with congenital heart disease. Circulation 2003;108(17):2099–106.

34. Weipert J, Noebauer C, Schreiber C, et al. Occurrence and management of atrial arrhythmia after long-term Fontan circulation. J Thorac Cardiovasc Surg 2004;127(2):457–64.

35. Moore JP, Shannon KM, Fish FA, et al. Catheter ablation of supraventricular tachyarrhythmia after extracardiac Fontan surgery. Heart Rhythm 2016;13(9):1891–7.

36. Mavroudis C, Backer CL, Deal BJ, et al. Fontan conversion to cavopulmonary connection and arrhythmia circuit cryoblation. J Thorac Cardiovasc Surg 1998;115(3):547–56.

37. Backer CL, Deal BJ, Mavroudis C, et al. Conversion of the failed Fontan circulation. Cardiol Young 2006;16(Suppl 1):85–91.

38. Bogers AJ, Kik C, de Jong PL, et al. Recovery of atrial transport function after a maze procedure for atrial fibrillation in conversion of a failing Fontan circulation. Neth Heart J 2008;16(5):170–2.

39. Teuwen CP, Ramdjan TT, Gotte M, et al. Non-sustained ventricular tachycardia in patients with congenital heart disease: an important sign? Int J Cardiol 2016;206:158–63.

Clinical Aspects and Ablation of Ventricular Arrhythmias in Tetralogy of Fallot

Katja Zeppenfeld, MD, PhD*,
Adrianus P. Wijnmaalen, MD, PhD

KEYWORDS

- Tetralogy of Fallot • Ventricular tachycardia • Risk stratification • Electroanatomical mapping
- Anatomic isthmus • Radiofrequency catheter ablation

KEY POINTS

- Changes in type and timing of surgical repair in tetralogy of Fallot (ToF) are likely to influence the potential substrate for late ventricular arrhythmias (VAs).
- Monomorphic ventricular tachycardia (MVT) is the most common arrhythmia subtype in repaired ToF (rToF).
- MVTs are usually fast and require a substrate-based ablation approach.
- Complete procedural success defined as noninducibility of any VT and transection of the slow conducting anatomic isthmus can be considered curative in patients with preserved cardiac function and no competing VA mechanism.
- The advances made in the understanding of the substrate for VT in rToF may have important implications for risk stratification and preventive treatment in contemporary patients with ToF.

INTRODUCTION

The reported incidence of tetralogy of Fallot (ToF) is approximately 0.42 per 1000 live births and has remained stable over time.[1] Life expectancy, however, has significantly improved over the last decades. Seventy-eight percent of all individuals born with ToF between 1990 and 1992 followed at one European center survived into adulthood, which is significantly better compared with patients born in preceding years.[2] The change in mortality, with favorable survival in infancy and a trend toward death at older age, is likely the result of earlier and improved surgical interventions and medical care. However, despite early repair, these patients are not cured and the improved long-term outcome generates new challenges.[3]

VENTRICULAR ARRHYTHMIAS

An age-dependent increase in the prevalence of atrial and ventricular arrhythmias (VAs) has been reported[4,5] with a high arrhythmia burden for both atrial and VAs. In contrast to other repaired congenital heart diseases, ventricular tachycardia (VT) is the most common arrhythmia subtype with a prevalence of 14.2%.[6] The prevalence of ventricular fibrillation (VF) was only 0.5% in a large North American collaboration study.[6] Although VF may be underestimated in this cohort, including adult survivors, with implantable cardioverter defibrillators (ICDs) being implanted in only 10.4%, the higher burden of monomorphic VT compared with polymorphic VT/VF has also been observed in ICD recipients. More than 80% of all VAs that triggered

Department of Cardiology, Leiden University Medical Center, Postal Zone: C-05-P, PO Box 9600, Leiden 2300 RC, The Netherlands
* Corresponding author.
E-mail address: K.Zeppenfeld@lumc.nl

Card Electrophysiol Clin 9 (2017) 285–294
http://dx.doi.org/10.1016/j.ccep.2017.02.010
1877-9182/17/© 2017 Elsevier Inc. All rights reserved.

cardiacEP.theclinics.com

ICD therapy in a cohort of 121 patients with TOF who had received an ICD for primary or secondary prevention were monomorphic VTs. Of note, treated VTs were fast with a median heart rate of 213 beats per minute (bpm) (interquartile range [IQR] 182–264 bpm).[7] The clinical importance of fast, monomorphic VTs has been confirmed by recent data from patients with repaired ToF (rToF) referred for risk stratification or VT ablation. The median VT cycle length of the 41 spontaneous and induced VTs recorded in 28 patients was only 252 ms (IQR 231–312).[8] These rapid VTs, if untreated, may be fatal even in the presence of a preserved biventricular function. Of concern, two-thirds of patients with rToF who died suddenly or experienced life-threatening VT, typically early to middle-aged adults, had a preserved or only moderately impaired cardiac function before the first event.[3,8,9] The average left ventricular (LV) ejection fraction of more than 50% and the only mildly impaired or normal right ventricular (RV) function in 75% of those who have experienced an arrhythmic event strongly suggest that non–heart failure–related substrates for VA play an important role in rToF.[3,6]

RISK STRATIFICATION AND VENTRICULAR ARRHYTHMIA SUBSTRATES

For risk stratification and treatment of VA in rToF, it is important to emphasize that different arrhythmia substrates and mechanisms may be encountered depending on the variation of the malformation, type and timing of repair, and residual lesions. ToF is characterized by a subpulmonary stenosis, a subaortic ventricular septal defect (VSD), dextroposition of the aortic orifice, and RV hypertrophy. The last characteristic is the consequence of the volume and pressure overload caused by the VSD and the subpulmonary stenosis.

The morphology of TOF, however, encompasses a broad spectrum, from a mild appearance with small VSDs and minimal pulmonary stenosis to severe forms of the disease with pulmonary atresia. The spectrum of the malformation, and the different types and timing of surgical interventions with variable hemodynamic outcomes, results in a heterogeneous population of adults with rToF. RV hypertrophy and interstitial fibrosis typically occur after long-standing cyanosis and high ventricular pressure overload due to repair at older age.[10]

Total repair usually includes (patch) closure of the perimembranous or muscular VSD, resection of the hypertrophic infundibulum, and insertion of an right ventricular outflow tract (RVOT) or a transannular patch to augment the restrictive RVOT or to relieve the stenosis of the pulmonary orifice. Surgery was initially performed through a vertical or transverse right ventriculotomy, often combined with the use of a large transannular patch with subsequent pulmonary regurgitation and RV dilatation and dysfunction.

Chronic volume and pressure overload can contribute to ventricular arrhythmogenesis due to nonreentrant mechanisms, such as triggered activity or abnormal automaticity typically observed in patients with nonischemic cardiomyopathies and end-stage heart failure.[11]

Accordingly, reported risk factors associated with any VA and/or sudden cardiac death in rToF are older age at repair, the presence of a transannular patch, the number of previous cardiac surgeries, moderate to severe pulmonary regurgitation, moderate to severe RV and LV systolic dysfunction, and a QRS duration of greater than 180 ms, which may be related to RV dilatation (**Box 1**). The number of prior cardiac surgeries, including prior palliative shunt operation, diastolic LV dysfunction, and, consistent with prior reports, QRS duration,[4] was independently associated with VT in a recent multicenter, cross-sectional study. Reasons why, in particular, diastolic LV dysfunction is associated with VA are unclear; the value of LV diastolic dysfunction in risk stratifying patients with rToF needs further evaluation.[6] Of note, most of the data on late morbidity, mortality, and risk stratification in rToF are based on patients who have undergone repair late in life, at a median age of 5 years (IQR 2.5, 7 years)[6] and 8 years (IQR 2, 9.4 years),[12] half of them after prior palliative shunt operation.

The detrimental effect of both late repair and right ventriculotomy on RV function and arrhythmogenecity has been recognized. As a consequence, the surgical strategy has evolved over time. Nowadays, patients often undergo repair early in life with a combined transatrial-transpulmonary approach. The RV incision is usually restricted to the pulmonary annulus; smaller patches are preferred, and effort is made to avoid or limit free pulmonary regurgitation. These changes are likely to positively influence the biventricular function and the occurrence of heart failure–related VA. In addition, they may also have significant impact on the substrate for monomorphic VT.

SUBSTRATE FOR MONOMORPHIC VENTRICULAR TACHYCARDIA IN REPAIRED TETRALOGY OF FALLOT

Intraoperative and catheter mapping studies have identified macro-reentry as the major underlying mechanism of spontaneous and induced

---

Box 1
Risk factors for ventricular arrhythmias in patients with repaired tetralogy of Fallot

Clinical parameter

Older age at total repair

Presence of transannular patch

Number of previous cardiac surgeries

Presyncope

History of atrial arrhythmias

History of nonsustained VT

ECG parameter

QRS duration ≥180 ms

QRS duration increase per year

QRS dispersion

QT duration

QT dispersion

JT(c) dispersion

LV parameter

LV longitudinal strain on echo

LV diastolic dysfunction/end-diastolic pressure

LV reduced systolic function

RV parameter

RV reduced systolic function

RV LGE

RV akinetic region length

RV dilatation

RV end systolic pressure (millimeter of mercury)

RV mass/volume ratio ≥0.3 g/mL

Moderate or severe PVR

Invasive parameter

Inducible for SMVT or SPVT

Abbreviations: ECG, electrocardiogram; LGE, late gadolinium enhancement; PVR, pulmonary valve regurgitation; SMVT, sustained monomorphic ventricular tachycardia; SPVT, sustained polymorphic ventricular tachycardia.

---

sustained monomorphic VT in rToF.[8,13–16] Reentry is facilitated by zones of fixed or functional conduction block protecting conducting isthmuses. Areas of dense fibrosis after surgical incisions, prosthetic patch material, and the valve annuli are typical regions of fixed conduction block in rToF. They create intervening isthmuses of myocardial bundles that might contain the critical reentry circuit isthmus of a VT. The malformation and type of repair are important determinants of

anatomic isthmuses (AIs). Four AIs related to VT in repaired TOF have been identified (**Fig. 1**)[14]: Isthmus 1 is bordered by the tricuspid annulus and the scar of a prior RV free wall incision, or an RV patch or a large transannular patch; isthmus 2 by the pulmonary annulus and an RV free wall incision or an RVOT patch sparing the pulmonary valve annulus; isthmus 3 by the pulmonary annulus and the VSD patch; and isthmus 4 by the VSD patch and the tricuspid annulus in patients with muscular VSDs.

In 2 postmortem series of rToF, isthmuses 1 and 3 were present in most specimens. In contrast, isthmuses 2 and 4 were observed in only 25% and 13%, respectively.[14,17] The low incidence of isthmus 4 is in line with the higher incidence of perimembranous VSDs compared with muscular VSDs in ToF. Isthmus 2 is the result of a transventricular approach and is usually prevented in contemporary patients with a transpulmonary access or a limited RV incision in continuity with the pulmonary annulus (see **Fig. 1**). Of interest, in one postmortem series, isthmus 1 was significantly wider and thicker with a smaller degree of interstitial and replacement fibrosis compared with isthmus 3 in subjects surviving the repair by 1 year or more.[17]

Earlier repair has been associated with less interstitial fibrosis.[10] However, specific AI characteristics, like narrow width and thinner myocardium, may be the decisive factors for remodeling over time. Progressive interstitial and replacement fibrosis interspersing and separating myocyte bundles are well-known substrates for slow conduction in patients with structural heart disease and have also been identified in patients with rToF with VT.[13,18] The coincidence of anatomic regions of conduction block and degenerative remodeling with conduction slowing over time may explain the high incidence of late monomorphic macro-reentrant VT.

CONTRIBUTION OF 3-DIMENSIONAL ELECTROANATOMICAL MAPPING FOR SUBSTRATE IDENTIFICATION AND RISK STRATIFICATION

The current cornerstone of catheter ablation for VT in rToF is the identification and delineation of those AIs that are related to VT.[8,14,16] Review of the surgical records provides important information on the presence and location of surgical incisions and patch material as potential borders of AIs. Preprocedural imaging is essential for evaluation of biventricular function and valvular competence. Patients who require surgery for residual lesions or pulmonary valve regurgitation may benefit from

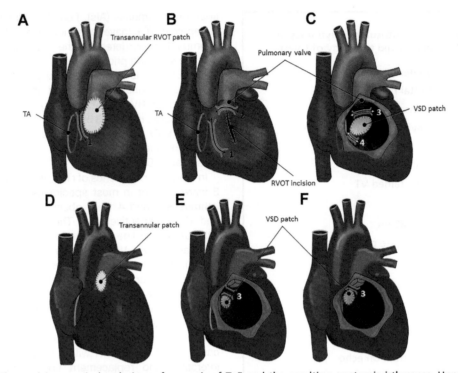

Fig. 1. The evolving surgical techniques for repair of ToF and the resulting anatomic isthmuses. Upper panel: Transventricular approach with (*A*) large transannular RVOT patch, (*B*) RV incision, and (*C*) patch closure of a muscular VSD. The 4 potential anatomic isthmuses for VT are indicated (*1–4*). Lower panel: Transatrial-transpulmonary approach with the use of a small transannular patch, thereby preventing isthmus 1 and 2 (*D*) and patch closure of a small perimembranous VSD (*E*). A perimembranous VSD excludes AI 4 as demonstrated in (*E, F*). Specific characteristics of anatomic isthmus 3, like isthmus width, depend on the size of the VSD (*E, F*) and may influence the arrhythmogenecity of the isthmus. TA, tricuspid annulus.

intraoperative cryoablation of AIs that are (potentially) related to VT.[19] Contrast-enhanced (CE) MRI is the current gold standard for detection of fibrosis. Preprocedural imaging and image integration have improved VT substrate identification in patients with scar-related VT and morphologic normal hearts.[20–24] The feasibility of 3-dimensional high-resolution CE MRI with semiautomated scar segmentation to visualize VSD repair sites and the RVOT incision has been recently demonstrated in a small series of 15 patients with rToF.[25] Whether this promising technique can noninvasively identify all AIs and most importantly those that are related to VT requires further studies.

Three-dimensional electroanatomical mapping may be considered as the current gold standard to reconstruct AIs.[8,14,16,26] Point-by-point electroanatomical contact mapping can be performed during stable sinus rhythm or RV pacing. All contact points can be saved together with the local bipolar and unipolar electrograms. Electroanatomical maps can be displayed as bipolar voltage maps (peak-to-peak bipolar amplitude) (**Fig. 2**, panel A) and as activation maps, based

on the local activation time (defined as sharp peak deflection of the local bipolar electrogram that coincides with the maximum down stroke of the local unipolar signal) (see **Fig. 2**, panel B). At low amplitude sites (<1.5 mV), pacing can be performed with high output (10 mA/2 ms). Sites with a pacing threshold greater than 10 mA are considered unexcitable tissue because of surgical scars or patch material, which together with the valve annuli determine the AIs (see **Fig. 2**). Contact force monitoring can be helpful to distinguish noncontact sites from true unexcitable scar.[27]

Of importance, AIs are present in almost all patients with rToF but not all AIs are related to VT. In a recent cohort of 74 consecutive patients with rToF who underwent programmed electrical stimulation and detailed electroanatomical mapping, at least one AI could be identified in all patients regardless of prior spontaneous or inducible VTs.[8] The most prevalent isthmuses were AI 1 and 3, which is in line with the postmortem studies.[14,17] Of importance, AIs in patients with spontaneous and/or inducible VT had distinct electroanatomical characteristics. These isthmuses were narrower and

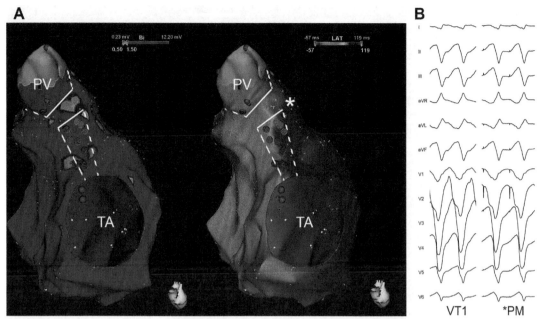

Fig. 2. Electroanatomical assessment of anatomic isthmus 3 (between the pulmonary valve [PV] and VSD patch). Examples of an RV electroanatomical bipolar (Bi) voltage map (*A, purple indicates normal voltages, coding according to color bar*) and activation map (*B, red indicates early activation, purple late activation*) obtained during sinus rhythm and displayed in a posterior view. The gray tags (electrically unexcitable tissue) correspond to the VSD patch. Isthmus 3 is located between the solid white lines. Isthmus 3 was related to the induced VT 1 based on pace mapping with a good pace map at the free wall site of the isthmus (indicated with the *asterisk*). LAT, local activation time; PM, pace map; TA, tricuspid annulus.

had a slower conduction velocity (CV) calculated from the electroanatomical activation map obtained during stable rhythm (**Fig. 3**).[8]

Of the 41 spontaneous and induced VTs in 28 patients, 37 were related to a slow conducting anatomic isthmus (SCAI) based on entrainment mapping, pace mapping, or VT termination during RF. Most VTs were related to AI 3, followed by isthmus 1. Of importance, all VT-related AIs had a calculated CV of less than 0.5 m/s. In contrast, 87 of 89 AIs in the 46 patients without VT had CV greater than 0.5 m/s. SCAIs were targeted by either catheter ablation or surgical cryoablation. During a follow-up of 50 ± 22 months, all 63 patients without SCAI either at baseline or after successful ablation remained free of any VT. In contrast, 5 of 10 patients with failed or not performed ablation experienced at least one episode of VT. Identification of an SCAI was a stronger predictor of spontaneous and inducible VT than traditional risk factors.[8]

The demonstrated strong link between SCAIs and monomorphic VT in rToF may have important implications for risk stratification, guidance of radiofrequency catheter or surgical cryoablation, and procedural end points. In patients who are scheduled for pulmonary valve replacement or other resurgery, preoperative electroanatomical mapping for SCAI can identify those with a substrate for VT, which can be targeted during surgery.[8]

VENTRICULAR TACHYCARDIA ABLATION: STRATEGIES, END POINTS, AND OUTCOME

Radiofrequency catheter ablation (RFCA) has been shown to be an effective treatment of monomorphic VT in patients with rToF. In early series, only slow and hemodynamically well-tolerated VTs were targeted using conventional techniques like activation and entrainment mapping during ongoing VT.[28–30] In more recent series, most of the included patients had rapid and hemodynamically poorly tolerated VT, which better reflects the arrhythmic presentation of contemporary patients with rToF.[7,14–16]

Point-by-point propagation mapping is usually not feasible to identify the critical isthmus of a poorly tolerated reentry VT. Noncontact mapping systems consisting of a multielectrode balloon array that allows simultaneous acquisition of virtual unipolar electrograms can be helpful to record the activation sequence of unstable and nonsustained VT. In a small series of 10 patients, the anatomic location of the critical part of the reentry circuit of 11 macro-reentrant VTs could be

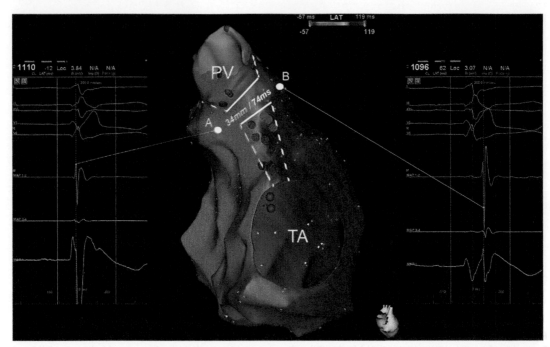

Fig. 3. Electroanatomical assessment of anatomic isthmus 3. Electroanatomical activation map during sinus rhythm (view as in **Fig. 2**). The isthmus width is the distance between the unexcitable borders. The isthmus length is measured as distance between the first sites with a normal bipolar electrogram at both sides of the isthmus (indicated by the *2 circles*, site A and site B). The length of the isthmus (from site A to site B) was 34 mm. Conduction time (difference between the local activation time at site A and site B) from site A to site B was 74 ms; the calculated conduction velocity over the isthmus was 0.46 m/s. LAT, local activation time; PV, pulmonary valve; TA, tricuspid annulus.

identified. The corresponding AI could be successfully targeted by a linear RF lesion during stable rhythm in 8 patients. In 2 patients, RF delivery was withheld because of the proximity of the His bundle. This approach still requires contact mapping to reconstruct the chamber of interest and inducibility of the clinical VT.[15]

With the identification of SCAI as a dominant substrate for VT, inducibility of the clinical arrhythmia and hemodynamic tolerance are no longer prerequisites for successful ablation. SCAI can be transected by a linear RF lesion during stable rhythm without prior VT induction. However, programmed ventricular stimulation to induce VT should not be abandoned. Although rare, focal sources for monomorphic sustained VT have been described requiring VT induction and activation mapping or pace mapping for those VTs that are poorly tolerated.[14–16,26]

Noninducibility of any sustained monomorphic VT after RFCA has been associated with favorable outcomes in patients with structural heart disease. However, despite achieved noninducibility, VTs may recur. In contrast to structural heart diseases with complex and often poorly understood scars and multiple reentry circuits, the well-

characterized and limited number of SCAIs as a substrate for monomorphic sustained VT in rToF allows an ablation approach with a well-defined end point.[8,16] Accordingly, a combined end point of noninducibility and transection of VT-related AI by connecting the unexcitable boundaries has been proposed.[14,16] In these studies, an attempt was still made to prove the relation of an induced VT to an identified AI by either entrainment mapping, pace mapping, or by VT termination during RF within the AI (see **Fig. 2**).[14,16] Considering the strong association between VT and SCAI,[8] transection of these SCAIs could be considered without the need to prove that the critical VT reentry circuit site is located within the SCAI. This strategy may positively impact procedural time and patient comfort.

Successful transection of an isthmus can be assumed if noncapture at high-output pacing along the ablation line has been achieved. Conduction block is further supported by a change in the activation sequence after completing the line.[8,14,16] However, as for cavotricuspid isthmus ablation, demonstration of bidirectional conduction block by differential pacing across the ablation line might be the optimal end point for the linear lesion (**Fig. 4**).

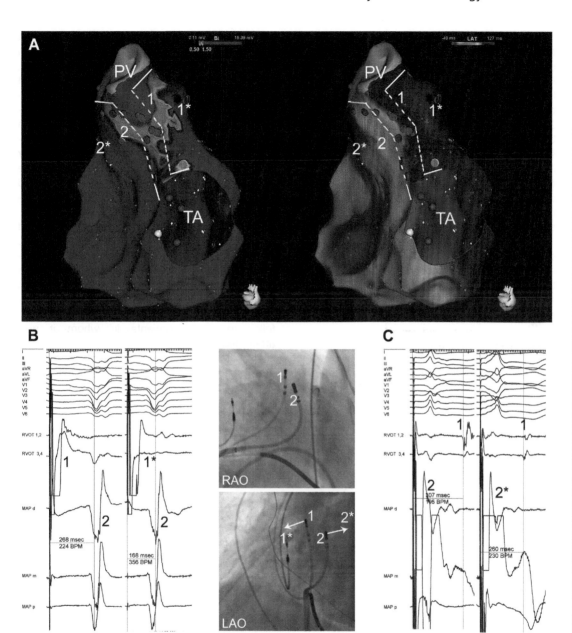

Fig. 4. Typical example of electroanatomical mapping after successful ablation of isthmus 3 and differential pacing to confirm conduction block over the isthmus. (*A*) RV electroanatomical bipolar (Bi) voltage map (*left, purple indicates normal voltages, coding according to color bar*) and activation map (*right, red indicates early activation, purple late activation*) obtained during sinus rhythm (posterior view, same patient as in **Figs. 2** and **3**). The gray tags (electrically unexcitable tissue) correspond to the VSD patch and the ablation line connecting the patch with the pulmonary valve (PV). Please note the change in the activation sequence after ablation of the isthmus. (*B, C*) Examples of differential pacing to confirm conduction block over the isthmus. (*B*) Pacing from the RVOT free wall site (*site 1*) of AI 3 close to the ablation line using a second steerable catheter (SC) and recording from the mapping catheter (map) located at the septal site of isthmus 3. The conduction time from the pacing site to the septal site of the isthmus (*site 2*) was long (268 ms). Moving the SC away from the AI 3 (*1**) resulted in a decrease of the conduction time between SC and septal isthmus site (168 ms). (*C*) Pacing from the mapping catheter close to the septal site of the AI line and recording from the SC located at the free wall site showed a long stimulus to electrograms distance of 307 ms; pacing at a site away from the line (*2**) results in a decrease of the conduction time to 260 ms. LAO, left anterior oblique; LAT, local activation time; RAO, right anterior oblique; TA, tricuspid annulus.

The first study reporting on the acute and long-term outcome after VT ablation applying the pre-defined combined procedural end point has included 34 patients with repaired congenital heart disease, most after rToF. VT-related AIs could be identified for 59 of 61 induced VTs. In 25 of 34 patients the combined end point could be reached; all VT-related isthmuses could be successfully transected resulting in noninducibility of any VT. Of importance, none of these patients experienced any monomorphic VT during a follow-up of 46 months. In contrast, VT recurred in 4 of the 9 patients without complete procedural success.[16]

In a recent study of 21 patients with various congenital heart disease, 48% with rToF, the induced VT was AI dependent in two-thirds of the patients.[26] In 8 out of these, 14 patients the AI could be successful transected; none of these patients experienced VT recurrence.

PROCEDURAL FAILURE

Failure to transect the SCAI can be due to the hypertrophied myocardium but also due to prosthetic material. Both VSD patch and pulmonary homograft cover parts of the clinically relevant isthmus 3. In patients with a muscular VSD, patch material can also prevent transection of isthmus 4. In 11 out of 28 patients with rToF who underwent VT ablation, an RV approach to transect the VT-related AI was not successful.[31] In 8 of the 11 patients, the VT was mapped to isthmus 3 or 4, both involving the outlet septum. The anterior and cranial displacement of the outlet or infundibular septum is the hallmark of ToF. In contrast to the normal heart, the outlet septum can be recognized as a separate and mostly muscular structure between the aortic valve and the RVOT (**Fig. 5**, panels 1 and 2). The outlet septum with AI 3 and 4 can be accessed from the RV and from the aortic root or LVOT (see **Fig. 5**, panels 4 and 5). A retrograde aortic approach with RF applications from the aortic root or LVOT after right-sided ablation failure has resulted in complete procedural success and freedom from VT recurrence during follow-up in all patients in whom it was attempted.[31]

The proximity of the His bundle has to be considered and can be another limitation if isthmus 4 is targeted by ablation. RF application may be withheld to avoid atrioventricular block.[31]

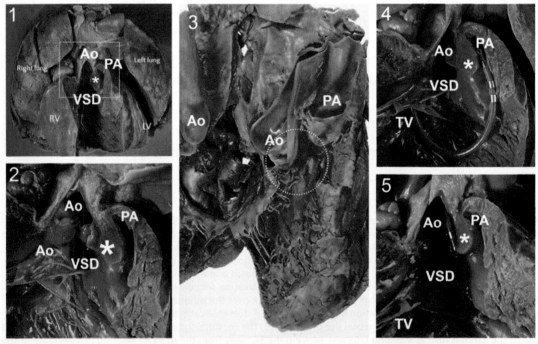

Fig. 5. Postmortem specimen of unrepaired ToF (overview in *1*, close up in *2–5*), and postmortem specimen of a normal heart in [*3*]). The anterior and cranial displacement of the outlet septum (*1, 2* indicated by the *asterisk*) results in malalignment with the ventriculo-infundibular fold and the trabecula septomarginalis with a subaortic VSD as a consequence. The relation between the aorta and outlet septum (*asterisk*) is shown in (*1, 2*). In contrast, in a normal heart, the outlet septum cannot be recognized as a separate structure (*3, dashed circle*). (*4, 5*) Catheter access to the outlet septum. (*4*) The catheter is positioned in a coronary cusp. (*5*) The catheter is positioned at the pulmonary side of the outlet septum. Ao, aorta; PA, pulmonary artery; TV, tricuspid valve.

In addition, aortic root enlargement and aortic valve calcification may prevent easy access. Although not reported, the risk of aortic valve and coronary artery damage needs to be considered in particular if multiple RF applications are needed for complete isthmus transection. The importance of AI 3 as a (potential) substrate for late VT, the difficulty to achieve conduction block if parts of the AI are protected by pulmonary homografts or percutaneous valves, and the potential risks of a left-sided approach justify incorporating electroanatomical mapping into the preoperative evaluation. Preventive catheter or intraoperative SCAI ablation should be considered in the many patients with rToF who require reinterventions.

SUMMARY

Life expectancy of patients with rToF has considerably improved over the last decades as a result of earlier and refined surgical interventions. Despite early repair, monomorphic and fast VTs are frequently encountered in adult patients with rToF. The dominant substrate of VT is related to anatomic isthmuses bordered by surgical incisions, patch material, and valve annuli. VT-related AIs are typically narrow with slow conduction velocities and specific characteristics, which can be determined by electroanatomical catheter mapping during stable sinus rhythm. Substrate-based catheter or surgical ablation strategies aim to transect all identified SCAIs. Complete procedural success of RFCA is currently defined as noninducibility of any VT and confirmed conduction block over the SCAI resulting in long-term VT-free survival in most patients. Reaching these end points may even be considered curative in patients with preserved cardiac function and without competing VA mechanisms. The identification of SCAIs as a dominant arrhythmogenic substrate in rToF may have important implications for risk stratification and preventive treatment.

REFERENCES

1. Hoffman JI, Kaplan S. The incidence of congenital heart disease. J Am Coll Cardiol 2002;39:1890–900.
2. Moons P, Bovijn L, Budts W, et al. Temporal trends in survival to adulthood among patients born with congenital heart disease from 1970 to 1992 in Belgium. Circulation 2010;122:2264–72.
3. Diller GP, Kempny A, Alonso-Gonzalez R, et al. Survival prospects and circumstances of death in contemporary adult congenital heart disease patients under follow-up at a large tertiary centre. Circulation 2015;132:2118–25.
4. Gatzoulis MA, Balaji S, Webber SA, et al. Risk factors for arrhythmia and sudden cardiac death late after repair of tetralogy of Fallot: a multicentre study. Lancet 2000;356:975–81.
5. Khairy P, Ionescu-Ittu R, Mackie AS, et al. Changing mortality in congenital heart disease. J Am Coll Cardiol 2010;56:1149–57.
6. Khairy P, Aboulhosn J, Gurvitz MZ, et al. Arrhythmia burden in adults with surgically repaired tetralogy of Fallot: a multi-institutional study. Circulation 2010; 122:868–75.
7. Khairy P, Harris L, Landzberg MJ, et al. Implantable cardioverter-defibrillators in tetralogy of Fallot. Circulation 2008;117:363–70.
8. Kapel GF, Sacher F, Dekkers OM, et al. Arrhythmogenic anatomical isthmuses identified by electroanatomical mapping are the substrate for ventricular tachycardia in repaired tetralogy of Fallot. Eur Heart J 2017;38(4):268–76.
9. Koyak Z, Harris L, de Groot JR, et al. Sudden cardiac death in adult congenital heart disease. Circulation 2012;126:1944–54.
10. Chowdhury UK, Sathia S, Ray R, et al. Histopathology of the right ventricular outflow tract and its relationship to clinical outcomes and arrhythmias in patients with tetralogy of Fallot. J Thorac Cardiovasc Surg 2006;132:270–7.
11. Pogwizd SM. Nonreentrant mechanisms underlying spontaneous ventricular arrhythmias in a model of nonischemic heart failure in rabbits. Circulation 1995;92:1034–48.
12. Diller GP, Kempny A, Liodakis E, et al. Left ventricular longitudinal function predicts life-threatening ventricular arrhythmia and death in adults with repaired tetralogy of fallot. Circulation 2012;125: 2440–6.
13. Misaki T, Tsubota M, Watanabe G, et al. Surgical treatment of ventricular tachycardia after surgical repair of tetralogy of Fallot. Relation between intraoperative mapping and histological findings. Circulation 1994;90:264–71.
14. Zeppenfeld K, Schalij MJ, Bartelings MM, et al. Catheter ablation of ventricular tachycardia after repair of congenital heart disease: electroanatomic identification of the critical right ventricular isthmus. Circulation 2007;116:2241–52.
15. Kriebel T, Saul JP, Schneider H, et al. Noncontact mapping and radiofrequency catheter ablation of fast and hemodynamically unstable ventricular tachycardia after surgical repair of tetralogy of Fallot. J Am Coll Cardiol 2007;50:2162–8.
16. Kapel GF, Reichlin T, Wijnmaalen AP, et al. Re-entry using anatomically determined isthmuses: a curable ventricular tachycardia in repaired congenital heart disease. Circ Arrhythm Electrophysiol 2015;8:102–9.
17. Moore JP, Seki A, Shannon KM, et al. Characterization of anatomic ventricular tachycardia isthmus

pathology after surgical repair of tetralogy of Fallot. Circ Arrhythm Electrophysiol 2013;6:905–11.

18. de Bakker JM, van Capelle FJ, Janse MJ, et al. Slow conduction in the infarcted human heart. 'Zigzag' course of activation. Circulation 1993;88:915–26.

19. Sabate Rotes A, Connolly HM, Warnes CA, et al. Ventricular arrhythmia risk stratification in patients with tetralogy of Fallot at the time of pulmonary valve replacement. Circ Arrhythm Electrophysiol 2015;8: 110–6.

20. Wijnmaalen AP, van der Geest RJ, van Huls van Taxis CF, et al. Head-to-head comparison of contrast-enhanced magnetic resonance imaging and electroanatomical voltage mapping to assess post-infarct scar characteristics in patients with ventricular tachycardias: real-time image integration and reversed registration. Eur Heart J 2011;32: 104–14.

21. Piers SR, Tao Q, van Huls van Taxis CF, et al. Contrast-enhanced MRI-derived scar patterns and associated ventricular tachycardias in nonischemic cardiomyopathy: implications for the ablation strategy. Circ Arrhythm Electrophysiol 2013;6:875–83.

22. Piers SR, van Huls van Taxis CF, Tao Q, et al. Epicardial substrate mapping for ventricular tachycardia ablation in patients with non-ischaemic cardiomyopathy: a new algorithm to differentiate between scar and viable myocardium developed by simultaneous integration of computed tomography and contrast-enhanced magnetic resonance imaging. Eur Heart J 2013;34:586–96.

23. Piers SR, Tao Q, de Riva Silva M, et al. CMR-based identification of critical isthmus sites of ischemic and nonischemic ventricular tachycardia. JACC Cardiovasc Imaging 2014;7:774–84.

24. Tao Q, Piers SR, Lamb HJ, et al. Preprocedural magnetic resonance imaging for image-guided catheter ablation of scar-related ventricular tachycardia. Int J Cardiovasc Imaging 2015;31:369–77.

25. Stirrat J, Rajchl M, Bergin L, et al. High-resolution 3-dimensional late gadolinium enhancement scar imaging in surgically corrected tetralogy of Fallot: clinical feasibility of volumetric quantification and visualization. J Cardiovasc Magn Reson 2014;16:76.

26. van Zyl M, Kapa S, Padmanabhan D, et al. Mechanism and outcomes of catheter ablation for ventricular tachycardia in adults with repaired congenital heart disease. Heart Rhythm 2016;13:1449–54.

27. Mizuno H, Vergara P, Maccabelli G, et al. Contact force monitoring for cardiac mapping in patients with ventricular tachycardia. J Cardiovasc Electrophysiol 2013;24:519–24.

28. Gonska BD, Cao K, Raab J, et al. Radiofrequency catheter ablation of right ventricular tachycardia late after repair of congenital heart defects. Circulation 1996;94:1902–8.

29. Morwood JG, Triedman JK, Berul CI, et al. Radiofrequency catheter ablation of ventricular tachycardia in children and young adults with congenital heart disease. Heart Rhythm 2004;1:301–8.

30. Furushima H, Chinushi M, Sugiura H, et al. Ventricular tachycardia late after repair of congenital heart disease: efficacy of combination therapy with radiofrequency catheter ablation and class III antiarrhythmic agents and long-term outcome. J Electrocardiol 2006;39:219–24.

31. Kapel GF, Reichlin T, Wijnmaalen AP, et al. Left-sided ablation of ventricular tachycardia in adults with repaired tetralogy of Fallot: a case series. Circ Arrhythm Electrophysiol 2014;7:889–97.

Management

Drug Therapy in Adult Congenital Heart Disease

Tahmeed Contractor, MD[a],*, Vadim Levin, MD[b], Ravi Mandapati, MD, FHRS, FACC[a]

KEYWORDS

• Drug therapy • Anticoagulation • Congenital heart disease • Arrhythmia

KEY POINTS

• Class I antiarrhythmic drugs (sodium channel blockers) should be used with caution in patients having ventricular scar, decreased ejection fraction, significant mitral regurgitation and significant PR prolongation.

• Flecainide and Propafenone are the most potent and commonly used class I antiarrhythmics; there are several differences between these 2 medications that are important to remember for day to day use.

• Class III antiarrhythmic drugs (potassium channel blockers) have been used in the setting of ventricular scar. Most of these also have negative inotropic effects.

• Amiodarone is the most commonly used antiarrhythmic drug which has significant long-term side effects including lung, liver, thyroid and neurological abnormalities.

• Sotalol and dofetilide are the other commonly used class III antiarrhythmics; these can result in a dose-dependent QTc prolongation requiring close monitoring at the time of initiation. There are several differences between these 2 medications that are important to remember for practical use.

INTRODUCTION

With advances in cardiology, patients born with moderate and even complex congenital heart disease are living well into adulthood.[1] Structural abnormalities predispose them to not only pump-related issues but also complex atrial as well as ventricular arrhythmias leading to significant morbidity and mortality.[2] These arrhythmias are not always amenable to ablation and many of these patients require antiarrhythmic drug therapy, sometimes in conjunction with ablative approaches. In addition, the risk of systemic thromboembolism is high in patients with moderate and severe forms of congenital heart disease who develop atrial arrhythmias.[3] Anticoagulation with warfarin and now the non—vitamin K antagonist oral anticoagulants (NOACs) is often required in these patients.

Although the principles of use of antiarrhythmic therapy in patients with adult congenital heart disease are similar to those in the general population, important differences exist:

1. The heart is structurally abnormal and there is presence of atrial as well as ventricular scar in many of these patients, which alters the pharmacodynamics of antiarrhythmic drugs.

2. Renal and hepatic function may be abnormal in these patients and may alter the pharmacokinetics of these medications.

3. Clinical data on the use of antiarrhythmic medications in this patient population are scant, and hence most recommendations are based on opinion.

This article summarizes the use of antiarrhythmic and anticoagulant drugs in patients with adult congenital heart disease and highlights features of these medications that are important for clinicians to remember when dealing with this patient population.

[a] Department of Cardiology, Arrhythmia Center, Loma Linda University International Heart Institute, 11234 Anderson Street, Loma Linda, CA 92354, USA; [b] Electrophysiology, Phoenixville Hospital, 1591 Medical Drive, Pottstown, PA 19464, USA
* Corresponding author.
E-mail address: TContractor@llu.edu

Card Electrophysiol Clin 9 (2017) 295–309
http://dx.doi.org/10.1016/j.ccep.2017.02.011
1877-9182/17/© 2017 Elsevier Inc. All rights reserved.

ANTIARRHYTHMIC DRUGS

The pharmacologic effects of each antiarrhythmic drug are highly variable. The widely used Vaughan-Williams[4] classification scheme does not adequately describe the antiarrhythmic effect of each of its classes and there is significant overlap. The Sicilian gambit classification[5] scheme, although more specific, is tedious and less practical to use on a daily basis.

Based on the more commonly used Vaugh-Williams[4] classification scheme, antiarrhythmic drugs are classified into 4 groups:

1. Class I agents: predominantly sodium channel blockers
2. Class II agents: β-blockers
3. Class III agents: predominantly potassium channel blockers
4. Class IV agents: calcium channel blockers

In addition to these, there are several medications, such as ranolazine, adenosine, digoxin, and magnesium, that have not found a place in this classification scheme.

A general description of antiarrhythmic drug is provided next that is applicable to all patients; recommendations are included (if available) for use in congenital heart disease populations.

CLASS I ANTIARRHYTHMIC AGENTS

The class 1 antiarrhythmic agents are predominantly sodium channel blockers and include 3 subclasses. These medications can be pro-arrhythmic in the presence of myocardial scar and should be avoided in patients with congenital heart disease and significant ventricular scarring. Additionally, most of the medications in the class have significant negative inotropic effects and should be avoided in patients with congestive heart failure. These medications can also worsen forward flow in patients with significant mitral regurgitation. Many patients with congenital heart disease can have a first degree AV block; Class 1 agents should generally be avoided if the PR interval is >250 to 300 ms to avoid AV dys-synchrony related side-effects. Class IA, 1B and 1C medications have intermediate, fast and slow kinetics, respectively. The slow kinetics of the class IC agents results in slow unbinding of these medications from the ion channels making these the most potent sodium channel blockers. Details regarding these medications are outlined in **Table 1**.

Class 1 Agents in Patients with Congenital Heart Disease

There are not many studies that have evaluated the safety and efficacy of class I antiarrhythmic agents in patients with adult congenital heart disease. There is a fear of proarrhythmic effects of these medications given the underlying scar. In a study in young patients who were administered class IC agents, proarrhythmic events were observed in close to 8% of patients, especially in those with underlying structural heart disease.[6] Class I agents were also associated with the increased risk of ventricular arrhythmias when used in patients with tetralogy of Fallot.[7] Although class I antiarrhythmics are usually not recommended in patients with so-called structural heart disease, they are used in patients with congenital heart disease with caveats (discussed later).

A brief description of these medications follows.

Class 1A antiarrhythmics

Quinidine This was one of the first antiarrhythmic drugs used. It has excellent oral absorption, and is predominantly excreted through the liver. It has fast sodium channel blocking properties; however, it also blocks the potassium channels (prolonging QT interval) and has autonomic effects. Over time, the dangers associated with its use have been recognized and hence it is rarely used in contemporary practice. Its most serious adverse effect is a dose-independent increase in the corrected QT (QTc) interval leading to torsades de pointes.[8]

Quinidine can potentially be used in patients with ventricular arrhythmias and simple congenital heart disease (especially if they have an implantable cardioverter defibrillator [ICD] as backup), but its only practical contemporary use is in patients with Brugada syndrome.[9] By blocking the Ito channel, quinidine can reduce the transmyocardial electrical gradient during the repolarization, preventing phase II reentry in patients with Brugada syndrome.[10]

Procainamide Procainamide also has potassium channel blocking as well as autonomic effects in addition to sodium channel blocking properties. It has good oral absorption but it is also available in the intravenous form. It has a complex metabolism whereby it is metabolized in the liver to N-acetyl procainamide (NAPA), which is then excreted renally. NAPA has predominantly potassium channel blocking properties and can accumulate in renal dysfunction, leading to QTc prolongation/torsades de pointes.[11] In contrast, slow acetylators of procainamide[12] (which can be up to 50% of the population) or patients with hepatic dysfunction generate less NAPA and hence have less class III action. Similar to quinidine, procainamide also causes dose-independent QTc prolongation. It can cause ANA (anti-nuclear antibody) positivity in up to 80% of the patients; however, systemic lupus erythematosus develops in only 30% of these patients.[13]

Table 1
Class 1 antiarrhythmic agents: properties, uses, doses, and adverse reactions

	Quinidine	Procainamide	Disopyramide	Lidocaine	Mexiletine	Flecainide	Propafenone
Absorption (%)	80–90	80–90[a]	80–90	Intravenous only	70	>90	>90
Half-life (h)/ Protein Binding (%)	8/90	5[b]/minimal	8/variable	1–4/70	8–16/70	12–24/40	6–8/70
Excretion	Hepatic	Hepatic and renal[c]	Hepatic and renal[d]	Hepatic	Hepatic	Hepatic 70% Renal 30%	Hepatic
Practical Uses	Brugada syndrome, VT	AF with WPW, VT	SVT in patients with HCM	VT	VT	Atrial arrhythmias PVCs/VT CPVT	Atrial arrhythmias PVCs/VT
Dose	300–600 mg every 6 h	IV: 15 mg/kg, then 1–6 mg/min. Oral: 500–1250 mg every 6 h	100–200 mg every 6 h	1.5 mg/kg loading; 1–4 mg/min drip	150–250 mg every 8 h	50–150 mg BID	150–300 mg TID ER: 225–325–425 BID
Adverse Reactions	GI side effects Dose-independent QTc prolongation	SLE dose-independent QTc prolongation	Anticholinergic side effects	CNS side effects Respiratory arrest	CNS side effects GI symptoms Thrombocytopenia	GI symptoms QRS prolongation proarrhythmia	Dizziness Metallic aftertaste Lupuslike rash QRS prolongation/ proarrhythmia

Abbreviations: AF, atrial fibrillation; BID, twice a day; CNS, central nervous system; CPVT, catecholaminergic polymorphic ventricular tachycardia; ER, extended release; GI, gastrointestinal; HCM, hypertrophic cardiomyopathy; IV, intravenous; PVC, premature ventricular contraction; SLE, systemic lupus erythematosus; SVT, supraventricular tachycardia; TID, 3 times a day; VT, ventricular tachycardia; WPW, Wolff-Parkinson-White syndrome.
[a] Also available in intravenous form.
[b] Intravenous form acts immediately.
[c] 50% is metabolized to N-acetyl procainamide, which is excreted renally.
[d] 40% hepatic and 60% renal excretion.

Its most common contemporary use is in the acute management of patients with atrial fibrillation who have evidence of antegrade accessory pathway conduction.[14] In these patients, atrioventricular (AV) nodal blocking agents are not recommended because they can result in uninhibited accessory pathway conduction. Procainamide blocks the accessory pathway in such patients and hence can control the ventricular rate. It is also often the last resort in patients with incessant ventricular arrhythmias after amiodarone and/or lidocaine have failed and when ablative therapies are not an option.

Disopyramide Disopyramide also has excellent oral absorption. It is excreted through both the liver and the kidney. Similar to other class IA agents, disopyramide also blocks sodium as well as a potassium channels. However, it has very strong vagolytic effects. Because of this, it has significant anticholinergic side effects (dry eyes, blurry vision, urinary retention) and is in general not well tolerated.[15]

Its contemporary use is limited to the treatment of atrial arrhythmias in patients with hypertrophic cardiomyopathy. It is also occasionally used as a third-line negative inotropic agent after β-blockers and calcium channel blockers have failed to decrease symptoms related to obstructive hypertrophic cardiomyopathy.[16]

Class 1B agents

The class Ib agents are available in an intravenous (lidocaine) and oral (mexiletine) form. Details of these medications are outlined in **Table 1**. A brief description is as follows:

Lidocaine Lidocaine is available only in an intravenous form and has a significant protein binding (70%). It is excreted mainly through the liver and has a half-life of 1 to 4 hours. It is rapidly acting and hence is often the drug of choice for acute treatment of ventricular arrhythmias. Its mechanism of action involves blocking the fast sodium channel especially in ischemic and diseased myocardium.[17] It is more effective in the presence of a higher potassium concentration (and hence hypokalemia must be corrected).

Given its significant protein binding and a rapid deethylation by liver microsomes, a high load (usually 2 boluses 30 minutes apart) followed by a low maintenance drip (2–4 mg/min) is generally recommended to prevent toxicities. The toxicities include central nervous system effects (slurred speech, paresthesias, perioral numbness, respiratory arrest) and asystole. Periodic monitoring of lidocaine levels is essential in patients who remain on this medication for a prolonged period of time, as can happen in patients in the intensive care unit with ventricular arrhythmias. If there is concern for toxicity, the medication should be stopped first when waiting for the levels to be measured in the laboratory. Poor hepatic blood flow (in patients with low cardiac output or beta-blockade) and liver disease predispose to lidocaine toxicity. Sinus arrest can occur with concomitant β-blocker usage.

Mexiletine Mexiletine is an oral class Ib agent that also has significant protein-binding activity and is excreted through the liver. It is used as an alternative, or in addition to, amiodarone for chronic suppression of ventricular arrhythmias. Common side effects include blurred vision, gastrointestinal (GI) symptoms, and thrombocytopenia.

Mexiletine for ventricular arrhythmias in patients with congenital heart disease A case series in patients with congenital heart disease reported favorable outcomes with mexiletine.[18] Mexiletine may be added to amiodarone to reduce ventricular arrhythmias and ICD therapies.[19]

Phenytoin Phenytoin is an antiepileptic medication that is rarely used in the current era. It has class Ib antiarrhythmic effects. It may be effective as an antiarrhythmic against ventricular arrhythmias occurring after congenital heart surgery. In patients with epilepsy and ventricular arrhythmias, it may serve a dual role.

Class 1C agents

Class IC agents are potent sodium channel blockers (resulting in QRS widening) that have minimal potassium channel blockade (inwardly rectifying K^+ conductance [I_{Kr}]). Although they have minimal effect on the action potential duration, they cause marked conduction slowing, resulting in electrical heterogeneity and proarrhythmia, with consequent development of ventricular arrhythmias and increased mortality when they are used in patients with structurally abnormal hearts. Similarly, slowing of conduction can organize atrial fibrillation into a slow atrial flutter[20] (which can potentially conduct in a 1:1 ratio to the ventricle) and hence AV nodal blocking agents should always be used with class IC agents.

These agents are predominantly used in the treatment of atrial arrhythmias, but are also effective in the treatment of ventricular arrhythmias when the benefits outweigh their proarrhythmic risks. Details about these agents are outlined in **Table 1**. Differences between flecainide and

Table 2
Practical differences between flecainide and propafenone

Flecainide	Propafenone
Kinetics less variable	Kinetics of non–sustained-release form variable
No beta-blockade	Variable beta-blockade[a]
Needs renal dose adjustment	Does not need renal dose adjustment
Levels can be measured[b]	Levels cannot be measured
Interaction with amiodarone (increased flecainide levels: half dose recommended)	Interaction with warfarin (reduced dose of warfarin required) and digoxin (reduced dose of digoxin required)

[a] Cytochrome PD6-deficient patients have higher β-blocker effect.
[b] Recommended to keep trough levels less than 1 μg/mL.

propafenone are outlined in **Table 2**. Important features are as follows:

Flecainide Flecainide is a class IC agent with excellent GI absorption. Aside from its class IC effects, flecainide also blocks calcium channels in the sarcoplasmic reticulum, making it a niche agent for catecholaminergic polymorphic ventricular tachycardia (VT).[21] It can result in blurred vision and GI side effects aside from its proarrhythmic toxicities.

Propafenone Similar to flecainide, propafenone also has excellent GI absorption. It is predominantly excreted through the liver. Aside from its class IC effects, it also has β-blocking activity. An important fact is that 7% of the population is deficient in cytochrome P-450 2D6,[22] an enzyme that converts propafenone (significant β-blocker effect) to 5-hydroxy propafenone (weak β-blocker effect). These patients have a higher β-blocker effect with propafenone and also have more central nervous system (CNS) side effects. Adverse effects of this medication include dizziness, metallic taste, and a lupuslike rash. It is relatively contraindicated in patients with bronchospastic disease.

CLASS II AGENTS

β-Blockers or commonly used medications that are included as class II agents in the antiarrhythmic classification. They predominantly block the adrenergic nervous system, including the supply to the sinoatrial (SA) node as well as the AV node. They also can homogenize the heterogeneous adrenergic supply to the heart postischemia and in advanced heart failure states (including patients with adult congenital heart disease).

These medications can be used for supraventricular tachycardia (SVT) as well as VT. They can terminate SA node–dependent and AV node–dependent arrhythmias such as SA node reentrant tachycardia, AV node reentrant tachycardia, and AV reentrant tachycardia. The arrhythmias that are not SA/AV node dependent (atrial tachycardia, atrial fibrillation, atrial flutter) can be slowed down by these medications. They can also be used in VT (usually in combination with other antiarrhythmics, such as amiodarone) because of their anti-ischemic and their antiadrenergic effects, including instances of so-called electrical storm. Class II agents are also the predominant medications used in several inherited arrhythmia conditions, such as long QT syndrome and catecholaminergic polymorphic VT.

A detailed discussion of the different β-blockers is beyond the scope of this article. Some important properties to consider while choosing these agents include:

Selectivity

In patients with asthma, a β1-selective β-blocker such as atenolol, esmolol, or metoprolol should be used. If patients have coexistent hypertension, alpha-and beta-blockers such as labetalol or carvedilol (much more alpha blockade with labetolol) should be used.

Lipophilic Versus Hydrophilic Properties

In patients with liver dysfunction or those experiencing CNS side effects, renally excreted β-blockers should be used (such as atenolol or nadolol). In contrast, if there is coexistent renal dysfunction, hydrophilic β-blockers such as propranolol or metoprolol should be used.

Intrinsic Sympathomimetic Activity

Medications such as pindolol or acebutolol have intrinsic symptomatic activity and can increase the incidence of arrhythmias. However, these medications may be useful in young patients with vasovagal syncope or postural orthostatic tachycardia syndrome. In contrast, propranolol has a membrane stabilizing effect and hence may have a stronger antiarrhythmic effect then the aforementioned β-blockers. In the Cardiac Arrest Study Hamburg (CASH), amiodarone and metoprolol had similar outcomes with regard to ventricular arrhythmias.

Half-life

Intravenous esmolol, which is a selective beta-1 antagonist, has a half-life of 9 minutes. It is quickly metabolized in the red blood cells and is independent of renal/hepatic function. In patients with arrhythmias who are unstable and/or have obstructive airway disease, esmolol is an excellent therapeutic option.

CLASS III AGENTS

The class III agents include 5 antiarrhythmic agents available in the United States: amiodarone, sotalol, dofetilide, dronedarone, and ibutilide.

Details about the pharmacokinetic and pharmacodynamic properties, adverse effects, and uses are given in **Table 3**. Important aspects of these agents are as follows:

Amiodarone

Amiodarone is likely the most commonly used antiarrhythmic agent in recent years. It has poor oral bioavailability with approximately 30% to 50% GI absorption and has a slow onset of action because of the loading required. Elimination is predominantly hepatic with a half-life of several weeks. Amiodarone is used for atrial as well as ventricular arrhythmias. It is not approved for the treatment of atrial fibrillation but it is used off label frequently.

From an electrophysiologic standpoint, amiodarone has class I, 2, 3, and 4 effects. However, acutely in the intravenous form, the predominant effects are class I, 2, and 4. The class III effect is seen after complete loading and usually results in

Table 3
Adverse effects and monitoring of amiodarone

Organ System	Adverse Effects (Incidence)	Monitoring	Treatment of Adverse Effects
Cardiac	QTc prolongation (risk of torsades <0.5%) Bradycardia (2%–5%)	Yearly ECG	Discontinue or decrease dose
Respiratory	Amiodarone lung toxicity (1%–17%)	Yearly chest radiograph or pulmonary function tests	Discontinue; consider steroid use
Thyroid gland	Hypothyroidism (6%) or hyperthyroidism (1%–2%)	Thyroid function tests every 6 mo	Discontinue (thyroid replacement for hypothyroidism can be considered)
Liver	Liver toxicity (increased liver enzymes in 15%–30%, hepatitis/cirrhosis <3%)	Liver function tests every 6 mo	Discontinue use
Eye	Corneal microdeposits (>90%) Optic neuropathy (<1%–2%)	Eye examination every year	Discontinue use[a]
Skin	Photosensitive rash (25%–75%) Bluish-gray discoloration (4%–9%)	History and physical examination	Use sunscreen for photosensitive rash Reduce dose or discontinue use for skin discoloration
CNS	Headache, ataxia, tremors, impaired memory, dyssomnia, bad dreams (variable)	History and physical examination	Discontinue use or reduced dose
Miscellaneous	Testicular dysfunction (rare) Nausea (25%)	History/gonadotropin level increase History	Discontinue or reduce dose

Abbreviation: ECG, electrocardiogram.
 [a] Corneal microdeposits are usually asymptomatic and amiodarone can usually be continued.

prolongation of action potential duration in all cardiac tissues, decreasing any electrical inhomogeneity in the heart. Amiodarone is usually loaded in its intravenous form for 1 to 2 g. It takes approximately 10 g for its complete load to have class III effects.

The biggest concern with amiodarone is its long-term toxicities. The toxicities associated with amiodarone and the monitoring that is required are highlighted in **Table 4**. Amiodarone levels can be measured (therapeutic range is 1–2.5 mg/mL) because higher levels have been associated with increased toxicity.[23] The common drug interactions of amiodarone include warfarin (warfarin dose is to be reduced) and digoxin (digoxin dose needs to be reduced). In the Sudden Cardiac Death in Heart Failure Trial (SCD-HeFT) there was an increased mortality in patients with amiodarone who had NYHA Class 3 symptoms[24] likely related to its negative inotropic effects; it should be used with caution in patients with advanced heart failure.

Amiodarone for supraventricular arrhythmias in patients with congenital heart disease

Although amiodarone is the most effective antiarrhythmic agent for maintaining sinus rhythm, its side effects should be strongly considered before committing a young adult with congenital heart disease to long-term amiodarone therapy; ablation may be a better option. The risk of thyrotoxicosis is especially high in women with congenital heart disease and cyanotic heart disease or univentricular heart with Fontan palliation.[25] The risk of thyrotoxicosis is also high in thin patients with low body mass index.[26] Amiodarone can be considered a first-line or second-line antiarrhythmic in patients with congenital heart disease and pathologic hypertrophy of the ventricle, ventricular dysfunction, or coronary artery disease (class IIa). It should be used with caution in those at high risk for adverse effects, such as cyanotic heart disease, or low body mass index and preexistent hepatic, pulmonary, or thyroid disease (class IIa).[19]

Amiodarone for ventricular arrhythmias in patients with congenital heart disease

Amiodarone is the most effective antiarrhythmic agent for chronic suppression of ventricular arrhythmias in patients with congenital heart disease[19]; long-term use is associated with adverse effects, as mentioned earlier. A study showed that, in patients with tetralogy of Fallot or double-outlet right ventricle that failed catheter ablation for VT, sotalol or amiodarone rendered them non-inducible for VT.[27]

Sotalol and Dofetilide

Sotalol (racemic mixture of dextro [class 3 effect] and levo [class 2 effect] isomers, clinically available) and dofetilide (class 3 effect only) are similar class III antiarrhythmic agents. They both have excellent GI absorption and are excreted renally. The half-life of both is approximately 12 hours. Both these medications can be used for atrial as well as ventricular arrhythmias. Anecdotally, sotalol is used more frequently for ventricular arrhythmias.

These medications can cause a dose-dependent prolongation in QTc and hence require electrocardiogram (ECG) monitoring. This requirement applies especially for dofetilide, which requires inpatient initiation of the medication. Based on the estimated glomerular filtration rate, the highest possible dose of dofetilide is initiated (500 µg orally twice a day). ECG is obtained 2 hours after every dose and QTc is closely monitored. If the QTc after the first dose increases to more than 500 milliseconds or more than 15% of the prior QTc, the dose is reduced. If the QTc remains prolonged or there is a further increase, dofetilide should be discontinued. Sotalol is usually started at the lowest possible dose (80 mg orally twice a day) and gradually increased to approximately 160 mg orally twice a day. QTc is monitored in a similar fashion. There is a variable practice regarding initiation of sotalol (inpatient vs outpatient); in our institution, sotalol is routinely started on an outpatient basis with close weekly QTc monitoring and uptitration of the dose. Practical differences between sotalol and dofetilide are outlined in **Table 5**.

Sotalol for supraventricular arrhythmias in congenital heart disease

Sotalol has been used with variable safety and efficacy in patients with congenital heart disease[28–31]; there is a concern for increased mortality in pediatric patients.[32] As such, the current guidelines give a class IIb recommendation for maintenance of sinus rhythm in patients with congenital heart disease and preserved systemic ventricular function (class 2B).[19]

Sotalol for ventricular arrhythmias in congenital heart disease

Sotalol can be used as a second-line agent after amiodarone for control of ventricular arrhythmias in patients with congenital heart disease.[19]

Dofetilide for supraventricular arrhythmias in congenital heart disease

There is at least 1 study that has shown the safety of dofetilide in patients with congenital heart

Table 4
Class 3 antiarrhythmics

	Amiodarone	Sotalol	Dofetilide	Dronedarone	Ibutilide
Absorption (%)	30–50	>90	100	>90	Only IV
Half-life	Weeks	12 h	12 h (variable)	30 h	10 h
Excretion	Hepatic	Renal	Renal (mainly)	Hepatic	Renal
Practical Uses	VT SVT	AF, VT	AF (not approved for VT)	AF	AF (acute conversion)
Dose	1 to 2 g acute loading; 200–400 mg once a day (maintenance)	80–320 mg PO BID • Interval 2–3 d • Watch QT	125–500 µg BID	400 mg PO BID	10 mg IV over 10 min; can repeat
Adverse Reactions	Thyroid abnormalities Lung toxicity Liver toxicity Optic neuropathy	CHF exacerbation Prolong QT and TdP Fatigue Bradycardia	Headache Prolong QT and TdP	Increased mortality in patients with CHF	Prolongs QT and TdP

Abbreviations: CHF, congestive heart failure; PO, by mouth; TdP, torsades de pointes.

Table 5
Practical differences between sotalol and dofetilide

Sotalol	Dofetilide
Has β-blocker effect	No significant β-blocker effect
Has a negative inotropic effect	No significant negative anti-inotropic effect
Used for atrial and ventricular arrhythmias	Used predominantly for atrial arrhythmias
Less drug interactions	More drug interactions because of complex pharmacokinetics
Can be initiated as outpatient	Requires inpatient initiation
Dose titrated from low to high	Highest dose started first and titrated lower if required
Considered unsafe in patients with systolic dysfunction/CHF symptoms	Considered safe in patients with systolic dysfunction or CHF symptoms
Can result in bronchospasm	Safe in patients with obstructive airway disease
Risk of torsades lower (<0.5% at 320 mg/d dose)	Risk of torsades higher (3%)

disease and atrial arrhythmias.[33] However, 2 of these patients had torsades. The current guidelines recommend dofetilide as a reasonable alternative to amiodarone as a first-line antiarrhythmic agent in patients with congenital heart disease and ventricular dysfunction (class 2A).[19]

Dronedarone

Dronedarone was initially introduced as an alternative to amiodarone. It was thought that it would be very similar to amiodarone except for its iodine moiety, which would result in a similar antiarrhythmic effect with much lesser side effects. However, dronedarone has not been as efficacious as amiodarone for treatment of arrhythmias.

It has an excellent GI absorption and is excreted predominantly through the liver. The half-life is close to 36 hours and it requires 10 days to achieve a steady state. It is mainly used for the treatment of atrial arrhythmias, with a typical dose of 400 mg orally twice a day. Dose-dependent diarrhea is a common side effect. Based on the Antiarrhythmic Trial with Dronedarone in Moderate to Severe CHF Evaluating Morbidity Decrease (ANDROMEDA)[34] and Permanent Atrial Fibrillation Outcome Study Using Dronedarone on Top of Standard Therapy (PALLAS)[35] trials, dronedarone should be avoided in patients with systolic congestive heart failure as well as those with permanent atrial fibrillation. It significantly increases digoxin concentrations and can result in toxicity.[35]

Dronedarone for supraventricular arrhythmias in congenital heart disease

Dronedarone can be used in patients with congenital heart disease. However, given the problems seen in patients with advanced heart failure, the current guidelines do not recommend its use in patients with heart failure, moderate or severe systemic ventricular dysfunction, or moderate and complex congenital heart disease.[19]

Ibutilide

Ibutilide is available only in the intravenous form and has a half-life of approximately 10 hours. It is excreted through the kidneys. Ibutilide is predominantly used for a pharmacologic cardioversion of atrial arrhythmias by inhibition of the delayed rectifier potassium current (I_{Kr}). It is usually given at the dose of 1 mg intravenously over 10 minutes (or 0.01 mg/kg if weight <60 kg). It can be repeated after a waiting period of 10 minutes. Its efficacy for acute termination is up to 50% with a mean termination time of 27 minutes[36]; it can also facilitate electrical cardioversion.[37] The medication should be stopped if there is QTc prolongation or if ventricular arrhythmias are seen (risk of torsades approximately 4%).[38] It should also obviously be stopped if the end point of cardioversion to normal sinus rhythm occurs. The patient should be monitored in the hospital for at least 4 hours for late development of QTc prolongation and ventricular arrhythmias. Other QTc-prolonging medications, such as class Ia or class III agents, should be avoided at the time of its use.

Ibutilide for supraventricular arrhythmias in congenital heart disease

There was 1 small series of using ibutilide in patients with congenital heart disease; the success rate was 70% with a rate of torsades less than 1%.[39] It is reasonable to use ibutilide for acute conversion of atrial arrhythmias in patients with congenital heart disease per the guidelines.[19]

CLASS VI ANTIARRHYTHMICS

Calcium channel blockers are another commonly used class of medications that are included as class IV agents in the antiarrhythmic classification. The nondihydropyridine calcium channel blockers (verapamil and diltiazem) have antiarrhythmic effects (as opposed to the dihydropyridine calcium channel blockers, such as amlodipine, which are vascular selective). The nondihydropyridine calcium channel blockers block the SA node and the AV node. They can also block early afterdepolarizations (EADs).

Calcium channel blockers can be used for SVTs as well as VTs. They can block the SA node–dependent and AV node–dependent arrhythmias and slow down the arrhythmias that are not SA node and AV node dependent (similar to β-blockers). They can be used for multifocal atrial tachycardia (which occurs because of EADs). They are also useful in the treatment of VT, especially those involving the Purkinje fibers (fascicular or Belhassen VT). These medications are usually not used in patients with depressed ejection fraction because of their hemodynamic effects.

Miscellaneous Antiarrhythmics

Ranolazine

Ranolazine is an anti-ischemic agent that has anti-arrhythmic properties. In the setting of advanced structural heart disease, there can be intracellular sodium overload from the late sodium current. This overload, in turn, can lead to an intracellular calcium overload caused by the sodium-calcium exchanger. This condition can further result in afterdepolarizations and transmural dispersion of repolarization, which can result in arrhythmias. Ranolazine, by virtue of blocking the late sodium channel, can decrease this sodium overload, resulting in an antiarrhythmic effect.

It is usually used in the dose range of 500 to 1000 mg orally twice a day. It can cause a modest QTc prolongation. It is usually excreted through the GI system and the liver. It has a half-life of 6 to 9 hours. It has been used for the treatment of both atrial and ventricular arrhythmias. There is an ongoing trial to study the effect of ranolazine versus placebo to reduce ICD shocks in patients who undergo ICD implantation at risk for shocks. Dronaderone (225 mg or 150 mg orally twice a day) and ranolazine (750 mg orally twice a day) in combination have been shown to be efficacious against atrial fibrillation.[40]

Adenosine

Adenosine is a commonly used and exclusively intravenous medication that is used to terminate AV nodal, SA nodal, and triggered activity–dependent arrhythmias. Its mechanism of action involves the opening of the adenosine-sensitive inward rectifier potassium channel. It can also slow down the AV node during arrhythmias that are not AV nodal dependent (such as atrial fibrillation, atrial flutter, and atrial tachycardia) revealing the underlying P or fibrillatory waves. It usually has no effect on ventricular tachycardia except outflow tract VT which is triggered-activity mediated.[41]

It has a peak effect in 10 seconds and its effect lasts for approximately 10 more seconds. It is usually given as a bolus of 6 mg followed by 12 mg if the first dose is not effective. It has a host of side effects, which are usually short lived and include flushing, bronchospasm, bradycardia, and chest pressure.

Digoxin

Digoxin is available in both oral and intravenous forms and is excreted through the kidneys. The predominant mechanism of action is an increased parasympathetic tone that blocks the AV as well as the SA node. It also increases intercellular calcium level, thus increasing inotropy. Similar to β-blockers and calcium channel blockers, it can potentially terminate arrhythmias that are AV and SA nodal dependent and can slow down the SVTs that are not SA/AV node dependent.

At higher levels, it can cause a host of side effects, including GI effects (nausea, vomiting), CNS effects (visual symptoms, delirium), and arrhythmias (sinus arrest, complete heart block, atrial tachycardia, junctional tachycardia, and fascicular ventricular arrhythmias). A detailed description of the treatment of digoxin toxicity is beyond the scope of this article but it includes correction of electrolyte levels (hypokalemia and hypomagnesemia enhance digoxin toxicity), pacing, lidocaine, and the use of digoxin-binding antibodies (Digibind). Amiodarone is not typically used because it further increases the digoxin level.

Magnesium

Intravenous magnesium also has antiarrhythmic effects by decreasing EADs and thus reducing the occurrence of torsades de pointes. It is especially useful in the setting of digoxin toxicity. Hypermagnesemia can prolong the PR and QT intervals. At much higher levels, it can lead to respiratory paralysis as well as cardiac arrest.

SPECIAL CONSIDERATIONS FOR ANTIARRHYTHMICS IN PATIENTS WITH ADULT CONGENITAL HEART DISEASE
Use of Class 1C Antiarrhythmics in Patients with Congenital Heart Disease

In general, flecainide and propafenone are contra-indicated in patients with structural heart disease and in patients with sick sinus syndrome/conduction abnormalities. These proarrhythmic effects were reported by the CAST[42] and CASH[43] trials. It has been hypothesized that nonuniform slowing of conduction in patients with myocardial scar may increase the risk of ventricular arrhythmias.

Patient's with moderate and complex congenital heart disease have a variable amount of myocardial scar. When ablative therapies are not an option or fail, antiarrhythmics may be the only option. In such circumstances, class IC agents can be used with the following cautions:

1. As recommended in the guidelines, the authors do not use it in patients with coexistent coronary artery disease or systemic ventricle dysfunction (PACES [Pediatric and Congenital Electrophysiology Society] guidelines).
2. Initiate at a low dose with slow uptitration and careful monitoring of the QRS duration.
3. Perform Holter monitoring and stress testing once medications have been loaded to ensure there are no proarrhythmic effects.

Use of Sotalol in Patients with Congenital Heart Disease

In the ESVEM trial,[44] sotalol was much more effective than other class I agents in the reduction of death and ventricular arrhythmias. However, D-sotalol, which is a pure class III agent, had increased mortality in postinfarct patients with a low ejection fraction (the SWORD study).[45] The current atrial fibrillation guidelines[46] thus do not recommend sotalol in patients with low ejection fraction, and some clinicians also extrapolate this to the management of ventricular arrhythmias.

Sotalol has been used with mixed results in patients with congenital heart disease. Some retrospective studies show reasonable safety and efficacy[28–30] but some showed high rates of proarrhythmia.[31] Meta-analyses of sotalol in pediatric patients have shown an increased all-cause mortality. This finding has led to reservation in the use of sotalol for patients with adult congenital heart disease. The guidelines give it a class IIb indication for first-line antiarrhythmic maintenance of sinus rhythm in the presence of preserved systemic ventricular function.

Similar to the use of flecainide, sotalol can be used in patients with structural heart disease. The authors recommend the following cautions:

1. Inpatient initiation and gradual uptitration.
2. The risk of ventricular arrhythmias/torsades is very low with a dose of 320 mg per day (0.3%) or less.
3. Avoid its use in patients with significant renal dysfunction (creatinine clearance <40 mL/min) or if the baseline QTc is greater than 450 milliseconds

Anticoagulants

Atrial arrhythmias, including typical and atypical atrial flutters as well as atrial fibrillation, are common in patients with adult congenital heart disease. The risk of systemic thromboembolism in these populations is higher than in the general population, especially in patients with moderate and complex congenital heart disease.[47] This article addresses some practical questions with regard to the use of anticoagulants in patients with congenital heart disease:

1. Which arrhythmia warrants consideration of anticoagulation?
2. Which patients need anticoagulation?
3. Which medication to use?
4. What about anticoagulation in the pericardioversion period?

Which arrhythmia warrants anticoagulation? From a pathophysiologic standpoint, it seems that arrhythmias without an effective atrial contraction (atrial fibrillation and atrial flutter) have a higher risk of clot formation resulting in stroke and systemic embolism. Slower atrial arrhythmias (such as focally emanating atrial tachycardias with tachycardia cycle lengths >400 milliseconds) seem to be associated with a lower risk of stroke. However, there are no prospective studies that have differentiated the risk between these arrhythmias. To further add to the complexity, there are several arrhythmias in the gray zone where it is impossible to differentiate between macroreentrant atrial flutter and focally emanating tachycardias based on surface ECG because of atrial scar. When in doubt, it may be best to err on the side of recommending anticoagulation given the implication of strokes on quality and quantity of life.

Who needs anticoagulation? The CHA_2DS_2-VASc score is the most commonly used contemporary scoring system to predict the risk of systemic thromboembolism in the general population.[48] In patients with adult congenital heart disease, a

Table 6
Properties of currently available anticoagulants

	Warfarin	Dabigatran	Rivaroxaban	Apixaban	Edoxaban
Pharmacology					
Mechanism of Action	Vitamin K epoxide reductase inhibitor	Direct thrombin inhibitor (reversible)	Factor Xa inhibitor	Factor Xa inhibitor	Factor Xa inhibitor
Prodrug/Converting Agent	None	Dabigatran etexilate (double prodrug)/esterase	None	None	None
Metabolism					
Oral Bioavailability (%)	80–100	6.5	80–100	~50	~50
Plasma Protein Binding (%)	~100	35	95	~90	40–60
Kidney Excretion (%)	Metabolized by liver; excreted by kidneys (92)	80	~35	25	35
Interactions					
Effect of Food on Absorption	None	Delays by 2 h	Increases bioavailability for doses ≥15 mg	None	None
CYP 450 Involvement	Present	None	Present	Present	Present
P-gP Interaction	No	Present	Present	Present	Present
Major Drug Interactions	Amiodarone, mexiletine, propafenone, verapamil, several others	Rifampin, quinidine	Ritonavir, ketoconazole	Ritonavir, ketoconazole	Ritonavir, ketoconazole
Pharmacokinetics					
Half-life (h)	20–60	12–17	7–11	8–15	8–10
T_{max} (h)	4	1–3	2–3	1–2	1–2
Clinical Use					
Dose	Variable (needs INR monitoring)	150 mg PO BID 75 mg PO BID[a]	20 mg PO QD 15 mg PO QD[a]	5 mg PO BID 2.5 mg PO BID[b]	60 mg PO QD[c] 30 mg PO QD[a,c]
Adverse Effects	Bleeding Rare skin necrosis	Dyspepsia Bleeding (especially GI)	Bleeding	Bleeding	Bleeding Rash and abnormal LFTs

Abbreviations: CYP, cytochrome P; INR, International Normalized Ratio; LFT, liver function test; P-gP, P-Glycoprotein; QD, every day; T_{max}, the time after administration of a drug when the maximum plasma concentration is reached.

[a] For creatinine clearance between 15 and 50 mL/min; contraindicated for use less than 15 mL/min.

[b] If 2 or 3 present: age more than 80 years, weight less than 60 kg, and creatinine level greater than 1.5 mg/dL; full dose recommended in dialysis patients.

[c] Avoid use of edoxaban if creatinine clearance greater than 95 mL/min.

high CHA_2DS_2-VASc score (≥2) warrants anticoagulation.[46] However, a low CHA_2DS_2-VASc score is not expected to be predictive of low-risk thromboembolic events in these patients, for 2 reasons:

1. These patients are young and hence are less likely to have risk factors, such as hypertension, diabetes mellitus, and coronary artery disease, that are components of the CHA_2DS_2-VASc score.
2. Based on the complexity of the congenital heart disease, there are varying degrees of myocardial scar and valvular abnormalities that increase the risk of stroke independent of the traditional risk factors.

There are no prospective studies evaluating the risk of systemic thromboembolism in patients with atrial arrhythmias and congenital heart disease. The current guidelines recommend full-dose anticoagulation as follows[19]:

1. Full-dose anticoagulation is recommended in patients with a CHA_2DS_2-VASc score greater than or equal to 2 and atrial arrhythmias that are known to be associated with stroke/thromboembolism (atrial fibrillation and flutter).
2. In patients with a low CHA_2DS_2-VASc score and the aforementioned atrial arrhythmias, full-dose anticoagulation is recommended in patients with moderate and severely complex congenital heart disease as well as simple congenital heart disease with prosthetic valves or hemodynamically significant valvular disease.

Which medication? Until the last few years, warfarin was the only available oral anticoagulant. However, there are currently 4 non–vitamin K antagonist oral anticoagulants (NOACs) that are US Food and Drug Administration approved for stroke prevention with atrial arrhythmias in patients with nonvalvular atrial fibrillation.[49] There are no prospective studies comparing warfarin with NOACs in patients with congenital heart disease. A detailed description of these medications is beyond the scope of this article but their essential properties are highlighted in **Table 6**. Aside from warfarin and the NOACs, antiplatelet agents such as aspirin have also been used for stroke prevention, although the data for its efficacy are controversial. Our approach is as follows:

1. In patients with mechanical valves or significant residual mitral/tricuspid valve disease as a part of the congenital heart disease, warfarin is recommended.
2. In patients with moderate or severely complex congenital heart disease, warfarin is

recommended given that pharmacokinetics are unknown in these patients (eg, Fontan physiology with hepatic dysfunction).

3. In patients with simple congenital heart disease and prior valve repair or bioprosthetic valves, or those with simple congenital heart disease and nonvalvular atrial fibrillation, warfarin or NOACs is recommended after discussion of the risks and benefits of these medications.
4. The authors do not believe that aspirin significant reduces the risk of stroke associated with atrial arrhythmias (related to atrium/appendage). Aspirin can be considered instead of anticoagulation in patients with CHA_2DS_2-VASc of 1.

What about anticoagulation in the pericardioversion period? As mentioned previously, there is a significant risk of thromboembolism in the patient population with atrial arrhythmias, especially in those with moderate and complex congenital heart disease. In small series, thrombi were found in ~37% of patients undergoing transesophageal echocardiography before cardioversion.[50] The authors recommend precardioversion anticoagulation (for 3 weeks at least) or transesophageal echocardiography to rule out clot irrespective of duration of atrial arrhythmias, unless emergent cardioversion is required. The only exception to the rule is new-onset (<48 hours) atrial flutter/fibrillation with simple congenital heart disease and no valvular abnormalities or prosthetic valves.

REFERENCES

1. Khairy P, Ionescu-Ittu R, Mackie AS, et al. Changing mortality in congenital heart disease. J Am Coll Cardiol 2010;56(14):1149–57.
2. Warnes CA, Williams RG, Bashore TM, et al. ACC/AHA 2008 guidelines for the management of adults with congenital heart disease: executive summary: a report of the American College of Cardiology/American Heart Association Task Force on Practice Guidelines (Writing Committee to Develop Guidelines for the Management of Adults with Congenital Heart Disease) developed in collaboration with the American Society of Echocardiography, Heart Rhythm Society, International Society for Adult Congenital Heart Disease, Society for Cardiovascular Angiography and Interventions, and Society of Thoracic Surgeons. J Am Coll Cardiol 2008;52(23):1890–947.
3. Khairy P. Thrombosis in congenital heart disease. Expert Rev Cardiovasc Ther 2013;11(12):1579–82.

4. Vaughan-Williams EM. Classification of antiarrhythmic actions. In: Vaughan-Williams EM, editor. Antiarrhythmic drugs. Berlin: Springer; 1989. p. 45–67.

5. Rosen MR, Schwartz PJ. The 'Sicilian Gambit'-A new approach to the classification of antiarrhythmic drugs based on their actions on arrhythmogenic mechanisms. Eur Heart J 1991;12(10):1112–31.

6. Fish FA, Gillette PC, Benson DW. Proarrhythmia, cardiac arrest and death in young patients receiving encainide and flecainide. J Am Coll Cardiol 1991; 18(2):356–65.

7. Khairy P, Harris L, Landzberg MJ, et al. Implantable cardioverter-defibrillators in tetralogy of Fallot. Circulation 2008;117(3):363–70.

8. Bauman JL, Bauernfeind RA, Hoff JV, et al. Torsade de pointes due to quinidine: observations in 31 patients. Am Heart J 1984;107(3):425–30.

9. Belhassen B, Glick A, Viskin S. Efficacy of quinidine in high-risk patients with Brugada syndrome. Circulation 2004;110(13):1731–7.

10. Alings M, Dekker L, Sadée A, et al. Quinidine induced electrocardiographic normalization in two patients with Brugada syndrome. Pacing Clin Electrophysiol 2001;24(9):1420–2.

11. Stevenson WG, Weiss J. Torsades de pointes due to n-acetylprocainamide. Pacing Clin Electrophysiol 1985;8(4):528–31.

12. Reidenberg MM, Drayer DE, Levy M, et al. Polymorphic acetylation of procainamide in man. Clin Pharmacol Ther 1975;17(6):722–30.

13. Reidenberg MM, Drayer DE. Procainamide, N-acetylprocainamide, antinuclear antibody and systemic lupus erythematosus. Angiology 1986;37(12 Pt 2): 968–71.

14. Fengler BT, Brady WJ, Plautz CU. Atrial fibrillation in the Wolff-Parkinson-White syndrome: ECG recognition and treatment in the ED. Am J Emerg Med 2007;25(5):576–83.

15. Bauman JL, Gallastegui J, Strasberg B, et al. Long-term therapy with disopyramide phosphate: side effects and effectiveness. Am Heart J 1986;111(4): 654–60.

16. Sherrid M, Delia E, Dwyer E. Oral disopyramide therapy for obstructive hypertrophic cardiomyopathy. Am J Cardiol 1988;62(16):1085–8.

17. Hondeghem LM. Effects of lidocaine, phenytoin and quinidine on the ischemic canine myocardium. J Electrocardiol 1976;9(3):203–9.

18. Moak JP, Smith RT, Garson A. Mexiletine: an effective antiarrhythmic drug for treatment of ventricular arrhythmias in congenital heart disease. J Am Coll Cardiol 1987;10(4):824–9.

19. Khairy P, Van Hare GF, Balaji S, et al. PACES/HRS expert consensus statement on the recognition and management of arrhythmias in adult congenital heart disease: developed in partnership between the Pediatric and Congenital Electrophysiology Society (PACES) and the Heart Rhythm Society (HRS). Endorsed by the governing bodies of PACES, HRS, the American College of Cardiology (ACC), the American Heart Association (AHA), the European Heart Rhythm Association (EHRA), the Canadian Heart Rhythm Society (CHRS), and the International Society for Adult Congenital Heart Disease (ISACHD). Can J Cardiol 2014;30(10):e1–63.

20. Feld GK, Chen PS, Nicod P, et al. Possible atrial proarrhythmic effects of class 1C antiarrhythmic drugs. Am J Cardiol 1990;66(3):378–83.

21. Watanabe H, Chopra N, Laver D, et al. Flecainide prevents catecholaminergic polymorphic ventricular tachycardia in mice and humans. Nat Med 2009; 15(4):380–3.

22. Rogers JF, Nafziger AN, Bertino JS. Pharmacogenetics affects dosing, efficacy, and toxicity of cytochrome P450-metabolized drugs. Am J Med 2002; 113(9):746–50.

23. Connolly SJ. Evidence-based analysis of amiodarone efficacy and safety. Circulation 1999;100(19): 2025–34.

24. Bardy GH, Lee KL, Mark DB, et al. Amiodarone or an implantable cardioverter–defibrillator for congestive heart failure. N Engl J Med 2005; 352(3):225–37.

25. Thorne SA, Barnes I, Cullinan P, et al. Amiodarone-associated thyroid dysfunction risk factors in adults with congenital heart disease. Circulation 1999; 100(2):149–54.

26. Stan MN, Ammash NM, Warnes CA, et al. Body mass index and the development of amiodarone-induced thyrotoxicosis in adults with congenital heart disease—a cohort study. Int J Cardiol 2013; 167(3):821–6.

27. Furushima H, Chinushi M, Sugiura H, et al. Ventricular tachycardia late after repair of congenital heart disease: efficacy of combination therapy with radiofrequency catheter ablation and class III antiarrhythmic agents and long-term outcome. J Electrocardiol 2006;39(2):219–24.

28. Koyak Z, Kroon B, de Groot JR, et al. Efficacy of antiarrhythmic drugs in adults with congenital heart disease and supraventricular tachycardias. Am J Cardiol 2013;112(9):1461–7.

29. Miyazaki A, Ohuchi H, Kurosaki K, et al. Efficacy and safety of sotalol for refractory tachyarrhythmias in congenital heart disease. Circ J 2008;72(12):1998–2003.

30. Beaufort-Krol GC, Bink-Boelkens MT. Sotalol for atrial tachycardias after surgery for congenital heart disease. Pacing Clin Electrophysiol 1997;20(8): 2125–9.

31. Pfammatter JP, Paul T, Lehmann C, et al. Efficacy and proarrhythmia of oral sotalol in pediatric patients. J Am Coll Cardiol 1995;26(4):1002–7.

32. Lafuente-Lafuente C, Mouly S, Longas-Tejero MA, et al. Antiarrhythmics for maintaining sinus rhythm after cardioversion of atrial fibrillation. Cochrane Database Syst Rev 2007;(4):CD005049.

33. Wells R, Khairy P, Harris L, et al. Dofetilide for atrial arrhythmias in congenital heart disease: a multi-center study. Pacing Clin Electrophysiol 2009; 32(10):1313–8.

34. Køber L, Torp-Pedersen C, McMurray JJ, et al. Increased mortality after dronedarone therapy for severe heart failure. N Engl J Med 2008;358(25): 2678–87.

35. Connolly SJ, Camm AJ, Halperin JL, et al. Dronedarone in high-risk permanent atrial fibrillation. N Engl J Med 2011;365(24):2268–76.

36. Stambler BS, Wood MA, Ellenbogen KA, et al. Efficacy and safety of repeated intravenous doses of ibutilide for rapid conversion of atrial flutter or fibrillation. Circulation 1996;94(7):1613–21.

37. Oral H, Souza JJ, Michaud GF, et al. Facilitating transthoracic cardioversion of atrial fibrillation with ibutilide pretreatment. N Engl J Med 1999;340(24): 1849–54.

38. Kowey PR, VanderLugt JT, Luderer JR. Safety and risk/benefit analysis of ibutilide for acute conversion of atrial fibrillation/flutter. Am J Cardiol 1996;78(8): 46–52.

39. Hoyer AW, Balaji S. The safety and efficacy of ibutilide in children and in patients with congenital heart disease. Pacing Clin Electrophysiol 2007;30(8): 1003–8.

40. Reiffel JA, Camm AJ, Belardinelli L, et al. The HARMONY Trial: combined ranolazine and dronedarone in the management of paroxysmal atrial fibrillation: mechanistic and therapeutic synergism. Circ Arrhythm Electrophysiol 2015. [Epub ahead of print].

41. Griffith MJ, Garratt CJ, Rowland E, et al. Effects of intravenous adenosine on verapamil-sensitive "idiopathic" ventricular tachycardia. Am J Cardiol 1994; 73(11):759–64.

42. Epstein AE, Hallstrom AP, Rogers WJ, et al. Mortality following ventricular arrhythmia suppression by encainide, flecainide, and moricizine after myocardial infarction: the original design concept of the Cardiac Arrhythmia Suppression Trial (CAST). JAMA 1993; 270(20):2451–5.

43. Kuck KH, Cappato R, Siebels J, et al. Randomized comparison of antiarrhythmic drug therapy with implantable defibrillators in patients resuscitated from cardiac arrest the Cardiac Arrest Study Hamburg (CASH). Circulation 2000;102(7): 748–54.

44. Wnuk-Wojnar AM, Giec L, Drzewiecki J, et al. Predictors of ventricular tachycardia inducibility in programmed electrical stimulation and the effectiveness of serial drug testing: Polish multicenter study. Pacing Clin Electrophysiol 1990;13(12): 2127–32.

45. Waldo AL, Camm AJ, deRuyter H, et al. Effect of d-sotalol on mortality in patients with left ventricular dysfunction after recent and remote myocardial infarction. Lancet 1996;348(9019):7–12.

46. January CT, Wann LS, Alpert JS, et al. 2014 AHA/ACC/HRS guideline for the management of patients with atrial fibrillation: a report of the American College of Cardiology/American Heart Association Task Force on Practice Guidelines and the Heart Rhythm Society. J Am Coll Cardiol 2014;64(21): e1–76.

47. Hoffmann A, Chockalingam P, Balint OH, et al. Cerebrovascular accidents in adult patients with congenital heart disease. Heart 2010;96(15): 1223–6.

48. Minamiguchi H, Okuyama Y, Minamino T, et al. The efficacy of CHA2DS2-VASc score to predict ischemic stroke in patients with atrial fibrillation in clinical practice: 4-year follow-up study-a report from the STACIN registry. Circulation 2013;128(22 Suppl):A16287.

49. Contractor T, Levin V, Martinez MW, et al. Novel oral anticoagulants for stroke prevention in patients with atrial fibrillation: dawn of a new era. Postgrad Med 2013;125(1):34–44.

50. Feltes TF, Friedman RA. Transesophageal echocardiographic detection of atrial thrombi in patients with nonfibrillation atrial tachyarrhythmias and congenital heart disease. J Am Coll Cardiol 1994; 24(5):1365–70.

Catheter Ablation
General Principles and Advances

Sabine Ernst, MD, PhD, FESC

KEYWORDS

- Catheter ablation • 3D image integration • Remote navigation • 3D mapping
- Simultaneous mapping • Sequential mapping

KEY POINTS

- The underlying anatomy can be understood through three-dimensional reconstruction of tomographic imaging.
- Choosing the most appropriate acquisition system (simultaneous vs sequential) is necessary for the given arrhythmia.
- Recognizing the need for close collaboration with cardiac anesthesia ensures good hemodynamic support and adequate analgesia.

INTRODUCTION

Cardiac arrhythmias are typically encountered after cardiac surgery and can occur in the immediate postsurgical period or, more often, decades after surgery. In the postoperative period, arrhythmias may complicate the patient's course and prolong the stay in the intensive care unit.[1,2] Late after surgery, cardiac arrhythmias are thought to stem mainly from the unavoidable scars left behind (eg, after an atriotomy, the cannulation sites for the cardiopulmonary bypass, or other scars inherent to the specific cardiac surgery [patch sutures]).[3–5] However, age and progression of the structural/congenital heart disease, resulting in pressure increase and dilation, can lead to pronounced fibrosis, which in itself can promote focal and/or reentrant arrhythmia.[6] The presence of frequently recurrent or sustained arrhythmias is associated with reduced quality of life, risk of development of heart failure symptoms caused by tachycardiomyopathy, higher thromboembolic risk, and reduced survival.[7–9]

Catheter ablation of postsurgical arrhythmias in patients with congenital heart disease is currently feasible and successful with the use of advanced image integration and ablation tools. This article reviews the general steps of preparation for such a procedure and discusses the available techniques as an alternative to long-term antiarrhythmic therapy. **Fig. 1** summarizes a stepwise approach that helps clinicians to perform even complex ablation procedure successfully.

GENERAL PREPARATION OF PATIENTS WITH CONGENITAL HEART DISEASE PRESENTING WITH ARRHYTHMIAS

In the first instance, 12-lead electrocardiogram (ECG) documentation is the key investigation to allow differentiation between atrial and ventricular, as well as regular (eg, atrial tachycardia) as opposed to irregular (eg, atrial fibrillation vs frequent atrial or ventricular ectopy or arrhythmias) arrhythmias. The 12-lead ECG allows a first localization of the origin of the documented arrhythmia, but, because of the possibly distorted cardiac

Disclosures: S. Ernst is consulting for Stereotaxis Inc, Biosense Webster, and Spectrum Dynamics.
Cardiology Department, National Heart and Lung Institute, Royal Brompton and Harefield Hospital, Imperial College, Sydney Street, London SW3 6NP, UK
E-mail address: S.Ernst@rbht.nhs.uk

Card Electrophysiol Clin 9 (2017) 311–317
http://dx.doi.org/10.1016/j.ccep.2017.02.012
1877-9182/17/© 2017 Elsevier Inc. All rights reserved.

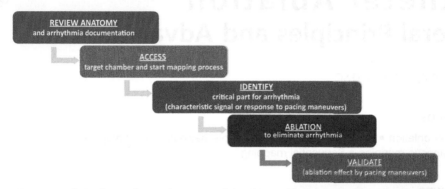

Fig. 1. Stepwise approach to plan and execute a successful catheter ablation procedure in patients with congenital heart disease.

anatomy, common ECG algorithms may not be sufficient. Holter recordings are especially valuable in intermittent arrhythmias and also allow documentation of the arrhythmias when more than 1 type of arrhythmia is present. Correlation with symptoms and potential consequences (eg, prolonged pauses after tachycardia termination) can be identified. However, the duration of Holter recordings (typically up to 7–14 days) may limit the yield of this diagnostic test if patients experience rare palpitations.[10] Implantable loop recorder systems are an alternative, but lack the accuracy of P-wave detection and therefore differentiation of various atrial tachycardias may be based on cycle length analysis only.[11,12]

Standard Imaging Studies

Because the arrhythmia could be an expression of worsening of the underlying congenital condition, careful transthoracic and, if necessary, transesophageal echocardiography should be performed to understand the relevant hemodynamic issues (eg, increase in pulmonary valve regurgitation in tetralogy of Fallot). Invasive hemodynamic studies may need to be considered either as stand-alone investigations or as part of the ablation procedure.

PREPARATION OF THE ABLATION PROCEDURE
Detailed Knowledge of Individual Anatomy

Understanding the individual three-dimensional (3D) anatomy is the cornerstone of any successful ablation procedure, even in patients without congenital conditions.[13,14] Information on the dimensions of the cardiac chambers, the spatial relationship and angulations between different cardiac structures, and the presence of a patent foramen ovale are some examples of necessary information that may facilitate any procedure. In patients with congenital heart disease, this

detailed understanding of the specific anatomy becomes vitally important, and is in the author's personal opinion an essential prerequisite for a successful ablation. Patients with congenital defects often have limited accessibility to their cardiac chambers because of complex intracardiac/extracardiac anomaly and/or presence of intra-atrial baffles or artificial materials. With this detailed knowledge of the individual anatomy and the use of advanced tools, these obstacles can be overcome and procedures can be performed as safely and successfully as possible with minimal fluoroscopy exposure.[15]

Review of Surgical Procedure Note

Although knowing the underlying 3D anatomy is a necessary guide to insertion and navigation of the catheters, knowing the location and extent of surgical incisions and suture placement is of paramount importance in order to unveil the arrhythmia origin. Review of the surgical operation reports, if available, is valuable to understand the exact procedure performed in each individual and obtain information about the technique used (on/off pump, cannulation sites, location of patches). Cardiac surgeons have modified their technique over the years, so surgically created scars may be variable and, in the absence of surgical records, it may be difficult to reconstruct what has been done. This uncertainty is especially likely if preventive measures such as surgical mazelike ablations or incisions have been performed.[16,17]

ADVANCED TECHNIQUES
Three-Dimensional Image Reconstruction

In order to obtain a 3D reconstruction of the individual anatomy, the authors routinely perform a cardiac magnetic resonance (CMR) scan or, alternatively, a computed tomography (CT) scan when CMR is contraindicated.

Limitation of contrast flow in CT caused by long transit times necessitate long scan times and prolonged contrast bolus injections.[18] In addition, patients with adult congenital heart disease (ACHD) are relatively young and most have already been exposed to several invasive (hemodynamic) procedures. Their lifetime burden with regard to radiation exposure is expected to be much higher than their peers who do not have ACHD, because they typically have had many hemodynamic studies in childhood and adulthood.[19]

For cardiac MRI, a free-breathing diaphragm–navigated balanced steady-state free-precession sequence with 3D reconstruction can be performed to image the whole heart.[20]

Three-Dimensional Imaging for Procedural Planning

All preacquired 3D imaging DICOM (Digital Imaging and Communications in Medicine) data can then be processed for 3D reconstructions and used during ablation procedures by integration with the mapping information (eg, using POLARIS software, Biosense Webster, Brussels, Belgium) (**Fig. 2**).

Careful 3D assessment and procedural planning are necessary to access the most likely target chamber. Asking for a larger field of view (particularly when using nonfluoroscopic techniques such as CMR) allows review of the whole vascular tree, which can be integrated in the overall 3D reconstruction. Obstruction of the iliac vessels can also be present with multiple collaterals too small to navigate a catheter through. In the presence of completely occluded femoral venous access, alternative routes (eg, a superior approach using jugular or subclavian veins) need to be considered. In case of inferior vena cava interruptions, vessels of the azygos system can be used, which is made easy using remote magnetic navigation (discussed later).[21]

Another example is the surgically created access limitation from a superior vein via the superior

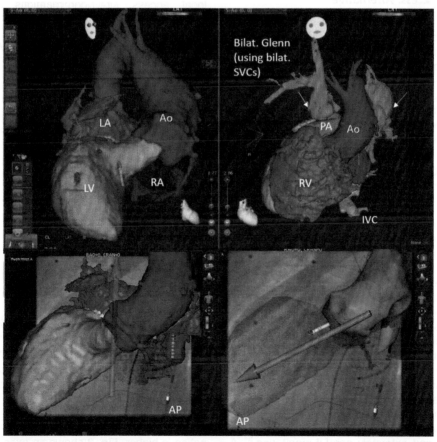

Fig. 2. Image integration from cardiac MRI during a magnetically remote controlled ablation procedure in a patient with atrial isomerism and situs inversus and transposition of the great arteries. Retrograde navigation across the aortic valve is shown with the soft magnetic catheter aligning parallel to the applied magnetic field vector (*yellow*). Ao, aorta; AP, anteroposterior; LA, left atrium; LV, left ventricle; IVC, inferior vena cava; PA, pulmonary artery; RA, right atrium; RV, right ventricle.

vena cava (SVC) after a Glenn operation. Careful review of 3D imaging with a wide imaging window allows assessment of the patency of the superior pathways.

Access planning for patients after baffle operations is also key, because the target chamber might be located behind the baffle, necessitating either transbaffle puncture or remote magnetic navigation.[22–26] Dimensions and, if available, scar/fibrosis information need to be reviewed carefully to predict reentrant circuits.

Vascular Access: Femoral

Vascular access in patients with complex ACHD can be challenging or even impossible using the standard femoral venous access because of extensive scarring (eg, after vascular cut-down procedures during/before surgery). Ultrasonography guidance for vascular access is helpful to gain safe and reliable access.

Vascular Access: Alternative

If unavoidable, alternative access such as transhepatic punctures to gain access to the right-sided atrium can be performed, but carry a high bleeding risk on sheath removal.[27] Careful risk/benefit assessment should be performed and alternatives like retrograde remote approaches should be considered. Transapical ventricular access could be another option, as well as access via punctures through the ventricular septum.[28,29]

INTRAPROCEDURAL CONSIDERATIONS
Dedicated Anesthetic Monitoring

Patients with ACHD conditions undergoing invasive electrophysiology (EP) studies are typically exposed to longer procedure times and more difficult or more numerous arrhythmias compared with their peers without ACHD. They also can have more hemodynamic consequences of sustained arrhythmias and, therefore, need careful intraprocedural monitoring.[30] A dedicated cardiac anesthetist who is well trained in the special requisites of complex EP procedures should be present throughout the ablation procedure to allow the operators to concentrate on the task of arrhythmia management. Depending on the nature of the arrhythmia, conscious sedation may be indicated rather than general anesthesia. Patients with high pulmonary artery pressure or changing shunting volumes need extremely careful monitoring.[31] A collaborative approach that is focused on the primary outcome of the ablation (ie, elimination of all arrhythmias by ablation) is key and communication of applied medications (including choice of sedative drugs, hemodynamic support, and so forth) is vital. At the end of the procedure, patients may need to be completely awake to expose them to enough sympathetic stimulation to exert further arrhythmias. In contrast, all 3D mapping systems require minimal patient movement, which can be difficult to obtain, especially in longer procedures when the patient is not fully sedated. In addition, monitoring of the fluid balance is another important feature that needs special consideration. Because most ablations are nowadays performed using irrigated-tip ablation catheters, patients can be exposed to a substantial amount of fluids during an invasive EP procedure. Diuretics may be necessary to avoid fluid overload, which may impair respiratory function in the periprocedural period. Adequate analgesia during and after an invasive EP procedure is equally important and helps the operator to perform an effective procedure without voluntary or involuntary movements of the patient on the catheter laboratory table. Postprocedural pain control is also mandatory to avoid local access site complications (extensive hematomas).

Three-Dimensional Electroanatomic Mapping

A 3D electroanatomic mapping system is used to (1) localize the catheters without the need for radiographs, (2) calculate 3D displays of electrical activation sequences (activation maps) and of local voltage (voltage maps), and (3) display in 3 dimensions the anatomy of a heart chamber using sequential localization of the catheter.[32] The 3D electroanatomic maps are superimposed on the reconstructed 3D surfaces of each cardiac structure (see **Fig. 2**). These point-by-point mapping systems require a stable arrhythmia and reaching all sites of interest, which then results in a meaningful 3D reconstruction of the activation sequence of a given arrhythmia. Inability to achieve a complete map may result in inconclusive maps and unsuccessful ablation attempts.

Multielectrode High-Resolution Mapping

In order to hasten the mapping process, multielectrode mapping has been introduced to shorten the time required for mapping of a given arrhythmia. However, critical for these systems is that the arrhythmia must be stable enough, with little cycle length variation.[33] Also, because direct contact is required, the risk of mechanical alteration or termination is higher. **Fig. 3** shows an example of the Rhythmia system (Boston Scientific), which collects a large number of points with a dedicated multielectrode basket catheter. Comparison of neighboring points and various other stability

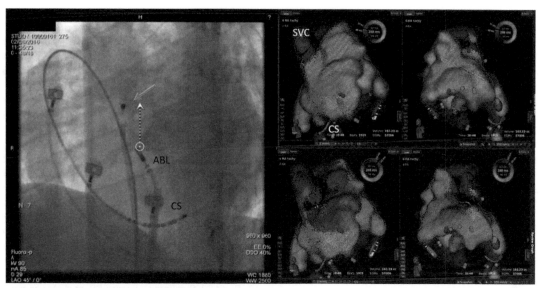

Fig. 3. A patient with enlarged RA after Fontan operation with multipolar sequential mapping of an atrial tachy-cardia (265 milliseconds cycle length). Note the enlarged RA shown on the fluoroscopy image and the multipolar catheter in the coronary sinus (CS) positioned in a large loop. The multielectrode basket is highlighted with a yel-low arrow. The critical part of the tachycardia is located between the superior vena cava (SVC) and the roof of the RA toward the pulmonary artery. ABL, ablation catheter.

criteria (including cycle length stability) allows rapid mapping of several thousand points on a 3D reconstruction. However, larger cohorts of pa-tients with ACHD have not yet been investigated with this system.

Simultaneous Mapping System

Simultaneous mapping systems have been intro-duced to the invasive EP arena: contact mapping using multielectrode baskets or noninvasive body surface mapping combined with 3D imaging. For the latter, data on patients with ACHD now exist.[34] This system records simultaneously from 252 surface ECG electrodes and displays the electrical information of each cardiac activa-tion on a 3D epicardial reconstruction of either the biatrial or biventricular chambers. This sys-tem allows the mapping of multiple arrhythmias or even very rare arrhythmias (eg, ventricular ectopy triggering ventricular fibrillation) while the patient is still on the ward. Mapping can be per-formed for several hours and provocation such as physical exercise on a stationary bike or with various common stimulants (food, social interac-tion, pharmacologic, and so forth) is performed on the ward, rather than in the catheter labora-tory. Because this system is an exclusive map-ping system, intraprocedural navigation to the site of origin can be challenging. However, compatibility with remote magnetic navigation has been shown.

Catheter Ablation Techniques

The thickness of a chronically volume-overloaded or scarred myocardium can present an insur-mountable obstacle to successful catheter abla-tion even in the presence of perfect 3D mapping and subsequent understanding of the underlying tachycardia substrate. Recently, the introduction of so-called irrigated tip catheters with increased lesion depth has improved the ability to create transmural lesions, but, in situations with limited catheter-tissue contact (eg, in the presence of a massively dilated atrial chamber) or increased/reduced blood flow, lesion formation continues to be problematic.[35]

Remote Navigation by Magnetic Navigation

In order to overcome the dominant problem in ACHD EP procedures, which is access to the target chamber, a remote controlled navigation system has been successfully used by several centers in patients with ACHD. Because the cath-eter tip is flexible and aligns in an outer magnetic field, the navigation of the mapping and ablation catheter, even through usual access vessels (eg, of the azygos system) or retrogradely across the aortic valve, can be achieved (see **Fig. 2**).[22] The magnetic navigation system (Niobe, Stereotaxis Inc, St Louis) consists of 2 computer-controlled permanent magnets (composed of the magnetic rare earth neodymium, Bor, and iron) positioned on either side of the fluoroscopy table resulting in a uniform magnetic field (0.08 T) of about 15 cm in diameter in the area of the patient's chest.[36] The flexible mapping catheter is equipped at its tip with small magnets that align parallel to the externally controlled direction of the magnetic field. In combination with a 3D mapping system such as CARTO RMT (Biosense Webster, Brussels, Belgium), the magnetic field directions (vectors) needed for sequential 3D reconstruction are applied from a remote position inside the control room. In addition, the magnetic navigation system allows integration of the preacquired 3D image directly on the reference fluoroscopy displays. Registration of all 3 systems (magnetic navigation, 3D mapping system [CARTO], and conventional fluoroscopy) allows superimposition of all information on the same reference image with depiction of the ablation catheter tip in real time.[21]

SUMMARY

A structured approach to arrhythmia ablation in patients with congenital heart disease involves the review of the anatomy and surgical notes, 3D reconstruction of the cardiac endocardial surfaces, 3D electroanatomic mapping, and (if necessary) facilitated access and movement of the ablation catheter using remote magnetic navigation technology. The recent advances in imaging and ablation tools can now offer solutions and successful ablation of even the most complex postsurgical arrhythmias.

REFERENCES

1. Chung MK. Cardiac surgery: postoperative arrhythmias. Crit Care Med 2000;28(10 Suppl):N136–44.
2. England MR, Gordon G, Salem M, et al. Magnesium administration and dysrhythmias after cardiac surgery. A placebo-controlled, double-blind, randomized trial. JAMA 1992;268(17):2395–402.
3. Mantovan R, Gatzoulis MA, Pedrocco A, et al. Supraventricular arrhythmia before and after surgical closure of atrial septal defects: spectrum, prognosis and management. Europace 2003;5(2):133–8.
4. Nabar A, Timmermans C, Medeiros A, et al. Radiofrequency ablation of atrial arrhythmias after previous open-heart surgery. Europace 2005;7(1):40–9.
5. Gatzoulis MA, Freeman MA, Siu SC, et al. Atrial arrhythmia after surgical closure of atrial septal defects in adults. N Engl J Med 1999;340(11):839–46.
6. de Jong S, van Veen TA, van Rijen HV, et al. Fibrosis and cardiac arrhythmias. J Cardiovasc Pharmacol 2015;57(6):630–8.
7. Gatzoulis MA, Balaji S, Webber SA, et al. Risk factors for arrhythmia and sudden cardiac death late after repair of tetralogy of Fallot: a multicentre study. Lancet 2000;356(9234):975–81.
8. Roubertie F, Thambo JB, Bretonneau A, et al. Late outcome of 132 Senning procedures after 20 years of follow-up. Ann Thorac Surg 2011;92(6):2206–13 [discussion: 2213–4].
9. von Olshausen K, Witt T, Schmidt G, et al. Ventricular tachycardia as a cause of sudden death in patients with aortic valve disease. Am J Cardiol 1987;59(12):1214–5.
10. Locati ET, Vecchi AM, Vargiu S, et al. Role of extended external loop recorders for the diagnosis of unexplained syncope, pre-syncope, and sustained palpitations. Europace 2014;16(6):914–22.
11. Volosin K, Stadler RW, Wyszynski R, et al. Tachycardia detection performance of implantable loop recorders: results from a large 'real-life' patient cohort and patients with induced ventricular arrhythmias. Europace 2013;15(8):1215–22.
12. Podd SJ, Sugihara C, Furniss SS, et al. Are implantable cardiac monitors the 'gold standard' for atrial fibrillation detection? A prospective randomized trial comparing atrial fibrillation monitoring using implantable cardiac monitors and DDDRP permanent pacemakers in post atrial fibrillation ablation patients. Europace 2016;18(7):1000–5.
13. Sithamparanathan S, Padley SP, Rubens MB, et al. Great vessel and coronary artery anatomy in transposition and other coronary anomalies: a universal descriptive and alphanumerical sequential classification. JACC Cardiovasc Imaging 2013;6(5):624–30.
14. Gerlis LM, Ho SY, Somerville J. A postmortem review of congenital cardiac malformations in a series of 180 adults, over the age of 16 years, born between 1865 and 1980. Cardiovasc Pathol 1999;8(5):263–72.
15. Ueda AS, Mantziari L, Gujic M, et al. Contribution of remote magnetic navigation to supraventricular tachycardia ablation in complex congenital heart diseases. Circ Arrhythm Electrophysiol 2013;6:606–13.
16. Uemura H. Surgical aspects of atrial arrhythmia: right atrial ablation and anti-arrhythmic surgery in congenital heart disease. Herzschrittmacherthe Elektrophysiol 2016;27(2):137–42.
17. Stulak JM, Dearani JA, Puga FJ, et al. Right-sided Maze procedure for atrial tachyarrhythmias in congenital heart disease. Ann Thorac Surg 2006;81(5):1780–4 [discussion: 1784–5].
18. Siripornpitak S, Pornkul R, Khowsathit P, et al. Cardiac CT angiography in children with congenital heart disease. Eur J Radiol 2013;82(7):1067–82.
19. Glatz AC, Purrington KS, Klinger A, et al. Cumulative exposure to medical radiation for children requiring surgery for congenital heart disease. J Pediatr 2014;164(4):789–94.e10.

20. Keegan J, Jhooti P, Babu-Narayan SV, et al. Improved respiratory efficiency of 3D late gadolinium enhancement imaging using the continuously adaptive windowing strategy (CLAWS). Magn Reson Med 2014;71(3):1064–74.

21. Ernst S, Chun JK, Koektuerk B, et al. Magnetic navigation and catheter ablation of right atrial ectopic tachycardia in the presence of a hemi-azygos continuation: a magnetic navigation case using 3D electroanatomical mapping. J Cardiovasc Electrophysiol 2009;20(1):99–102.

22. Ueda A, Suman-Horduna I, Mantziari L, et al. Contemporary outcomes of supraventricular tachycardia ablation in congenital heart disease: a single-center experience in 116 patients. Circ Arrhythm Electrophysiol 2013;6(3):606–13.

23. Krause U, Backhoff D, Klehs S, et al. Transbaffle catheter ablation of atrial re-entrant tachycardia within the pulmonary venous atrium in adult patients with congenital heart disease. Europace 2016;18(7):1055–60.

24. Schwagten B, Cuypers J, Szili-Torok T. The magnetic navigation system allows avoidance of puncturing a baffle during ablation of a postincisional macroreentrant tachycardia. Cardiol Young 2009;19(2):216–9.

25. El-Said HG, Ing FF, Grifka RG, et al. 18-year experience with transseptal procedures through baffles, conduits, and other intra-atrial patches. Catheter Cardiovasc Interv 2000;50(4):434–9 [discussion: 440].

26. Dave AS, Aboulhosn J, Child JS, et al. Transconduit puncture for catheter ablation of atrial tachycardia in a patient with extracardiac Fontan palliation. Heart Rhythm 2010;7(3):413–6.

27. Singh SM, Neuzil P, Skoka J, et al. Percutaneous transhepatic venous access for catheter ablation procedures in patients with interruption of the inferior vena cava. Circ Arrhythm Electrophysiol 2011;4(2):235–41.

28. Kliger C, Jelnin V, Sharma S, et al. CT angiography-fluoroscopy fusion imaging for percutaneous transapical access. JACC Cardiovasc Imaging 2014;7(2):169–77.

29. Vaseghi M, Macias C, Tung R, et al. Percutaneous interventricular septal access in a patient with aortic and mitral mechanical valves: a novel technique for catheter ablation of ventricular tachycardia. Heart Rhythm 2013;10(7):1069–73.

30. Seal R. Adult congenital heart disease. Paediatr Anaesth 2011;21(5):615–22.

31. Bennett JM, Ehrenfeld JM, Markham L, et al. Anesthetic management and outcomes for patients with pulmonary hypertension and intracardiac shunts and Eisenmenger syndrome: a review of institutional experience. J Clin Anesth 2014;26(4):286–93.

32. Knackstedt C, Schauerte P, Kirchhof P. Electroanatomic mapping systems in arrhythmias. Europace 2008;10(suppl 3):iii28–34.

33. Anter E, McElderry TH, Contreras-Valdes FM, et al. Evaluation of a novel high-resolution mapping technology for ablation of recurrent scar-related atrial tachycardias. Heart Rhythm 2016;13(10):2048–55.

34. Ernst S, Saenen J, Rydman R, et al. Utility of noninvasive arrhythmia mapping in patients with adult congenital heart disease. Card Electrophysiol Clin 2015;7(1):117–23.

35. Everett TH 4th, Lee KW, Wilson EE, et al. Safety profiles and lesion size of different radiofrequency ablation technologies: a comparison of large tip, open and closed irrigation catheters. J Cardiovasc Electrophysiol 2008;20(3):325–35.

36. Faddis MN, Blume W, Finney J, et al. Novel, magnetically guided catheter for endocardial mapping and radiofrequency catheter ablation. Circulation 2002;106(23):2980–5.

Cardiac Arrhythmias in Adults with Congenital Heart Disease
Pacemakers, Implantable Cardiac Defibrillators, and Cardiac Resynchronization Therapy Devices

Frank Cecchin, MD*, Daniel G. Halpern, MD

KEYWORDS

- Adult congenital heart disease • Pacemaker • Defibrillator • Cardiac resynchronization

KEY POINTS

- Important issues regarding device implantation in adult congenital heart disease are venous access to chambers, venous obstruction, coronary sinus location, venous anomalies, cardiac position, dilated chambers, comorbidities, high capture thresholds or poor sensing due to fibrosis, oversensing due to chamber hypertrophy, and valve-related issues.
- Epicardial pacing systems are used for more than a third of the adult congenital heart disease population requiring pacemaker implantation.
- For those individuals who are neither a candidate for a transvenous or a subcutaneous ICD, another option is a nontransvenous system composed of a rate-sensing lead attached directly to the epicardium and coils placed in the subcutaneous tissue and/or pericardial space.
- The types of patients requiring cardiac resynchronization therapy can be divided into 4 groups based on the type ventricular arrangement. The groups are systemic left ventricle, subpulmonary right ventricle, systemic right ventricle, and single ventricle.

INTRODUCTION

As the number of adults living with congenital heart disease (CHD) continues to increase due to improving surgical outcomes and survival, it is expected that cardiac rhythm device utilization will increase also. Data from the US Nationwide Inpatient Sample on hospital admissions, for those with adult congenital heart disease (ACHD), document an increase in device-related procedures from 2003 to 2012.[1] Implantable cardiac defibrillator (ICD) and pacemaker procedures increased 10% and 30%, respectively.

There is both growing evidence and consensus that ongoing care and interventions in the ACHD population are best performed by those with expertise in ACHD and in specialized ACHD centers. Data from the Quebec Congenital Heart Disease database demonstrated that specialized ACHD care was independently associated with reduced mortality and reduced odds of death, which was predominantly driven by patients with severe CHD.[2] In an analysis of the Healthcare Cost and Utilization Project database for the 7-year period 2005 to 2011, CHD was associated

NYU Langone Medical Center, 550 First Avenue, New York, NY 10016, USA
* Corresponding author.
E-mail address: frank.cecchin@nyumc.org

Card Electrophysiol Clin 9 (2017) 319–328
http://dx.doi.org/10.1016/j.ccep.2017.02.013
1877-9182/17/© 2017 Elsevier Inc. All rights reserved.

with a higher risk of implant-related complications for ICDs but not for pacemakers.[3] However, this dataset may not represent the type of patients cared for at specialized ACHD centers because 94% of the dataset patients had noncomplex CHD, with atrial septal defect being the most common defect. Complex CHD accounted for 0.1% of the device implants. The low incidence of complex CHD at generic hospitals illustrates how difficult it can be for nonspecialized centers to gain enough experience to care for this unique group of patients because it only represents a very small percentage of the total patient volume.

PACEMAKER IMPLANTATION

The presence of CHD increases the level of complexity for device implantation. In those with CHD, there are issues regarding venous access to chambers, venous obstruction, coronary sinus location, venous anomalies, cardiac position, dilated chambers, comorbidities, high capture thresholds or poor sensing due to fibrosis, oversensing due to chamber hypertrophy, and valve-related issues.

In 2014, the Pediatric And Congenital Electrophysiology Society (PACES) and Heart Rhythm Society (HRS) released an expert consensus statement on the recognition and management of arrhythmias in ACHD.[4] That statement includes not only general pacemaker implant recommendations for ACHD patients based primarily on heart rate and symptoms but also specific recommendations regarding anatomy, surgical repair and its consequences, implant site, and pacing mode.

The general recommendations can be summarized as follows:

Class I: Permanent pacing is recommended for symptomatic bradycardia due to sinus and/or atrioventricular (AV) node dysfunction; or heart block with a wide QRS escape rhythm, complex ventricular ectopy, or ventricular dysfunction; or postoperative high-grade second- or third-degree AV block that is not expected to resolve.

Class IIa: Permanent pacing is reasonable for bradycardia or loss of AV synchrony associated with impaired hemodynamics; or for correction of sinus or junctional bradycardia to prevent recurrent intra-atrial re-entrant tachycardia; or in those with congenital complete AV block and an average daytime resting heart rate less than 50 bpm; or those with complex CHD and an awake resting heart rate (sinus or junctional) less than 40 bpm or ventricular pauses greater than 3 seconds.

Class IIb: Permanent pacing may be reasonable in those with CHD of moderate complexity and an awake resting heart rate (sinus or junctional) less than 40 bpm or ventricular pauses greater than 3 seconds; or those with a history of transient postoperative complete AV block, and residual bifascicular block.

Class III: Pacing is not indicated in those without symptoms and bifascicular block with or without first-degree AV block in the absence of a history of transient complete AV block.

In addition, the guidelines lay out core principles that need to be adhered to in order to successfully implant a pacemaker in those with ACHD. The most basic of these is to "know the anatomy." The operator must understand the patient's anatomic defect, including any known or anticipated associated anomalies. Reviewing all prior surgical and device procedures is essential because that information provides the groundwork to "determine venous access before any incisions." In these individuals, there are often synthetic septal patches, atrial baffles, conduits, obstructed venous channels, persistent left superior vena cava (SVC), and extensive surgical fibrosis that have to be planned for. Advanced imaging, such as computed tomography (CT), MRI, and vascular Doppler, can be helpful in understanding the anatomy and in mapping out potential vascular routes and obstacles. However, old leads and devices might cause significant artifact that will limit the diagnostic value of advanced imaging. It is for this reason that the authors always obtain venography at any cardiac catheterization or generator change in those with implanted devices or if an implant is anticipated to demonstrate the venous anatomy so that any obstacles are known before any further device implant or revision procedure. The exact route should be mapped out beforehand. Venous patency cannot be assumed.

Once all the background data have been reviewed and procedural plan created, the first step is venography. If the venous channels are obstructed, passing through occluded veins should always be attempted initially because floppy tipped hydrophilic guide wires can often be threaded through the stenotic areas. Placing a guide wire which can function as a rail through the obstruction allows subsequent placement of sheaths over these wires and pacing wires through these sheaths. If the venous pathway is completely impassable, then alternative venous access sites, such as supraclavicular access of the internal jugular vein, transhepatic, transatrial, transthoracic, transiliac, or transfemoral routes, can be used.[5–9] If a lead is present, then another option is to extract a lead and use the old tract to access the chamber. Once access to the desired chamber is obtained, then active fixation leads are the lead of choice and the lumenless leads with a wide array of delivery sheaths allow for lead placement in the optimal anatomic location.[10–12] Finally, in the patient with transient AV block in which backup ventricular pacing is indicated, a leadless pacing system might be appropriate.[13]

It is necessary to determine not only what type of pacing is possible but also most importantly what the pacing need is. Thus, the next step is to "evaluate sinus and AV nodal function." Pacing may be required due to congenital deficiencies in sinus or AV node dysfunction, postoperative heart block, progressive loss of sinus or AV node dysfunction from surgery, and/or poor hemodynamics or antiarrhythmic-induced bradycardia. In general, most individuals benefit from dual-chamber pacing, but there are individuals with pure sinus node dysfunction that only need atrial pacing. Ventricular demand pacing is not recommended in those with CHD that need a high percentage of ventricular pacing.[14]

The final step is to "choose the optimal pacing site." Traditionally, the apex or free wall of the subpulmonary ventricle was used for pacing. It is now known that pacing at these sites is associated with dyssynchronous ventricular activation that adversely affects ventricular function and can cause a pacing-induced cardiomyopathy that is most pronounced in those with impaired hemodynamics before pacing.[15,16] If the subpulmonary ventricle is chosen for pacing, then a cardiac resynchronization therapy (CRT) upgrade is needed at the first sign of progressive ventricular enlargement or dysfunction. Another strategy is one called prosynchronization, in which the systemic ventricle is preferentially paced with a lead placed apically or on the midposterior wall.[17]

Epicardial pacing systems are often used for the ACHD population: more than a third of the time in one single-center study with 38 years of ACHD pacemaker implantation.[18] These epicardial systems are used for various reasons, which include lack of venous access, intracardiac shunts, prosthetic valve, severe valvular regurgitation, and placement at the time of congenital heart surgery. The last issue is important because it requires planning and coordination with the cardiac surgical team. It is usually easiest for the surgeon to place the pacing lead on the anterior ventricular surface, but this is often the right ventricular (RV) outflow tract, which is likely to produce the most ventricular dyssynchrony. The cardiologist needs to emphasize to the surgeon that the systemic ventricle is the best location for lead placement

and will result in the best long-term surgical outcome. It may require more extensive dissection of pericardial adhesions, lifting the heart, or even adding a thoracotomy to get the right exposure. Finally, if pacing is anticipated in the future, then epicardial leads can be placed at the time of surgery with a pulse generator implanted at a later date.

Pacing in Specific Anatomic Variants

Sinus node dysfunction is common in those individuals with dextro-transposition of the great arteries (D-TGA) and postoperative atrial switch. The original surgical correction (Mustard, Senning procedures) involves creating an intra-atrial baffle to direct the venous return to the proper ventricular chamber, resulting in the left atrium becoming the systemic venous atrium. The atrial lead passes through the baffle and secures to the roof or posterior wall of the left atrium. The left atrial appendage should be avoided as a pacing site because the phrenic nerve drapes across the appendage and may result in inadvertent diaphragmatic pacing. In those patients wherein ventricular pacing is also indicated, the systemic venous ventricle is a morphologic smooth-walled left ventricle and will require an active fixation lead. Systemic venous baffle stenosis is common in these, and stents may be needed to enlarge the atrial baffle.[19]

Corrected transposition of the great arteries (L-TGA) is associated with a 2% per year incidence of complete heart block due to a superiorly displaced AV conduction system.[20] The systemic venous ventricle is a smooth-walled morphologic left ventricle (LV) in which the apex is rotated rightward. A ventricular angiogram at the time of implant is helpful to ensure proper lead placement.

The most complex anatomic variant to implant a pacing system is in the individual with single-ventricle anatomy, status post the Fontan operation. In long-term follow-up, 20% to 53% of these individuals require pacing.[21,22] The type of Fontan operation performed determines which if any chamber can be approached by endocardial access.[23] Endocardial pacing has been performed in patients after the extracardiac conduit Fontan procedure, but it requires either transhepatic puncture or atrial access via SVC to right pulmonary artery to right atrial puncture.[24] Otherwise, an epicardial approach is needed. In the lateral tunnel, Fontan atrial access can be obtained for pacing through the systemic veins, and both chambers may be accessible in the classic atriopulmonary form of the Fontan procedure. Access to the ventricle in the latter can be obtained via a coronary sinus vein.[25] Dual-chamber pacing may require a hybrid approach with a transvenous atrial and epicardial ventricular lead. The sluggish venous pooling associated with Fontan physiology increases the risk of thrombi and anticoagulation is advised.[26]

In tetralogy of Fallot, the anatomic arrangement is normal, but if severe tricuspid regurgitation is present, it may be difficult to keep a lead in stable position across the tricuspid valve to obtain fixation. In that situation, a long peel-away sheath should be used to stabilize the lead and allow for fixation in the ventricle.

Congenital anomalies of the caval veins are common cardiac malformations in those with CHD (5%–10%). Heterotaxy or isomerism is the prototypical disorder associated with venous anomalies. It is a laterality defect in which there is isomerism present in multiple organ systems. Those with left isomerism may have absence of a sinoatrial node and are at greater risk for developing AV block. In addition to heterotaxy, situs anomalies are frequently associated with anomalies of the systemic venous return.[27] There are many types of SVC anomalies, and they include connection of a right SVC to the left atrium, absence of the right caval vein with a persistent left superior caval vein (PLSVC), or bilateral SVCs. If a right and left SVC are present, this is called bilateral SVCs, which represent 80% to 90% of the anomalies. About 90% of PLSVCs drain into the coronary sinus; alternative sites include the inferior vena cava, hepatic vein, azygous, and left atrium. When bilateral SVCs are present, 30% have a bridging vein.[28,29] A left-sided implant using a PLSVC to coronary sinus requires a very long lead length or long peel-away sheath because the leads tend to bunch up in the atrium.[30]

IMPLANTABLE CARDIAC DEFIBRILLATOR IMPLANTATION

The indications for ICD implantation in ACHD were recently published in the 2014 PACES and HRS expert consensus statement on the recognition and management of arrhythmias in ACHD.[4] They are summarized as the following:

Class I: ICD therapy is indicated in survivors of cardiac arrest due to ventricular fibrillation or hemodynamically unstable ventricular tachycardia after evaluation excludes any completely reversible cause; or those with spontaneous sustained ventricular tachycardia who have undergone hemodynamic and electrophysiologic evaluation; or those with a systemic LV ejection fraction less than 35%, biventricular physiology, and New York Heart Association (NYHA) class II or III symptoms. Catheter ablation or surgery may offer a reasonable alternative or adjunct to ICD therapy in carefully selected patients.

Class IIa: ICD therapy is reasonable in tetralogy of Fallot and multiple risk factors for sudden cardiac death, such as LV systolic or diastolic dysfunction, nonsustained ventricular tachycardia, QRS duration greater than 180 milliseconds, extensive RV scarring, or inducible sustained ventricular tachycardia at electrophysiologic study.

Class IIb: ICD therapy may be reasonable in those with a single or systemic RV ejection fraction less than 35%, particularly in the presence of additional risk factors, such as complex ventricular arrhythmias, unexplained syncope, NYHA functional class II or III symptoms, QRS duration greater than 140 milliseconds, or severe systemic AV valve regurgitation; or in those with a systemic ventricular ejection fraction less than 35% in the absence of overt symptoms (NYHA class I) or other known risk factors; or in those with syncope of unknown origin with hemodynamically significant sustained ventricular tachycardia or fibrillation inducible at electrophysiologic study; or in outpatients awaiting heart transplantation; or those with syncope and moderate or complex CHD in whom there is a high clinical suspicion of ventricular arrhythmia and in whom thorough invasive and noninvasive investigations have failed to define a cause.

Class III: ICD therapy is not indicated for those with life expectancy less than 1 year; or incessant ventricular tachycardia or ventricular fibrillation; or significant psychiatric illness that may be aggravated by ICD implantation or preclude systematic follow-up; or drug-refractory NYHA class IV symptoms who are not candidates for cardiac transplantation or CRT; or advanced pulmonary vascular disease (Eisenmenger syndrome).

The type of system used can be either transvenous, epicardial, subcutaneous, or hybrid. The choice depends on cardiac position, ventricular mass, pacing indications, body habitus, previous hardware, vascular access, intracardiac shunt, valvular competency, and whether concomitant heart surgery is needed. Before ICD implantation, venography, echocardiography, and either cardiac CT or MRI is needed to assess the above factors.

Transvenous ICD implantation is straightforward in most patients with 2 septated ventricles and normal AV relationships. The most common septated lesions are tetralogy of Fallot, atrial septal defect, ventricular septal defect, and left-sided valvular disease. Standard implantation techniques used in adults with normal anatomy can be used.

In all patients the authors always perform a ventricular angiogram before ICD lead placement to ensure placement of the lead in the true ventricular apex. Obtaining an angiogram is especially important in those with TGA or heterotaxy because the sub-pulmonary ventricular apex will not be in the anticipated location. The authors always perform an RV angiogram before ICD lead placement to ensure placement of the lead in the true ventricular apex. This is especially important in those with TGA and heterotaxy because the subpulmonary ventricular apex will not be in the anticipated location.

A subcutaneous ICD is another type of implant choice for those with ACHD.[31] The main advantage of the subcutaneous ICD is that it minimizes all of the complications related to endocardial leads. The physical stresses exerted on the lead are fewer than for an endocardial lead. The lower lead stress is due to the fact that the lead is stationary and not moving with the heart. The primary limitation of this surgical route is that a certain number of patients cannot benefit from this approach, including those with a negative screening test, low body mass index or small body habitus, or a need for antibradycardia, biventricular, or antitachycardia pacing. In order to limit the risk of inappropriate therapies due to T-wave oversensing, a screening is performed before implantation to confirm the existence of at least one vector obtaining an acceptable R-wave/T-wave amplitude ratio, both at rest and during exercise, and in different positions. If the patient fails the screening test, it is not advisable to implant the ICD because it is not possible to ensure the proper functioning of the device. In a study specifically addressing this issue involving 30 patients with CHD, eligibility was 87% versus 100% in those with normal cardiac anatomy.[32] In another study of 100 ACHD patients including some with pacemakers, it was found that the use of right parasternal electrode positioning, reduced screening failure rate from 21% to 12%.[33]

For those individuals who are a candidate for neither a transvenous or a subcutaneous ICD, the only option is a nontransvenous system composed of a rate-sensing lead attached directly to the epicardium and coils placed in the subcutaneous tissue and/or pericardial space.[34] Various configurations have been used for nontransvenous ICD systems. Based on a finite element model used to predict defibrillation efficacy and risk of myocardial injury for different single- and 2-electrode subcutaneous configurations and epicardial electrodes, the best configurations involved placement of electrodes on contralateral sides of the heart.[35] The model found that the 2 most important principles in lowering defibrillation were placement of the electrodes to align the interelectrode shock vector as closely as possible to the center of mass of the ventricular myocardium, and the use of longer electrode coil lengths. Commercially available coils have electrode lengths of 5 cm (SVC coil) or 25 cm (subcutaneous coil). However, it is possible to cut the 25 cm to any smaller length and cap the cut tip. Placing the coil in the pericardial space will lower the defibrillation, but increase the risk of myocardial injury from electroporation when voltage gradients are greater than 30 V/cm. The risk of injury from high voltage gradients can be mitigated by using a coil length of 10 to 25 cm, depending on the size of heart.

When subcutaneous coils are used, it is important to understand that during transthoracic defibrillation in humans, approximately 4% of the total current traverses the heart. For transthoracic defibrillation, only current traversing the myocardium has physiologic importance.[36] Because current flow through the chest cavity is determined by geometric factors as well as by the relative resistivity of the thoracic tissues, it is not unexpected that defibrillation could change significantly when thoracic resistances are altered by clinical conditions, such as pleural effusion, pneumothorax, or any change in lung volume.

CARDIAC RESYNCHRONIZATION THERAPY VIA BIVENTRICULAR OR MULTISITE PACING

CRT has been thoroughly studied as a proven therapy for adults without CHD and LV failure, but there are no prospective randomized controlled trials evaluating CRT in those with ACHD. Instead, the knowledge of CRT in ACHD has been extracted from single-center case series and multicenter registries in those with CHD who have undergone CRT.[15,16,37,38] The larger series were mixed with pediatric and ACHD cases. CRT in CHD holds promise because the CRT studies in patients with CHD demonstrate a lower nonresponder rate to CRT (11%–23%) compared with the 30% nonresponse rate reported for CRT in adults without CHD. CRT can also be safely used in patients with CHD, with similar complication rates as in the adult population (10%–29%). Coronary sinus lead issues were the most common major complication, occurring in 5% to 18% of all transvenous systems. The types of patients requiring CRT can be divided into 4 groups based on the type ventricular arrangement. The groups are systemic left ventricle, subpulmonary right ventricle, systemic right ventricle, and single ventricle. Anomalies of the coronary sinus should always be looked for in those with CHD.

Biventricular pacing technology can also be used to provide "backup" pacing for the individual who is pacemaker dependent. Lead fractures are common in young adults and those with epicardial systems. Having a second lead has been shown to reduce the incidence of cardiovascular events (syncope and hypotension) in association with lead fracture in pacemaker-dependent individuals with biventricular pacing versus those with single ventricular pacing.[39]

Cardiac Resynchronization Therapy for the Systemic Left Ventricle

The failing systemic left ventricle represents ~50% of ACHD patients in CRT studies. Classically, anti-bradycardia pacing is easily achieved by RV apical pacing, given the procedural ease of accessing the venous ventricle and the proven long-term lead stability; however, chronic RV apical pacing results in both interventricular and intraventricular dyssynchrony and may in fact be the least favorable place to pace.[40,41] Those with ACHD can develop ventricular dyssynchrony and ventricular dysfunction related to conventional RV pacing or dilated cardiomyopathy associated with left bundle branch block. The presence of a systemic LV was the strongest multivariable predictor of improvement in cardiac function with CRT. CRT in this patient subgroup resulted in major clinical improvement, LV reverse remodeling, and a significant decrease in QRS duration representing successful correction of electrical dyssynchrony. The best response to CRT in patients with a systemic LV occurred in those with pacing-related dyssynchrony who were upgraded to biventricular pacing. Thus, in the individual with conventional RV pacing, at the first signs of LV dilation and dysfunction, the goal should be to move either to LV pacing or to biventricular pacing.

Cardiac Resynchronization Therapy for the Subpulmonary Right Ventricle

RV heart failure is an important cause of late morbidity in ACHD, with 30% to 40% of CRT implants targeting the right ventricle. Several pacing strategies exist for CRT in patients with RV failure, which has been most extensively studied in patients with tetralogy of Fallot wherein the right ventricle is chronically damaged by a combination of pressure and volume overload resulting in myocardial scarring. These individuals also have surgically induced right bundle branch block resulting in electrical dyssynchrony.[42–44]

Similar to LV pacing for left bundle branch block, it is possible to improve dyssynchrony via single-site or even dual-site RV pacing. In single-site RV pacing, the goal is to pre-excite the right ventricle with an appropriately timed AV interval, allowing merging of the native conduction through the left bundle with that of the paced right ventricle.[45–47] Although this is technically feasible, it may be difficult to achieve chronic electrical fusion because of variations in intrinsic AV conduction over a wide range of activities and heart rates. Thus, CRT with biventricular pacing may be necessary to resynchronize the subpulmonary right ventricle. Some of these individuals also have LV dysfunction, which occurs in 5% to 10% of patients after repair of tetralogy of Fallot.[48,49] Despite promising results in the adult, the implanter is still challenged with determining the optimal sites to pace. In contrast to those with a systemic left ventricle, there are little data on the effectiveness of noninvasive imaging to guide the implanter to the optimal site to pace and resynchronize a right ventricle. One approach is to target the latest site of RV activation or place the LV lead first and then look for the site that results in the shortest QRS duration.

Cardiac Resynchronization Therapy for the Systemic Right Ventricle

Patients with systemic RVs (such as L-TGA and D-TGA status post an atrial switch) represent another CHD population at risk for developing dyssynchrony-induced ventricular dysfunction. Results of CRT in this patient population have been mixed. Some of the discrepancy in response may relate to older age at the time of CRT with less favorable responses seen in older patients. The smaller benefit of CRT in the systemic RV population may be attributed to suboptimal myocardial fiber arrangement and abnormal ventricular contraction patterns when compared with both subpulmonary RVs and systemic LVs.[50,51]

Mechanical dyssynchrony is more important than electrical dyssynchrony for those with systemic RV dysfunction. One approach that shows promise is determining with 3-dimensional imaging whether the mechanical delay is on the longitudinal or short axis. Leads should be placed at the furthest sites along a longitudinal direction in those with longitudinal delay, and for those with short-axis delay, they should be placed laterally on opposite sides of both ventricles.[52]

In L-TGA, if the LV lead is going to be placed via the coronary sinus, it is essential that preprocedural imaging of the coronary sinus be performed, because the coronary sinus anatomy is always atypical, and coronary sinus atresia occurs in up to 20% of patients.[53] The coronary sinus ostium is otherwise normally located in most patients with L-TGA, but the ventricular veins that drain the morphologic RV tend to be small and short, which may not be adequate for lead implantation. However, large thebesian veins can be cannulated directly from the anterior right atrium. These thebesian vessels often connect to inter-ventricular collateral vessels. Angiography of these collateral vessels via the thebesian veins can provide a roadmap for the entire coronary venous system.[54,55]

In the patient with D-TGA status post atrial switch, 3 different approaches are possible: a complete epicardial system, hybrid system with transvenous atrial and LV lead, and epicardial or transbaffle RV lead. The last configuration has not been rigorously studied, and chronic anticoagulation is needed.[56,57]

Cardiac Resynchronization Therapy for the Single Ventricle

Patients with single-ventricle physiology, by definition, do not have 2 separate ventricles; thus, resynchronization must be achieved by pacing 2 sites of the functional single ventricle (multisite pacing). This strategy of multisite pacing was first evaluated in the acute postoperative setting in which temporary multisite epicardial pacing resulted in improvement in systolic blood pressure, cardiac index, indices of dyssynchrony by echocardiography, and QRS duration.[58] Three studies of chronic CRT in patients with CHD have included a small number of patients with single-ventricle physiology demonstrating mixed results.[15,37,38] Although the small number of patients in these studies are insufficient to draw firm conclusions about the effect of CRT in patients with single-ventricle physiology, inconsistent responses may reflect the complex and heterogeneous structural abnormalities in this population and nonstandardized techniques used. There have been well-described case reports of a strong response to CRT in young children, but little data in older adults.[59]

The first step in achieving CRT in a single-ventricle patient is putting together a team that is committed to intensive review of the clinical data. The team will consist of a CHD specialist, electrophysiologist, cardiac imager with CHD experience, and a cardiac surgeon. First, 3D imaging is obtained via CT or MRI and a 3D virtual model is created with musculoskeletal structures in place to plan the surgical approach. Next, an evaluation of mechanical dyssynchrony is needed to find the area of latest mechanical activation. In order to

succeed in this endeavor, the electrophysiologist needs to be in the operating room with the cardiac surgeon, and both need to have a thorough understanding of the anatomy and ventricular position. The posterior or apical lead is implanted first with the target being the area of latest ventricular activation or mitral apparatus. Then, a second diametrically opposed lead is placed. Another option is to pace from the first lead and target the area of latest activation or greatest shortening in QRS duration. It may require 2 surgical approaches, such as a thoracotomy and then a sternotomy. Significant pericardial adhesions are usually present, making it a bloody and tedious procedure, thus the importance of choosing precisely where to make a thoracotomy incision for the posterior lead.

SPECIAL SITUATIONS: LEAD EXTRACTION, VENOUS OCCLUSIONS, AND INTRACARDIAC SHUNTS

As individuals with transvenous leads age, they will inevitably require lead extraction in order to maintain vascular patency and valvular competence.[60,61] Venous occlusion is a known long-term complication of permanent transvenous pacing leads.[62] Risk factors for venous thrombosis after lead placement have been described, and they include the absence of anticoagulant therapy, a history of prior venous thrombosis, use of female hormone therapy, and the presence of multiple pacing leads.[63] If venous access is needed in the setting of a complete venous occlusion, a variety of techniques for recanalization and venous dilation are now available.[64,65] Baffle obstruction is fairly common in those with D-TGA after an atrial switch and may require endovascular stent placement before lead placement.[66]

Embolic stroke in those with implanted leads can occur from an intracardiac right to left shunt or inadvertent lead placement in the systemic circulation.[67,68] These shunts can be located at the atrial or ventricular level, ranging from a patent foramen ovale to large residual septal defects and patch leaks. Fontan patients with high central venous pressure can develop direct connections between the supracardiac veins and pulmonary venous atrium through venovenous collaterals.[69] Trivial shunts that are predominately left to right are probably not absolute contraindications to transvenous leads, but larger shunts, particularly if right to left, need to be evaluated carefully by angiography or echocardiography before a final decision is made on the route for lead implantation. If transvenous leads are strongly preferred in such cases, shunt closure should be performed beforehand with interventional techniques such as septal occluders, covered stents, or coils.[70–72] If intracardiac shunting cannot be eliminated satisfactorily, epicardial lead placement is probably the best course of action. If there are still compelling indications for a transvenous system, then a transvenous implant can be performed in conjunction with strict anticoagulation.

SUMMARY

Cardiac rhythm device management in adults with CHD can be a complex endeavor that requires training and experience in the treatment of CHD. Implantation of devices in these individuals is best done by those with experience in ACHD-specific established techniques and the latest innovations. These procedures are best performed in specialized ACHD centers where a team of specialized providers can be assembled. The team typically includes an ACHD-certified physician, electrophysiologist, cardiac surgeon, and cardiac catheterization interventionalist; all of whom are trained in CHD treatment.

REFERENCES

1. Agarwal S, Sud K, Menon V. Nationwide hospitalization trends in adult congenital heart disease across 2003-2012. J Am Heart Assoc 2016;5(1) [pii:e002330].
2. Mylotte D, Pilote L, Ionescu-Ittu R, et al. Specialized adult congenital heart disease care: the impact of policy on mortality. Circulation 2014;129(18):1804–12.
3. Hayward RM, Dewland TA, Moyers B, et al. Device complications in adult congenital heart disease. Heart Rhythm 2015;12(2):338–44.
4. Khairy P, Van Hare GF, Balaji S, et al. PACES/HRS expert consensus statement on the recognition and management of arrhythmias in adult congenital heart disease: developed in partnership between the Pediatric and Congenital Electrophysiology Society (PACES) and the Heart Rhythm Society (HRS). Endorsed by the governing bodies of PACES, HRS, the American College of Cardiology (ACC), the American Heart Association (AHA), the European Heart Rhythm Association (EHRA), the Canadian Heart Rhythm Society (CHRS), and the International Society for Adult Congenital Heart Disease (ISACHD). Can J Cardiol 2014;30(10):e1–63.
5. Adwani SS, Sreeram N, DeGiovanni JV. Percutaneous transhepatic dual chamber pacing in children with Fontan circulation. Heart 1997;77(6):574–5.
6. Fishberger SB, Camunas J, Rodriguez-Fernandez H, et al. Permanent pacemaker lead implantation via the transhepatic route. Pacing Clin Electrophysiol 1996;19(7):1124–5.
7. Emmel M, Sreeram N, Pillekamp F, et al. Transhepatic approach for catheter interventions in infants and children with congenital heart disease. Clin Res Cardiol 2006;95(6):329–33.
8. Costa R, Filho MM, Tamaki WT, et al. Transfemoral pediatric permanent pacing: long-term results. Pacing Clin Electrophysiol 2003;26(1 Pt 2):487–91.
9. Molina JE. Surgical options for endocardial lead placement when upper veins are obstructed or nonusable. J Interv Card Electrophysiol 2004;11(2):149–54.
10. Garnreiter J, Whitaker P, Pilcher T, et al. Lumenless pacing leads: performance and extraction in pediatrics and congenital heart disease. Pacing Clin Electrophysiol 2015;38(1):42–7.
11. Bharmanee A, Zelin K, Sanil Y, et al. Of lumenless versus stylet-delivered pacing leads in patients with and without congenital heart. Pacing Clin Electrophysiol 2015;38(11):1343–50.
12. Lapage MJ, Rhee EK. Alternative delivery of a 4Fr lumenless pacing lead in children. Pacing Clin Electrophysiol 2008;31:543–7.
13. Wilson DG, Morgan JM, Roberts PR. "Leadless" pacing of the left ventricle in adult congenital heart disease. Int J Cardiol 2016;209:96–7.
14. Fishberger SB, Wernovsky G, Gentles TL, et al. Long-term outcome in patients with pacemakers following the Fontan operation. Am J Cardiol 1996;77(10):887–9.
15. Janousek J, Gebauer RA, Abdul-Khaliq H, et al, Working Group for Cardiac Dysrhythmias and Electrophysiology of the Association for European Paediatric Cardiology. Cardiac resynchronisation therapy in paediatric and congenital heart disease: differential effects in various anatomical and functional substrates. Heart 2009;95(14):1165–71.
16. Khairy P, Fournier A, Thibault B, et al. Cardiac resynchronization therapy in congenital heart disease. Int J Cardiol 2006;109:160–8.
17. Janoušek J, Kubuš P. Cardiac resynchronization therapy in congenital heart disease. Herzschrittmacherther Elektrophysiol 2016;27(2):104–9.
18. McLeod CJ, Attenhofer Jost CH, Warnes CA, et al. Epicardial versus endocardial permanent pacing in adults with congenital heart disease. J Interv Card Electrophysiol 2010;28(3):235–43.
19. Patel S, Shah D, Chintala K, et al. Atrial baffle problems following the Mustard operation in children and young adults with dextro-transposition of the great arteries: the need for improved clinical detection in the current era. Congenit Heart Dis 2011;6(5):466–74.
20. Huhta JC, Maloney JD, Ritter DG, et al. Complete atrioventricular block in patients with atrioventricular discordance. Circulation 1983;67(6):1374–7.
21. Pundi KN, Johnson JN, Dearani JA, et al. 40-Year follow-up after the fontan operation: long-term outcomes of 1,052 patients. J Am Coll Cardiol 2015;66(15):1700–10.
22. Van Dorn CS, Menon SC, Johnson JT, et al. Lifetime cardiac reinterventions following the Fontan procedure. Pediatr Cardiol 2015;36(2):329–34.

23. Takahashi K, Cecchin F, Fortescue E, et al. Permanent atrial pacing lead implant route after Fontan operation. Pacing Clin Electrophysiol 2009;32(6):779–85.

24. Arif S, Clift PF, De Giovanni JV. Permanent transvenous pacing in an extra-cardiac Fontan circulation. Europace 2016;18(2):304–7.

25. Lopez JA. Transvenous right atrial and left ventricular pacing after the Fontan operation: long-term hemodynamic and electrophysiologic benefit of early atrioventricular resynchronization. Tex Heart Inst J 2007;34(1):98–101.

26. Shah MJ, Nehgme R, Carboni M, et al. Endocardial atrial pacing lead implantation and midterm follow-up in young patients with sinus node dysfunction after the fontan procedure. Pacing Clin Electrophysiol 2004;27(7):949–54.

27. Loomba RS, Aggarwal S, Gupta N, et al. Arrhythmias in adult congenital patients with bodily isomerism. Pediatr Cardiol 2016;37(2):330–7.

28. Lendzian T, Vogt J, Krasemann T. Are anomalies of the caval veins more common in complex congenital heart disease? Herz 2007;32(8):657–64.

29. Irwin RB, Greaves M, Schmitt M. Left superior vena cava: revisited. Eur Heart J Cardiovasc Imaging 2012;13(4):284–91.

30. Biffi M, Bertini M, Ziacchi M, et al. Clinical implications of left superior vena cava persistence in candidates for pacemaker or cardioverter-defibrillator implantation. Heart Vessels 2009;24(2):142–6.

31. Bordachar P, Marquié C, Pospiech T, et al. Subcutaneous implantable cardioverter defibrillators in children, young adults and patients with congenital heart disease. Int J Cardiol 2016;203:251–8.

32. Zeb M, Curzen N, Veldtman G, et al. Potential eligibility of congenital heart disease patients for subcutaneous implantable cardioverter-defibrillator based on surface electrocardiogram mapping. Europace 2015;17(7):1059–67.

33. Okamura H, McLeod CJ, DeSimone CV, et al. Right parasternal lead placement increases eligibility for subcutaneous implantable cardioverter defibrillator therapy in adults with congenital heart disease. Circ J 2016;80(6):1328–35.

34. Cannon BC, Friedman RA, Fenrich AL, et al. Innovative techniques for placement of implantable cardioverter-defibrillator leads in patients with limited venous access to the heart. Pacing Clin Electrophysiol 2006;29(2):181–7.

35. Jolley M, Stinstra J, Tate J, et al. Finite element modeling of subcutaneous implantable defibrillator electrodes in an adult torso. Heart Rhythm 2010;7(5):692–8.

36. Lerman BB, Deale OC. Relation between transcardiac and transthoracic current during defibrillation in humans. Circ Res 1990;67(6):1420–6.

37. Dubin AM, Janousek J, Rhee E, et al. Resynchronization therapy in pediatric and congenital heart disease patients: an international multicenter study. J Am Coll Cardiol 2005;46(12):2277–83.

38. Cecchin F, Frangini PA, Brown DW, et al. Cardiac resynchronization therapy (and multisite pacing) in pediatrics and congenital heart disease: five years experience in a single institution. J Cardiovasc Electrophysiol 2009;20(1):58–65.

39. Ceresnak SR, Perera JL, Motonaga KS, et al. Ventricular lead redundancy to prevent cardiovascular events and sudden death from lead fracture in pacemaker-dependent children. Heart Rhythm 2015;12(1):111–6.

40. Janousek J, Gebauer RA, Abdul-Khaliq H, et al. Cardiac resynchronisation therapy in paediatric and congenital heart disease: differential effects in various anatomical and functional substrates. Heart 2009;95:1165–71.

41. Tantengco MV, Thomas RL, Karpawich PP. Left ventricular dysfunction after long-term right ventricular apical pacing in the young. J Am Coll Cardiol 2001;37:2093–100.

42. Vogel M, Sponring J, Cullen S, et al. Regional wall motion and abnormalities of electrical depolarization and repolarization in patients after surgical repair of tetralogy of Fallot. Circulation 2001;103:1669–73.

43. Abd El Rahman MY, Hui W, Yigitbasi M, et al. Detection of left ventricular asynchrony in patients with right bundle branch block after repair of tetralogy of Fallot using tissue-Doppler imaging-derived strain. J Am Coll Cardiol 2005;45:915–21.

44. Pedersen TA, Andersen NH, Knudsen MR, et al. The effects of surgically induced right bundle branch block on left ventricular function after closure of the ventricular septal defect. Cardiol Young 2008;18:430–6.

45. Dubin AM, Feinstein JA, Reddy VM, et al. Electrical resynchronization: a novel therapy for the failing right ventricle. Circulation 2003;107:2287–9.

46. Janousek J, Vojtovic P, Hucín B, et al. Resynchronization pacing is a useful adjunct to the management of acute heart failure after surgery for congenital heart defects. Am J Cardiol 2001;88(2):145–52.

47. Plymen CM, Finlay M, Tsang V, et al. Haemodynamic consequences of targeted single- and dual-site right ventricular pacing in adults with congenital heart disease undergoing surgical pulmonary valve replacement. Europace 2015;17(2):274–80.

48. Thambo JB, De Guillebon M, Dos Santos P, et al. Electrical dyssynchrony and resynchronization in tetralogy of Fallot. Heart Rhythm 2011;8(6):909–14.

49. Merchant FM, Kella D, Book WM, et al. Cardiac resynchronization therapy in adult patients with repaired tetralogy of Fallot and left ventricular systolic dysfunction. Pacing Clin Electrophysiol 2014;37:321–8.

50. Ishizu T, Horigome H. Assessment and treatment of systemic right ventricular dyssynchrony. Circ J 2015; 79(3):519–21.

51. Sakaguchi H, Miyazaki A, Yamada O, et al. Cardiac resynchronization therapy for various systemic ventricular morphologies in patients with congenital heart disease. Circ J 2015;79(3):649–55.

52. Miyazaki A, Sakaguchi H, Kagisaki K, et al. Optimal pacing sites for cardiac resynchronization therapy for patients with a systemic right ventricle with or without a rudimentary left ventricle. Europace 2016;18(1):100–12.

53. Ruckdeschel ES, Quaife R, Lewkowiez L, et al. Pre-procedural imaging in patients with transposition of the great arteries facilitates placement of cardiac resynchronization therapy leads. Pacing Clin Electrophysiol 2014;37(5):546–53.

54. Manchanda M, McLeod CJ, Killu A, et al. Cardiac resynchronization therapy for patients with congenital heart disease: technical challenges. J Interv Card Electrophysiol 2013;36(1):71–9.

55. Bottega NA, Kapa S, Edwards WD, et al. The cardiac veins in congenitally corrected transposition of the great arteries: delivery options for cardiac devices. Heart Rhythm 2009;6(10):1450–6.

56. Michael KA, Paisey JR, Mayosi BM, et al. A hybrid form of cardiac resynchronisation therapy in patients with failing systemic right ventricles. J Interv Card Electrophysiol 2008;23(3):229–33.

57. Chakrabarti S, Szantho G, Turner MS, et al. Use of radiofrequency perforation for lead placement in biventricular or conventional endocardial pacing after Mustard or Senning operations for D-transposition of the great arteries. Pacing Clin Electrophysiol 2009; 32(9):1123–9.

58. Havalad V, Cabreriza SE, Cheung EW, et al. Optimized multisite ventricular pacing in postoperative single-ventricle patients. Pediatr Cardiol 2014; 35(7):1213–9.

59. Materna O, Kubuš P, Janoušek J. Right ventricular resynchronization in a child with hypoplastic left heart syndrome. Heart Rhythm 2014;11(12):2303–5.

60. Cecchin F, Atallah J, Walsh EP, et al. Lead extraction in pediatric and congenital heart disease patients. Circ Arrhythm Electrophysiol 2010;3(5):437–44.

61. Atallah J, Erickson CC, Cecchin F, et al. (PACES). Multi-institutional study of implantable defibrillator lead performance in children and young adults: results of the Pediatric Lead Extractability and Survival Evaluation (PLEASE) study. Circulation 2013; 127(24):2393–402.

62. Bar-Cohen Y, Berul CI, Alexander ME, et al. Age, size, and lead factors alone do not predict venous obstruction in children and young adults with transvenous lead systems. J Cardiovasc Electrophysiol 2006;17(7):754–9.

63. van Rooden CJ, Molhoek SG, Rosendaal FR, et al. Incidence and risk factors of early venous thrombosis associated with permanent pacemaker leads. J Cardiovasc Electrophysiol 2004;15:1258–62.

64. McCotter CJ, Angle JF, Prudente LA, et al. Placement of transvenous pacemaker and ICD leads across total chronic occlusions. Pacing Clin Electrophysiol 2005;28:921–5.

65. Pflaumer A, Chard R, Davis AM. Perspectives in interventional electrophysiology in children and those with congenital heart disease: electrophysiology in children. Heart Lung Circ 2012;21(6–7):413–20.

66. Hill KD, Fleming G, Curt Fudge J, et al. Percutaneous interventions in high-risk patients following Mustard repair of transposition of the great arteries. Catheter Cardiovasc Interv 2012;80(6):905–14.

67. Khairy P, Landzberg MJ, Gatzoulis MA, et al. Epicardial versus endocardial pacing and thromboembolic events investigators. Transvenous pacing leads and systemic thromboemboli in patients with intracardiac shunts: a multicenter study. Circulation 2006; 113(20):2391–7.

68. Van Gelder BM, Bracke FA, Oto A, et al. Diagnosis and management of inadvertently placed pacing and ICD leads in the left ventricle: a multicenter experience and review of the literature. Pacing Clin Electrophysiol 2000;23:877–83.

69. Weber HS. Incidence and predictors for the development of significant supradiaphragmatic decompressing venous collateral channels following creation of Fontan physiology. Cardiol Young 2001; 11:289–94.

70. Knauth AL, Lock JE, Perry SB, et al. Transcatheter device closure of congenital and postoperative residual ventricular septal defects. Circulation 2004; 110:501–7.

71. Khairy P, O'Donnell CP, Landzberg MJ. Transcatheter closure versus medical therapy of patent foramen ovale and presumed paradoxical thromboemboli: a systematic review. Ann Intern Med 2003;139:753–60.

72. Poddar KL, Nagarajan V, Krishnaswamy A, et al. Risk of cerebrovascular events in patients with patent foramen ovale and intracardiac devices. JACC Cardiovasc Interv 2014;7(11):1221–6.

Arrhythmia Surgery for Adults with Congenital Heart Disease

Barbara J. Deal, MD[a],*, Constantine Mavroudis, MD[b]

KEYWORDS

- Atrial fibrillation • Atrial flutter • Atrial septal defect • Ebstein anomaly • Univentricular physiology

KEY POINTS

- As survival following initial surgical repairs of congenital heart disease has improved, the late sequelae of heart failure and arrhythmias for patients with severe forms of congenital heart disease are increasingly recognized.
- Successful arrhythmia surgery requires a clear understanding of tachycardia mechanisms present in an individual patient, the specific operative techniques for each mechanism, and cooperation between the electrophysiologist and surgeon.
- Surgical repair of congenital heart disease can be viewed as both an anatomic and an electrical intervention, with the combined goals of improving hemodynamic status and minimizing morbidity from the development of later arrhythmias.

INTRODUCTION

The purpose of this article is to review arrhythmia surgical techniques that may be incorporated into concomitant repairs for congenital heart surgery patients. As survival to adulthood following initial surgical repairs of congenital heart disease has improved for most patients, the late sequelae of heart failure and arrhythmias for patients with severe forms of congenital heart disease are increasingly recognized.[1] The median age of adults with severe congenital heart disease was reported as 29 years, and one recent review described tachyarrhythmias as their "inevitable destiny."[2] Atrial arrhythmias negatively impact ventricular function, functional assessment, and long-term survival.[3–5] Among adults with congenital heart disease, atrial arrhythmia development results in a 50% increase in early mortality, a 2-fold increase in stroke and congestive heart failure,

and a 3-fold increase in the need for cardiac interventions.[4]

Understanding the mechanisms of arrhythmias is essential to determine appropriate catheter or surgical intervention and have been summarized in recent publications.[2,5,6] For adult patients with arrhythmias undergoing cardiac surgery, the options are transcatheter ablation of arrhythmias preoperatively or postoperatively, or incorporation of arrhythmia procedure into the cardiac surgery. Patients with unsuccessful or difficult catheter ablations (Ebstein anomaly), complex anatomy including markedly thickened atrial walls with multiple reentrant circuits, difficult venous access, or those requiring atrial reduction or treatment of atrial fibrillation (AF) are most suitable for arrhythmia surgical procedures. As the pioneer arrhythmia surgeon James Cox stated in 1983, "The selection of patients for the surgical treatment of cardiac arrhythmias is based on several

The authors have no commercial or financial conflicts of interest and no funding sources to declare.
[a] Feinberg School of Medicine, Northwestern University, 303 East Chicago Avenue, Chicago, IL 60611, USA;
[b] Johns Hopkins Children's Heart Surgery, Florida Hospital for Children, 2501 N Orange Avenue, Suite 540, Orlando, FL 32804, USA
* Corresponding author.
E-mail address: bdeal@northwestern.edu

Card Electrophysiol Clin 9 (2017) 329–340
http://dx.doi.org/10.1016/j.ccep.2017.02.014

cardiacEP.theclinics.com

variables. These variables include the patient's age and general condition, the nature of the presenting arrhythmia, its response to medical treatment, and the presence of associated anomalies that may require the additional surgical correction."[7] These original guidelines are particularly important for adults undergoing repair or reoperations for congenital heart disease presently.

STRUCTURAL CONGENITAL HEART DISEASE AND ARRHYTHMIAS

Diagnostic substrates associated with the highest prevalence of supraventricular tachycardia (SVT) include Ebstein anomaly, atrial repairs of transposition of the great arteries, univentricular hearts, atrial septal defects (ASDs), and right heart obstructive lesions, such as tetralogy of Fallot (TOF) and double outlet right ventricle.[2,4–6] **Table 1** summarizes the prevalence of arrhythmias and incidence of reoperation for congenital heart disease.[8] ASD closure in childhood is associated with late atrial flutter (AFL) and AF in as many as 20% to 35% of patients,[9–11] whereas patients undergoing ASD repair as adults have a 30% to 50% incidence of atrial arrhythmias, particularly AF.[9–13] The development of arrhythmias following TOF repair was initially concentrated on the risk of ventricular tachycardia (VT)[14–19]; more commonly, atrial arrhythmias are recognized in as many as 12% to 43% of older TOF patients, contributing to morbidity and hospitalizations.[4,20] Ebstein anomaly of the tricuspid valve is associated with SVT in up to 42% of patients, which is related to accessory connections, AF, and AFL.[21–23] Older

Fontan patients with atriopulmonary anastomoses have an increasing incidence of atrial tachycardia (AT) over time, exceeding 40% by 20 years postoperatively and steadily increasing to more than 70% by 25 years postoperatively.[24–30] Fontan modifications have decreased the incidence of AT to approximately 8% to 15% in extracardiac connections, and 13% to 60% in lateral tunnel connections,[24,30] yet is likely to increase with longer durations of follow-up.[25–27] The development of AT in Fontan patients is associated with right atrial thrombus formation, congestive heart failure, atrioventricular valve regurgitation, thromboembolic events, increased hospitalizations, and mortality.[4,28,29] Catheter ablation in the Fontan patient is associated with acute success of about 50% with at least 70% recurrence of tachycardia within 2 years.[12,31–33]

Mechanisms of Supraventricular Tachycardia

In adult patients with congenital heart disease, the most common mechanism of SVT is macro-reentrant AT, which accounts for at least 75% of SVT and involves the cavotricuspid isthmus in more than 60% of circuits.[13,34–36] AT is a slower form of AFL, with isoelectric periods between successive P waves; AFL is characterized by sawtooth flutter waves at more rapid atrial rates, without intervening isoelectric periods. AT develops most commonly in patients with TOF or right heart conduit repairs, ASDs, Ebstein anomaly, atrial baffle repairs for transposition of the great arteries, and in patients with univentricular hearts following Fontan surgery.[2,4–6] In addition

---

Table 1
Reoperation rates and estimated prevalence of arrhythmias in adults with congenital heart disease

Congenital Heart Disease	Reoperation (%)	Atrial Arrhythmias (%)	Ventricular Tachycardia (%)
ASD	<2	16–50	<2
Ebstein anomaly	30–50	33–60	>2
Single ventricle	>25	>40–70	>5
TOF	26–50	12–43	10–15
Transposition of the great arteries, atrial switch	15–27	26–50	7–9
Transposition of the great arteries, arterial switch	12–20	<2	1–2
Congenitally corrected transposition of the great arteries	25–35	>30	>2
Truncus arteriosus	55–89	>25	>2
Atrioventricular septal defect	19–26	5–10	<2

Modified from Khairy P, Van Hare GF, Balaji S, et al. PACES/HRS Expert Consensus Statement on the recognition and management of arrhythmias in adult congenital heart disease. Heart Rhythm 2014;11:e35; with permission.

to isthmus-dependent AT are right atrial macro-reentrant circuits, commonly referred to as "non-isthmus"-dependent tachycardia.[2,5,6,34–36] The lateral right atrial wall at the inferior aspect of the crista terminalis is frequently an area of unexcitable atrial tissue with low-voltage electrograms and is categorized as "scar." Ablation of the isthmus of slow conduction between these incisions, patches, or electrical scars forms the basis of treatment strategies for non-isthmus–dependent right AT.

Focal AT originates from a discrete area of atrial tissue, conducting in a centrifugal manner, and represents either a micro-reentrant or automatic circumscribed area of electrical activity.[35,37] Extracardiac Fontan repairs may result in an increase in focal AT as opposed to atrial reentry/AFL in atriopulmonary Fontan repairs and is particularly difficult to recognize on electrocardiogram.

Atrioventricular nodal reentry tachycardia (AVNRT) involves functionally distinct pathways of fast and slow conduction approaching the compact atrioventricular node, and targeting the slow pathway between the os of the coronary sinus and below the compact atrioventricular node is usually successful in terminating tachycardia. Patients with atrial baffle repairs of transposition of the great arteries frequently have AVNRT in addition to macro-reentrant AT or AF.[38] In patients with atrial baffles, the slow pathway may be partitioned to the pulmonary venous atrium, and in patients with heterotaxy syndrome, twin atrioventricular nodes may be present.[5]

Accessory pathway-mediated tachycardia, usually orthodromic reciprocating tachycardia, accounts for less than about 8% of SVT in adult congenital heart disease (ACHD). Approximately 20% to 30% of patients with Ebstein anomaly of the tricuspid valve or congenitally corrected transposition of the great arteries have accessory connections associated with the abnormal valve, which may be concealed or manifest on electrocardiogram (Wolff-Parkinson-White syndrome). Atrial reentrant tachycardia, AFL, orthodromic reciprocating tachycardia, or AF develops in ≥50% of patients with Ebstein anomaly and significant tricuspid regurgitation.[21–23] Preoperative electrophysiology studies with potential catheter ablation of accessory connections are recommended in patients with Ebstein anomaly before surgical interventions.[8,39]

The incidence of AF is about 10% in ACHD and increases with age and following ablation procedures for AT.[40–42] Patients with ASDs, patients with transposition of the great arteries following atrial baffle repairs, and Fontan patients have the highest incidence of AF. In Fontan patients, the mechanism of AT is macro-reentrant (AFL or atrial reentrant tachycardia) in about 75% of patients, with focal AT present in 3% to 15%; the incidence of AF is steadily increasing.[4,32,35,41–43]

Most mechanisms of SVT can be successfully ablated using a transcatheter approach.[5,6,12,31–35,37,38,40–42] Surgical ablation is recommended for patients undergoing concomitant repairs in whom catheter access is challenging, or unsuccessful.[8,39,43]

Ventricular Tachycardia

Because TOF was one of the earliest forms of more complex congenital heart disease undergoing complete repair, recognition of late VT in TOF patients received focused attention in the 1980s and 1990s.[14–19] Because patients with other congenital heart lesions underwent intracardiac repairs and are surviving into adulthood, VT is recognized with increasing frequency in other lesions, including ventricular septal defects, lesions with right ventricular (RV) conduit repairs such as truncus arteriosus and double outlet right ventricle, transposition of the great arteries, and univentricular hearts. Predisposition to VT may be prior surgical scar, hypertrophy, ventricular dysfunction, neonatal cyanosis impacting gap junctions, or genetic programming for myocardial apoptosis (**Table 2**). The mechanism of VT is typically a macro-reentrant circuit with a critical anatomically defined isthmus, which 3-dimensional electroanatomic mapping can help define.[44,45] Sustained VT is predominantly seen in patients with prior ventriculotomies or ventricular septal defect patches, and monomorphic VT may be ablated successfully using a transcatheter approach.[17,44–46] In patients requiring reoperations, mapping-guided surgical VT ablation has success rates ranging from 50% to 75%.[15,17,47–51] Limitations to the surgical treatment of VT are related to an inability to map under general anesthesia, late epicardial breakthrough remote from the critical isthmus, deep septal origin of VT, or left ventricular origin limiting appropriate resection or cryoablation.[50,51] Currently, very few patients with TOF with sustained VT are candidates for a surgical approach, because the catheter approach and defibrillator implantation are more likely to be used.

The development of atrial or ventricular arrhythmias in ACHD patients is often an indicator of progressive hemodynamic changes, which require in-depth functional and hemodynamic assessment. Intervention for residual hemodynamic/structural defects may need to be planned as part of chronic arrhythmia management. Patients

Table 2
Risk factors for arrhythmia development in congenital heart disease

Supraventricular Tachycardia	Ventricular Tachycardia
Older age at initial repair	Older age at initial repair
QRS duration >160 ms	QRS duration >180 ms
Longer duration of follow-up	Longer duration of follow-up
Reoperation for hemodynamic abnormalities does not eliminate SVT	Reoperation for hemodynamic problems may decrease risk of VT
Prior atrial surgery	Residual hemodynamic problems
Loss of sinus rhythm	RV hypertension
Preoperative arrhythmias	Pulmonary regurgitation
Residual hemodynamic problems	Cardiomegaly
	LVEF <40%

Abbreviation: LVEF, left ventricular ejection fraction.

with Ebstein anomaly or repaired TOF may have significant pulmonary regurgitation, tricuspid regurgitation, or both, which might benefit from reoperation. Surgical treatment of the hemodynamic problems does not eliminate atrial arrhythmias, and ablation of atrial arrhythmias alone could allow significant hemodynamic issues to progress and potentially deteriorate. Successful treatment involves assessing both the arrhythmia and the contributing hemodynamic changes and addressing both when indicated and feasible.[47–50] Preoperative transcatheter ablation is generally performed in patients with appropriate substrates and vascular access, as most mechanisms of SVT, and some monomorphic forms of VT, are amenable to transcatheter ablation. In selected settings, integration of operative ablation techniques with hemodynamic repair may be optimal.

ARRHYTHMIA SURGERY

The innovative advances of arrhythmia surgery include therapeutic application of specific lesion sets that were developed to treat existing refractory arrhythmias with or without associated intracardiac repair (**Table 3**).[8] Sealy and colleagues[52] demonstrated that surgical treatment of accessory connections could be successfully performed,

Table 3
Operative techniques for arrhythmia surgery

Type of Arrhythmia	Surgical Techniques
Supraventricular	
Accessory connection	Endocardial or epicardial dissection and division; cryoablation
Focal AT	Map-guided resection; cryoablation
AV nodal reentrant tachycardia	Slow pathway modification with cryoablation
RA macro-reentry	
Cavotricuspid isthmus dependent	Cavotricuspid isthmus ablation
Multiple reentrant circuits	Modified right atrial maze
Left atrial macro-reentry	Left atrial Cox-maze III lesions
AF	Left atrial Cox-maze III lesions with cavotricuspid isthmus ablation ± right atrial maze ± left atrial appendectomy
VT	
Scar related	Scar or endocardial fibrosis resection; focal ablation; lines of ablation between anatomic landmarks; map-guided resection or ablation

Abbreviation: AV, atrioventricular.
Modified from Khairy P, Van Hare GF, Balaji S, et al. PACES/HRS Expert Consensus Statement on the recognition and management of arrhythmias in adult congenital heart disease. Heart Rhythm 2014;11:e37; with permission.

before development of transcatheter techniques. Guiraudon and colleagues[53] expanded surgical ablation to patients with AFL using an isthmus lesion from the coronary sinus to the inferior vena cava (IVC). Cox and colleagues[54,55] developed the surgical technique for AF after extensive animal studies. The right-sided atrial maze technique was applied to patients with congenital heart disease and atrial arrhythmias.[22,23,47,56–58] Deal and colleagues[43,48,50,59,60] and Mavroudis and colleagues[49,61] expanded the surgical ablation techniques to treat both AFL and AF in patients with congenital heart disease of all ages, including neonates, and to patients with univentricular physiology. Giamberti and colleagues[62,63] reported their aggregate experience in 50 adults with congenital heart disease using irrigated radiofrequency ablation.

Recommendations for Arrhythmia Surgery

Because of the increasing awareness that arrhythmias contribute to long-term morbidity, recent guidelines and consensus statements have included recommendations for concomitant arrhythmia surgery in patients with existing arrhythmias undergoing planned cardiac surgery (**Table 4**).[8,39,64] The American College of Cardiology/American Heart Association/Heart Rhythm Society guidelines for the management of SVT in adults include a class I recommendation for assessment of associated hemodynamic abnormalities for potential repair in adults with congenital heart disease as part of therapy for SVT.[39] In the consensus statement for arrhythmia management in adults with congenital heart disease, surgical ablation of associated AT is recommended in patients undergoing planned surgical repair.[8] A left atrial Cox-maze III procedure with right atrial cavotricuspid isthmus ablation is recommended for adults with congenital heart disease and AF.[8]

ARRHYTHMIA SURGERY TECHNIQUES

Because the predominant mechanisms of SVT in congenital heart disease are macro-reentrant AT and AF, knowledge of these lesions sets is essential for successful arrhythmia surgery. Focal AT and accessory connections can usually be successfully treated with a transcatheter approach before surgical repair and can reduce the risk of acute postoperative tachycardia compromising hemodynamics. Infrequently, patients with Ebstein anomaly of the tricuspid valve have broad bands of accessory connections that may be approached surgically if the transcatheter approach fails.[22,23,48–50] Focal AT can be mapped to a discrete area of the atrium and targeted with

ablation energy or resection. The operative techniques for accessory connections, including endocardial and epicardial dissection and additional cryoablation, have been summarized previously.[65,66]

ATRIAL REENTRY TACHYCARDIA AND ATRIAL FLUTTER

The "cut and sew" or "classical right-sided maze" procedure as originally introduced[54,55] encompasses a linear incision from the superior vena cava (SVC) to the IVC, right atrial appendectomy, incision from the base of the resected right atrial appendage to the midpoint of the right atrial anterior wall not in communication with the SVC-IVC incision, an incision posteriorly from the base of the right atrial appendage to the anterior tricuspid valve annulus, and a communicating incision from the SVC-IVC incision to the posterior tricuspid valve annulus. These lesions were developed from animal models without congenital heart disease, without inherent arrhythmias, and without previous operations, and they were designed before recognition of the importance of the right atrial isthmus to maintaining AFL/atrial macroreentrant circuits.[34–36]

The design of surgical ablation lesions in Fontan patients was developed following preoperative electrophysiologic studies that identified 3 dominant reentrant circuits for AT.[59,60] These findings led to the development of the modified right atrial maze procedure (**Fig. 1**),[60,67,68] which differs significantly from the original lesions described by Cox. The "modified" right atrial maze procedure includes lesions between the SVC and IVC, between the coronary sinus and the tricuspid valve, and between the IVC and the coronary sinus, with lesions from the lateral atrial wall to the posterior rim of an ASD when present. The distinctive lesions of the modified right atrial maze procedure are instrumental in eliminating right atrial macroreentry tachycardia in patients with complex congenital heart disease, and are essential to eliminate reentry in the isthmus region.[43,59,60]

The Fontan conversion surgery refers to the replacement of an atriopulmonary anastomosis with an extracardiac total cavopulmonary connection, usually in association with arrhythmia surgery. Right atrial macro-reentry tachycardia is addressed using a modified right-sided maze procedure.[43,60,61,67] In the presence of either AF or left atrial reentry tachycardia, or in patients with significant left-sided atrioventricular valve regurgitation, the left atrial Cox-maze IV procedure is performed in addition to the modified right atrial maze

Table 4
Consensus statements and guideline recommendations for surgical treatment of arrhythmias

Class of Recommendation	Level of Evidence	Recommendation
2014 PACES/HRS Consensus statement for arrhythmia management in ACHD		
I	B	A modified right atrial maze procedure is indicated in adults undergoing Fontan conversion with symptomatic right atrial IART
I	B	A modified right atrial maze procedure in addition to a left atrial Cox maze III procedure is indicated in patients undergoing Fontan conversion with documented AF
IIa	B	Concomitant atrial arrhythmia surgery should be considered in adults with Ebstein anomaly undergoing cardiac surgery
IIa	B	A (modified) right atrial maze procedure can be useful in adults with CHD and clinical episodes of sustained typical or atypical right AFL
IIa	B	A left atrial Cox maze III procedure with right atrial cavotricuspid isthmus ablation can be beneficial in adults with CHD and AF
2014 ACC AHA Guidelines for the management of AF		
IIa	C	An AF surgical ablation procedure is reasonable for selected patients with AF undergoing cardiac surgery for other indications
IIb	B	A stand-alone AF surgical ablation procedure may be reasonable for selected patients with highly symptomatic AF not well managed with other approaches
2016 ACC AHA Guidelines for the management of SVT in adults		
I	C-LD	Assessment of associated hemodynamic abnormalities for potential repair of structural defects is recommended in ACHD patients as part of therapy for SVT
IIa	B-NR	Preoperative catheter ablation or intraoperative surgical ablation of accessory pathways or AT is reasonable in patients with SVT who are undergoing surgical repair of Ebstein anomaly
IIa	B-NR	Surgical ablation of AT or AFL can be effective in ACHD patients undergoing planned surgical repair
2014 PACES/HRS consensus statement for arrhythmia management in ACHD: Prophylactic arrhythmia surgery recommendations		
IIa	B	A modified right atrial maze procedure should be considered in adults undergoing Fontan conversion or revision surgery without documented atrial arrhythmias
IIa	B	Concomitant atrial arrhythmia surgery should be considered in adults with Ebstein anomaly undergoing cardiac surgery
IIb	C	Adults with CHD undergoing surgery to correct a structural heart defect associated with atrial dilatation may be considered for prophylactic atrial arrhythmia surgery
IIb	B	Adults with CHD and inducible typical or atypical right AFL without documented clinical sustained AT may be considered for (modified) right atrial maze surgery or cavotricuspid isthmus ablation
IIb	C	Adults with CHD and left-sided valvar heart disease with severe left atrial dilatation or limitations of venous access may be considered for left atrial maze surgery in the absence of documented or inducible AT
IIb	C	Closure of the left atrial appendage may be considered in adults with CHD undergoing atrial arrhythmia surgery

(continued on next page)

Table 4 *(continued)*		
Class of Recommendation	**Level of Evidence**	**Recommendation**
III	C	Prophylactic arrhythmia surgery is not indicated in adults with CHD at increased risk of surgical mortality from ventricular dysfunction or major comorbidities, in whom prolongation of cardiopulmonary bypass or cross-clamp times owing to arrhythmia surgery might negatively impact outcomes
III	C	Empiric ventricular arrhythmia surgery is not indicated in adults with CHD and no clinical or inducible sustained VT

Abbreviations: ACC, American College of Cardiology; AHA, American Heart Association; CHD, congenital heart disease; HRS, Heart Rhythm Society; IART, intra-atrial reentrant tachycardia; LD, limited data; NR, nonrandomized; PACES, Pediatric And Congenital Electrophysiology Society.
Reproduced from Refs.[8,39,64]; with permission.

(**Fig. 2**).[43,61,67,69,70] Implantation of an epicardial dual-chamber antitachycardia pacing system is performed to achieve atrial pacing with intact atrioventricular conduction, with programming to minimize ventricular pacing.[43,61,71] In 1994, when the authors performed their first such surgery, alternative therapy such as catheter ablation had been ineffective for Fontan patients and did not address the hemodynamic abnormalities imposed by the enlarged, boggy right atrium. Fontan patients with arrhythmias and exercise intolerance at that time had not been considered candidates for reoperations and would otherwise have died. In the subsequent 22 years, this surgery has been performed in centers around the world in more than 540 patients, with perioperative mortality of 1.4% to 6% as summarized recently.[43] The Fontan conversion surgery extended the durability of the Fontan circulation and resulted in significantly improved quality of life as well as life expectancy. As the number of patients with atriopulmonary Fontan physiology suitable for Fontan conversion declines, it may be anticipated that patients with extracardiac total cavopulmonary anastomoses performed in early childhood may similarly come to require conduit revisions in adolescence with potential arrhythmia interventions.

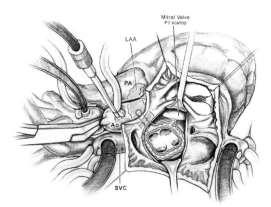

Fig. 2. Right and left atrial views of potential prophylactic ablative lesions that comprise the left-sided maze procedure without performing a left atrial appendectomy. Shown in the left atrium are circumferential isolation of the pulmonary vein confluence, connection of the pulmonary vein confluence with the P3 location of the posterior mitral valve annulus, and connection of the pulmonary vein confluence with the base of the left atrial appendage (LAA). (*Reproduced from* Mavroudis C, Stulak JM, Ad N, et al. Prophylactic atrial arrhythmia surgical procedures with congenital heart operations: review and recommendations. Ann Thorac Surg 2015;99:355; with permission from Elsevier.)

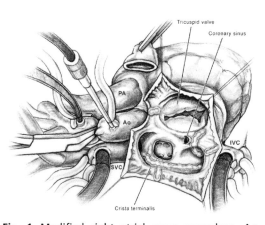

Fig. 1. Modified right atrial maze procedure. Ao, aorta; PA, pulmonary artery. (*Reproduced from* Mavroudis C. Arrhythmia surgery and pacemaker placement not associated with Fontan conversion. In: Mavroudis C, Backer CL, editors. Atlas of pediatric cardiac surgery. London: Springer Verlag; 2015. p. 268; with permission from Springer.)

ATRIAL FIBRILLATION

The Cox-maze I, II, and III procedures for AF ablation were characterized as "cut and sew" operations that had considerable cross-clamp time and risk of bleeding.[54,55] Subsequently, energy ablative sources were introduced (Cox-maze IV operation) to shorten the procedure and limit bleeding complications. The lesion sets were designed to preserve normal conduction from the sinoatrial node to the atrioventricular node, to maintain atrioventricular synchrony, to preserve left atrial transport function, and to reduce thromboembolism. The left atrial maze procedure has proved to be effective owing to specific lesions that are applied to encircle the pulmonary veins and to limit reentry circuits that would occur in the left atrioventricular valve isthmus, reentry via the coronary sinus, and reentry via the Bachmann bundle in the dome of the left atrium.[54,55] In the original description, the Cox-maze procedure included left atrial appendectomy to limit thrombus formation, and an incision to the confluence of pulmonary vein encircling lesions.

Surgeons who endeavored to shorten and simplify the operation made subsequent modifications to the maze procedure to allow epicardial approaches without cardiopulmonary bypass and facilitate transcatheter ablation.[72] Efforts were made to minimize the pulmonary vein and left atrial lesions, which resulted in procedures labeled as "mini-maze" and "modified" maze. "Maze" became synonymous with any modified lesion set that was applied to the atria as therapy for reentrant atrial arrhythmias. Energy sources including radiofrequency, microwave, laser, and cryoablation have been introduced to minimize the need for incisions and attendant bleeding complications. It is clear that depth of lesion by whatever method is essential to achieve the resultant transmural ablation. Unlike most patients with acquired heart disease, individuals with congenital heart disease have varying degrees of atrial thickness owing to specific heart defects and the adaptive changes over a lifetime of abnormal hemodynamic conditions. For example, patients with tricuspid atresia have thick atrial walls, whereas patients with double inlet left ventricle tend to have thin atrial walls. These anatomic variances become important when a transmural lesion needs to be accomplished.

The long-term freedom from AF recurrence with the original "cut and sew" Cox-maze III procedure was more than 97%.[73] All subsequent modifications and revisions have attained 65% to 90% arrhythmia-free follow-up; a comprehensive meta-analysis has demonstrated superior outcomes with the biatrial maze ablation procedure.[74] The application of the Cox-maze III/IV for patients with complex congenital heart surgery has been highly successful, resulting in freedom from AF in greater than 95% of patients, although atrial reentry tachycardia has recurred in approximately 15% of patients.[43,60,70]

PROPHYLACTIC ARRHYTHMIA SURGERY

At the present time, consensus has supported surgical indications for prophylactic arrhythmia surgery in association with specific congenital heart repairs.[8,69] The prophylactic lesion set should be simple to perform, should be attended by a minimum of complications, and should have a high chance of efficacy over the long term (see **Table 5**).[68,69] Justifiably, one must select those forms of congenital heart disease that are associated with a sufficiently high risk of developing arrhythmia to support the indications for concomitant prophylactic arrhythmia surgery.[8] Appeal of bioethical principles of nonmaleficence,

Table 5		
Lesion sets for surgical treatment of atrial tachycardia associated with congenital heart disease		
Congenital Heart Disease	**Type of Arrhythmia at Risk**	**Lesion Set**
Ebstein anomaly	Atrial reentry, large right atrium	Cavotricuspid isthmus ablation; atrial reduction
	Atrial reentry, large right and left atria	Cavotricuspid isthmus ablation; atrial reduction, left atrial maze
	Accessory connections	Endocardial or epicardial dissection; cryoablation
Univentricular hearts	Atrial reentry	Modified right atrial maze (see **Fig. 1**)[68]
	AF	Left atrial maze plus modified right atrial maze
ASD	AF	Left atrial maze (see **Fig. 2**)[69]
TOF	Atrial reentry	Cavotricuspid isthmus ablation or modified right atrial maze

beneficence, patient autonomy, and justice comes to mind and apply.

General application of these principles requires understanding of the techniques of a standard prophylactic maze procedure and the need to avoid injury to the sinus node, which may occur after a standard maze procedure. **Fig. 3** shows a lesion set that ablates the area of slow conduction at the isthmus.[69] This area is the first area that is approached for therapeutic transcatheter radiofrequency ablation in patients with atrial reentry tachycardia, which is successful in 75% of cases.[34–36] The area of interest is easy to locate, is easy to ablate, and has minimal risks. When considering prophylactic lesions sets, a limited isthmus lesion is favored over the more extensive modified right atrial maze.

Prophylactic arrhythmia surgery targeted against atrial reentry tachycardia can be applied to specific anatomic substrates: patients older than 40 years of age presenting for repair of ASD, patients with Ebstein anomaly undergoing tricuspid valve surgery, TOF patients presenting for pulmonary valve insertion, and single-ventricle patients who present for Fontan operations or revisions.[8,23,47,69] Prophylactic arrhythmia surgery for AF is considered for patients with significant left-sided atrioventricular disease and severe left atrial dilatation undergoing planned surgery, with lesions including left atrial maze and right-sided cavotricuspid isthmus ablation.[69]

Successful arrhythmia surgery requires a clear understanding of tachycardia mechanisms present in an individual patient as well as the specific operative techniques for each mechanism, and most importantly, an intense degree of cooperation and collaboration between the electrophysiologist and surgeon. Using these arrhythmia techniques, surgical repair of congenital heart disease can be viewed as both an anatomic and an electrical intervention, with the combined goals of improving hemodynamic status and minimizing morbidity from the development of later arrhythmias.

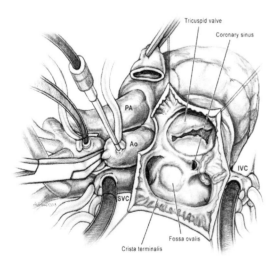

Fig. 3. A right atrial view of potential prophylactic ablative lesions that connect (1) the tricuspid annulus with the coronary sinus, (2) the coronary sinus with the os of the IVC, (3) and the inferior end of the atriotomy incision with the anterior os of the IVC. (*Reproduced from* Mavroudis C, Stulak JM, Ad N, et al. Prophylactic atrial arrhythmia surgical procedures with congenital heart operations: review and recommendations. Ann Thorac Surg 2015;99:355; with permission from Elsevier.)

REFERENCES

1. Marelli AJ, Mackie AS, Ionescu-Ittu R, et al. Congenital heart disease in the general population: changing prevalence and age distribution. Circulation 2007;115:163–72.
2. Teuwen CP, Taverne YJ, Houck C, et al. Tachyarrhythmia in patients with congenital heart disease: inevitable destiny? Neth Heart J 2016;24:161–70.
3. Khairy P, Ionescu-Ittu R, Mackie AS, et al. Changing mortality in congenital heart disease. J Am Coll Cardiol 2010;56:1149–57.
4. Bouchardy J, Therrien J, Pilote L, et al. Atrial arrhythmias in adults with congenital heart disease. Circulation 2009;120:1679–86.
5. Walsh EP, Cecchin F. Arrhythmias in adult patients with congenital heart disease. Circulation 2007; 115:534–45.
6. Brouwer C, Hazekamp MG, Zeppenfeld K. Anatomical substrates and ablation of reentrant atrial and ventricular tachycardias in repaired congenital heart disease. Arrhythm Electrophysiol Rev 2016;5:150–60.
7. Cox JL. Surgery for cardiac arrhythmias. Curr Probl Cardiol 1983;8:1–60.
8. Khairy P, Van Hare GF, Balaji S, et al. PACES/HRS expert consensus statement on the recognition and management of arrhythmias in adult congenital heart disease. Heart Rhythm 2014;11:e102–65.
9. Murphy JG, Gersh BJ, McGoon MD, et al. Long-term outcome after surgical repair of isolated atrial septal defect. Follow-up at 27 to 32 years. N Engl J Med 1990;323:1645–50.
10. Gatzoulis MA, Freeman MA, Siu SC, et al. Atrial arrhythmia after surgical closure of atrial septal defects in adults. N Engl J Med 1999;340:839–46.
11. Van De Bruaene A, Delcroix M, Pasquet A, et al. The importance of pulmonary artery pressures on late atrial arrhythmia in transcatheter and surgically closed ASD type secundum. Int J Cardiol 2011; 152:192–5.

12. Yap SC, Harris L, Silversides CK, et al. Outcome of intra-atrial re-entrant tachycardia catheter ablation in adults with congenital heart disease: negative impact of age and complex atrial surgery. J Am Coll Cardiol 2010;56:1589–96.

13. Wasmer K, Köbe J, Dechering DG, et al. Isthmus-dependent right atrial flutter as the leading cause of atrial tachycardias after surgical atrial septal defect repair. Int J Cardiol 2013;168:2447–52.

14. Deanfield JE, McKenna WJ, Presbitero P, et al. Ventricular arrhythmia in unrepaired and repaired tetralogy of Fallot. Relation to age, timing of repair, and haemodynamic status. Br Heart J 1984;52:77–81.

15. Downar E, Harris L, Kimber S, et al. Ventricular tachycardia after surgical repair of tetralogy of Fallot: results of intraoperative mapping studies. J Am Coll Cardiol 1992;20:648–55.

16. Gatzoulis MA, Till JA, Somerville J, et al. Mechanoelectrical interaction in tetralogy of Fallot. QRS prolongation relates to right ventricular size and predicts malignant ventricular arrhythmias and sudden death. Circulation 1995;92:231–7.

17. Harrison DA, Harris L, Siu SC, et al. Sustained ventricular tachycardia in adult patients late after repair of tetralogy of Fallot. J Am Coll Cardiol 1997;30:1368–73.

18. Gatzoulis MA, Balaji S, Webber SA, et al. Risk factors for arrhythmia and sudden cardiac death late after repair of tetralogy of Fallot: a multi-centre study. Lancet 2000;356:975–81.

19. Khairy P, Aboulhosn J, Gurvitz MZ, et al. Arrhythmia burden in adults with surgically repaired tetralogy of Fallot: a multi-institutional study. Circulation 2010;122:868–75.

20. Harrison DA, Siu SC, Hussain F, et al. Sustained atrial arrhythmias in adults late after repair of tetralogy of Fallot. Am J Cardiol 2001;87:584–8.

21. Khositseth A, Danielson GK, Dearani JA, et al. Supraventricular tachyarrhythmias in Ebstein anomaly: management and outcome. J Thorac Cardiovasc Surg 2004;128:826–33.

22. Bockeria L, Golukhova E, Dadasheva M, et al. Advantages and disadvantages of one-stage and two-stage surgery for arrhythmias and Ebstein's anomaly. Eur J Cardiothorac Surg 2005;28:536–40.

23. Stulak JM, Sharma V, Cannon BC, et al. Optimal surgical ablation of atrial tachyarrhythmias during correction of Ebstein anomaly. Ann Thorac Surg 2015;99:1700–5.

24. Deal BJ. Late arrhythmias following Fontan surgery. World J Pediatr Cong Heart Surg 2012;3:194–200.

25. d'Udekem Y, Iyengar AJ, Galati JC, et al. Redefining expectations of long-term survival after the Fontan procedure: twenty-five years of follow-up from the entire population of Australia and New Zealand. Circulation 2014;130:S32–8.

26. Song MK, Bae EJ, Kwon BS, et al. Intra-atrial reentrant tachycardia in adult patients after Fontan operation. Int J Cardiol 2015;187:157–63.

27. Quinton E, Nightingale P, Hudsmith L, et al. Prevalence of atrial tachyarrhythmia in adults after Fontan operation. Heart 2015;101:1672–7.

28. Diller GP, Giardini A, Dimopoulos K, et al. Predictors of morbidity and mortality in contemporary Fontan patients: results from a multicenter study including cardiopulmonary exercise testing in 321 patients. Eur Heart J 2010;31:3073–83.

29. Giannakoulas G, Dimopoulos K, Yuksel S, et al. Atrial tachyarrhythmias late after Fontan operation are related to increase in mortality and hospitalization. Int J Cardiol 2012;157:221–6.

30. Balaji S, Daga A, Bradley DJ, et al. An international multicenter study comparing arrhythmia prevalence between the intracardiac lateral tunnel and the extracardiac conduit type of Fontan operations. J Thorac Cardiovasc Surg 2014;148:576–81.

31. Collins KK, Love BA, Walsh EP, et al. Location of acutely successful radiofrequency catheter ablation of intraatrial reentrant tachycardia in patients with congenital heart disease. Am J Cardiol 2000;86:969–74.

32. de Groot NM, Lukac P, Blom NA, et al. Long-term outcome of ablative therapy of postoperative supraventricular tachycardias in patients with univentricular heart: a European multicenter study. Circ Arrhythm Electrophysiol 2009;2:242–8.

33. Correa R, Sherwin ED, Kovach J, et al. Mechanism and ablation of arrhythmia following total cavopulmonary connection. Circ Arrhythm Electrophysiol 2015;8:318–25.

34. Chan DP, Van Hare GF, Mackall JA, et al. Importance of atrial flutter isthmus in postoperative intra-atrial reentrant tachycardia. Circulation 2000;102:1283–9.

35. Lukac P, Pedersen AK, Mortensen PT, et al. Ablation of atrial tachycardia after surgery for congenital and acquired heart disease using an electroanatomic mapping system: which circuits to expect in which substrate? Heart Rhythm 2005;2:64–72.

36. Cosio FG. Understanding atrial arrhythmia mechanisms by mapping and ablation. Europace 2013;15:315–6.

37. de Groot NM, Zeppenfeld K, Wijffels MC, et al. Ablation of focal atrial arrhythmia in patients with congenital heart defects after surgery: role of circumscribed areas with heterogeneous conduction. Heart Rhythm 2006;3:526–35.

38. Kanter RJ, Papagiannis J, Carboni MP, et al. Radiofrequency catheter ablation of supraventricular tachycardia substrates after Mustard and Senning operations for d-transposition of the great arteries. J Am Coll Cardiol 2000;35:428–41.

39. Page RL, Joglar JA, Caldwell MA, et al. 2015 ACC/AHA/HRS guideline for the management of adult

patients with supraventricular tachycardia: a report of the American College of Cardiology/American Heart Association Task Force on Clinical Practice Guidelines and the Heart Rhythm Society. J Am Coll Cardiol 2016;67:e27–115.

40. de Groot NM, Atary JZ, Blom NA, et al. Long-term outcome after ablative therapy of postoperative atrial tachyarrhythmia in patients with congenital heart disease and characteristics of atrial tachyarrhythmia recurrences. Circ Arrhythm Electrophysiol 2010;3:148–54.

41. Ueda A, Suman-Horduna I, Mantziari L, et al. Contemporary outcomes of supraventricular tachycardia ablation in congenital heart disease: a single-center experience in 116 patients. Circ Arrhythm Electrophysiol 2013;6:606–13.

42. Anguera I, Dallaglio P, Macías R, et al. Long-term outcome after ablation of right atrial tachyarrhythmias after the surgical repair of congenital and acquired heart disease. Am J Cardiol 2015;115:1705–13.

43. Deal BJ, Costello JM, Webster G, et al. Intermediate-term outcome of 140 consecutive Fontan conversions with arrhythmia operations. Ann Thorac Surg 2016;101:717–24.

44. Kapel GF, Sacher F, Dekkers OM, et al. Arrhythmogenic anatomical isthmuses identified by electroanatomical mapping are the substrate for ventricular tachycardia in repaired tetralogy of Fallot. Eur Heart J 2016;38:268–76.

45. Zeppenfeld K, Schalij MJ, Bartelings MM, et al. Catheter ablation of ventricular tachycardia after repair of congenital heart disease: electroanatomic identification of the critical right ventricular isthmus. Circulation 2007;116:2241–52.

46. Kapel GF, Reichlin T, Wijnmaalen AP, et al. Left-sided ablation of ventricular tachycardia in adults with repaired tetralogy of Fallot: a case series. Circ Arrhythm Electrophysiol 2014;7:889–97.

47. Karamlou T, Silber I, Lao R, et al. Outcomes after late reoperation in patients with repaired tetralogy of Fallot: the impact of arrhythmia and arrhythmia surgery. Ann Thorac Surg 2006;81:1786–93.

48. Deal BJ, Mavroudis C, Backer CL. Beyond Fontan conversion: surgical therapy of arrhythmias including patients with associated complex congenital heart disease. Ann Thorac Surg 2003;76:542–54.

49. Mavroudis C, Deal BJ, Backer CL, et al. Arrhythmia surgery in patients with and without congenital heart disease. Ann Thorac Surg 2008;86:857–68.

50. Deal BJ, Mavroudis C, Backer CL. The role of concomitant arrhythmia surgery in patients undergoing repair of congenital heart disease. Pacing Clin Electrophysiol 2008;31(Suppl 1):S13–6.

51. Stevenson WG, Couper GS. A surgical option for ventricular tachycardia caused by nonischemic cardiomyopathy. Circ Arrhythm Electrophysiol 2011;4:429–31.

52. Sealy WC, Hattler BG Jr, Blumenschein SD, et al. Surgical treatment of Wolff-Parkinson-White syndrome. Ann Thorac Surg 1969;8:1–11.

53. Guiraudon GM, Klein GJ, Sharma AD, et al. Surgical treatment of supraventricular tachycardia: a five-year experience. Pacing Clin Electrophysiol 1986; 9:1376–80.

54. Cox JL. The surgical treatment of atrial fibrillation. IV. Surgical technique. J Thorac Cardiovasc Surg 1991; 101:584–92.

55. Cox JL, Jaquiss RD, Schuessler RB, et al. Modification of the maze procedure for atrial flutter and atrial fibrillation. II. Surgical technique of the maze III procedure. J Thorac Cardiovasc Surg 1995;110:485–95.

56. Theodoro DA, Danielson GK, Porter CJ, et al. Right-sided maze procedure for right atrial arrhythmias in congenital heart disease. Ann Thorac Surg 1998;65: 149–54.

57. Stulak JM, Dearani JA, Burkhart HM, et al. The surgical treatment of concomitant atrial arrhythmias during redo cardiac operations. Ann Thorac Surg 2012;94:1894–9.

58. Stulak JM, Dearani JA, Puga FJ, et al. Right-sided maze procedure for atrial tachyarrhythmias in congenital heart disease. Ann Thorac Surg 2006; 81:1780–5.

59. Deal BJ, Mavroudis C, Backer CL, et al. Impact of arrhythmia circuit cryoablation during Fontan conversion for refractory atrial tachycardia. Am J Cardiol 1999;83:563–9.

60. Deal BJ, Mavroudis C, Backer CL, et al. Comparison of anatomic isthmus block with the modified right atrial maze procedure for late atrial tachycardia in Fontan patients. Circulation 2002;106:575–9.

61. Mavroudis C, Deal BJ, Backer CL, et al. J. Maxwell Chamberlain Memorial Paper for congenital heart surgery. 111 Fontan conversions with arrhythmia surgery: surgical lessons and outcomes. Ann Thorac Surg 2007;84:1457–65.

62. Giamberti A, Chessa M, Foresti S, et al. Combined atrial septal defect surgical closure and irrigated radiofrequency ablation in adult patients. Ann Thorac Surg 2006;82:1327–31.

63. Giamberti A, Chessa M, Abella R, et al. Surgical treatment of arrhythmias in adults with congenital heart defects. Int J Cardiol 2008;129:37–41.

64. January CT, Wann LS, Alpert JS, et al. 2014 AHA/ACC/HRS guidelines for the management of patients with atrial fibrillation: a report of the American College of Cardiology/American Heart Association Task Force on Practice Guidelines and the Heart Rhythm Society. J Am Coll Cardiol 2014;64:e1–76.

65. Mavroudis C, Deal BJ, Backer CL. Surgical therapy of cardiac arrhythmias. In: Mavroudis C, Backer CL, editors. Pediatric cardiac surgery. 4th edition. London: Wiley Blackwell; 2013. p. 769–812.

66. Mavroudis C, Deal BJ, Backer CL, et al. Operative techniques in association with arrhythmia surgery in patients with congenital heart disease. World J Pediatr Cong Heart Surg 2013;4:85–97.

67. Mavroudis C, Backer CL, Deal BJ, et al. Evolving anatomic and electrophysiologic considerations associated with Fontan conversion. Semin Thorac Cardiovasc Surg Pediatr Card Surg Annu 2007;10:136–45.

68. Mavroudis C. Arrhythmia surgery and pacemaker placement not associated with Fontan conversion. In: Mavroudis C, Backer CL, editors. Atlas of pediatric cardiac surgery. London: Springer Verlag; 2015. p. 255–72.

69. Mavroudis C, Stulak JM, Ad N, et al. Prophylactic atrial arrhythmia surgical procedures with congenital heart operations: review and recommendations. Ann Thorac Surg 2015;99:352–9.

70. Backer CL, Tsao S, Deal BJ, et al. Maze procedure in single ventricle patients. Semin Thorac Cardiovasc Surg Pediatr Card Surg Annu 2008; 11:44–8.

71. Tsao S, Deal BJ, Backer CL, et al. Device management of arrhythmias after Fontan conversion. J Thorac Cardiovasc Surg 2009;138:937–40.

72. Dewire J, Calkins H. Update on atrial fibrillation catheter ablation technologies and techniques. Nat Rev Cardiol 2013;10:599–612.

73. Cox JL, Schuessler RB, Lappas DG, et al. An 8 1/2-year clinical experience with surgery for atrial fibrillation. Ann Surg 1996;224:267–73.

74. Phan K, Xie A, La Meir M, et al. Surgical ablation for treatment of atrial fibrillation in cardiac surgery: a cumulative meta-analysis of randomised controlled trials. Heart 2014;100:722–30.

Moving?

Make sure your subscription moves with you!

To notify us of your new address, find your **Clinics Account Number** (located on your mailing label above your name), and contact customer service at:

Email: journalscustomerservice-usa@elsevier.com

800-654-2452 (subscribers in the U.S. & Canada)
314-447-8871 (subscribers outside of the U.S. & Canada)

Fax number: 314-447-8029

Elsevier Health Sciences Division
Subscription Customer Service
3251 Riverport Lane
Maryland Heights, MO 63043

*To ensure uninterrupted delivery of your subscription, please notify us at least 4 weeks in advance of move.

Moving?

Make sure your subscription moves with you!

To notify us of your new address, find your Clinics Account Number (located on your mailing label above your name), and contact customer service at

Email: journalscustomerservice-usa@elsevier.com

800-654-2452 (subscribers in the U.S. & Canada)
314-447-8871 (subscribers outside of the U.S. & Canada)

Fax number: 314-447-8029

Elsevier Health Sciences Division
Subscription Customer Service
3251 Riverport Lane
Maryland Heights, MO 63043

Printed and bound by CPI Group (UK) Ltd, Croydon, CR0 4YY

03/10/2024

01040302-0019